BASIC CONCEPTS OF PSYCHIATRIC-MENTAL HEALTH NURSING

LOUISE REBRACA SHIVES, R.N., B.S.N.

Head Nurse, Department of Psychiatry, Florida Hospital, Orlando, Florida
Formerly Assistant Professor of Nursing, North Central Technical College,
Mansfield, Ohio

A   D A V I D   T.   M I L L E R   B O O K

BASIC CONCEPTS OF

PSYCHIATRIC –

MENTAL

HEALTH

NURSING

J. B. LIPPINCOTT COMPANY

Philadelphia · London · Mexico City · New York
St. Louis · São Paulo · Sydney

Sponsoring Editor: David T. Miller
Manuscript Editor: Mary K. Smith
Indexer: Alberta Morrison
Design Director: Tracy Baldwin
Design Coordinator: Earl Gerhart
Designer: Adrianne Onderdonk Dudden
Production Supervisor: Kathleen P. Dunn
Production Assistant: Susan Hess
Compositor: University Graphics, Inc.
Printer/Binder: R. R. Donnelley & Sons

6 5 4 3 2 1

Library of Congress Cataloging-in-Publication Data

Shives, Louise Rebraca.
   Basic concepts of psychiatric-mental health nursing.

   "A David T. Miller Book."
   Includes bibliographies and index.
   1. Psychiatric nursing.   I. Title.
[DNLM: 1. Psychiatric Nursing. WY 160 S558b]
RC440.S487   1986   610.73'68   85–23671
ISBN 0–397–54512–6

The author and publisher have exerted every effort to ensure that drug selection and dosage set forth in this text are in accord with current recommendations and practice at the
time of publication. However, in view of ongoing research, changes in government regulations, and the constant flow of information relating to drug therapy and drug reactions,
the reader is urged to check the package insert for each drug for any change in indications
and dosage and for added warnings and precautions. This is particularly important when the
recommended agent is a new or infrequently employed drug.

PREFACE

sychiatric–mental health nursing requires the use of a therapeutic interpersonal process and a problem-solving approach in meeting the biopsychosocial needs of individuals and groups of individuals. To achieve this goal, the psychiatric–mental health nurse must be able to provide a therapeutic setting in which the patient feels accepted, learns positive coping skills, and is the recipient of holistic and humanistic health care. Clinical experience provides a valuable foundation in the preparation of the graduate nurse because it enables him or her to develop a problem-solving approach while assessing patients, as well as planning and implementing appropriate nursing interventions. It was my intent to write a basic textbook for use in both the classroom setting and clinical area. It is written for students and educators who prefer a "core" book with brief and succinct coverage of the concepts used in psychiatric–mental health nursing. Information is presented in such a manner that it can be used by students in a variety of clinical areas, including pediatrics, obstetrics, emergency room, crisis center, and other settings while caring for patients with biopsychosocial needs. Nursing professionals who have reviewed *Basic Concepts of Psychiatric–Mental Health Nursing* have described the content as relevant, informative, essential information that is presented logically, clearly, and concisely.

The basic chapter format consists of 1) learning objectives; 2) a description of psychiatric disorders using the third edition of *The Diagnostic and Statistical Manual of Mental Disorders* (DSM-III) as well as current reference books to cite diagnostic criteria and presenting symptoms; 3) clinical examples of various psychiatric disorders; 4) a summary at the end of each chapter; 5) learning activities; 6) self-tests; and 7) a current reference list. Examples of student reactions to various conditions in the clinical setting are given as a means of reassurance and support, to make students aware that their reactions are fairly typical and that they are not alone.

Two books that were relied on heavily as references to the official list of nursing diagnoses and examples of the nursing process were *Nursing Diagnoses and Applications to Clinical Practice* by Lynda Juall Carpenito (J. B. Lippincott, 1983) and *The American Handbook of Psychiatric Nursing* by Suzanne Lego (J. B. Lippincott, 1984). Official nursing diagnoses and appropriate nursing interventions are listed in tabular form as guides for clinical nursing practice. Other examples of quick reference material in tabular form include characteristics of mental health and mental illness, milestones influencing psychiatric nursing, therapeutic communication techniques, the stages of various theories of personality development, descriptions of various disciplines composing the mental health team, a summary of neurologic side-effects of psychotropic drugs, and the daily dosage of commonly used psychotropic drugs. A glossary is included to familiarize the student with psychiatric terminology.

The pronoun "she" has been used for nurse and "he" for the patient only for the sake of convenience for the reader; these have no other significance, nor any sexist intent.

Louise Rebraca Shives, R.N., B.S.N.

ACKNOWLEDGMENTS

I would like to thank all my friends and colleagues for their continued support during the time I was committed to this project.

A special thanks goes to my three lovely daughters, Debbie, Lorrie, and Terri, for their unending faith in my ability to write a scholarly text while at the same time attending graduate school.

The following people were of invaluable assistance during the completion of this book:

Debbie Shives, my daughter, who typed and proofread at least 1000 pages of manuscript with much diligence and patience;

Lou Everett, R.N., M.S.N.
Assistant Professor,
Mental Health Nursing in the Community
East Carolina University
Greenville, North Carolina; and

Barbara Van Droof, R.N., M.N.
Professor of Nursing
Shoreline Community College
Seattle, Washington, who reviewed the entire manuscript;

Mary K. Smith
Manuscript Editor,
J. B. Lippincott Co.,

and

David T. Miller
Vice President and Editor
Nursing Division
J. B. Lippincott Co., who offered professional editorial guidance.

CONTENTS

PSYCHIATRIC NURSING

IN THE

MENTAL HEALTH SETTING

1

MENTAL HEALTH AND

MENTAL ILLNESS

LEARNING OBJECTIVES

1. Define mental health.
2. Differentiate between mental health and mental illness.
3. State factors that influence the development of mental health.
4. Cite misconceptions or myths about mental illness.
5. Explain how one maintains mental health.
6. Describe the levels of communication by which a person communicates with others.
7. State positive ways of dealing with one's emotions.
8. Define *ego defense mechanism.*
9. Cite examples of defense mechanisms and the purpose that each serves.
10. Explain the role of a significant other or support person in maintaining mental health.

THE concepts of mental health and mental illness are discussed in psychological, sociological, and psychiatric nursing texts under various headings including

The health–illness phenomenon

The health–illness continuum

Stress and mental health

Aspects of mental health

Healthy adjustment

Concepts of health and illness

Authors including John Powell, Sidney Jourard, Eric Berne, Jess Lair, and Virginia Satir have written best-selling books such as *Why Am I Afraid To Tell You Who I Am, The Transparent Self, What Do You Say After You Say Hello, I Ain't Well But I Sure Am Better,* and *Making Contact* focusing on self-awareness, personal growth, and interpersonal communication. These dynamics play an important part in the development of emotional maturity and mental health.

DEFINING MENTAL HEALTH

The American Psychiatric Association defines mental health in *A Psychiatric Glossary* as "simultaneous success at working, loving, and creating with the capacity for mature and flexible resolution of conflicts between instincts, conscience, important other people and reality" (1980, p. 89). Marmor and Pumpion (1950) describe mental health as "that state in the interrelationship of the individual and his environment in which the personality structure is relatively stable, and the environmental stresses are within its absorptive capacity" (p. 30). Other definitions refer to the ability to 1) solve problems; 2) fulfill one's capacity for love and work; 3) cope with crises without assistance beyond the support of family or friends; and 4) maintain a state of well-being by enjoying life, setting goals and realistic limits, and becoming independent, interdependent, or dependent as the need arises without permanently losing one's independence. Although there is no universal definition, helping people seem to agree that mental health is a positive state in which the person is responsible, self-directive, and displays self-awareness. His behavior is generally accepted within a group.

FACTORS INFLUENCING MENTAL HEALTH

Three factors influence the development of mental health. They include inherited characteristics, nurturing during childhood, and life circumstances. Some theorists feel that no one is completely normal and that the ability to maintain a mentally healthy outlook on life is, in part, due to one's genes, just as genetic defects may predispose a person to mental retardation, schizophrenia, or manic–depressive illness. Such persons have innate differences in sensitivity and temperament that prompt various responses to their environment. Nurturing during childhood refers to parent–child interactions, which also affect the development of mental health. Positive nurturing starts with bonding at childbirth and includes feelings of love, security, and acceptance. The child experiences positive interactions with parents and siblings. Negative nurturing includes circumstances such as maternal deprivation, parental rejection, sibling rivalry, and early communication failures. Life circumstances can influence one's mental health from birth. Examples of positive circumstances are success in school, financial security, good physical health, an enjoyable occupation, and a successful marriage. Negative circumstances include poverty, poor physical health, unemployment, or an unsuccessful marriage.

DEFINING MENTAL ILLNESS

If a person is unsuccessful in dealing with environmental stresses because of faulty inherited characteristics, poor nurturing during childhood, or negative life circumstances, mental illness may develop. The American Psychiatric Association's definition of mental illness or a mental disorder is an "illness with psychologic or behavioral manifestations and/or impairment in functioning due to a social, psychologic, genetic, physical/chemical, or biologic disturbance. The disorder is not limited to relations between the person and society. The illness is characterized by symptoms and/or impairment in functioning." (1980, p. 89). Other definitions refer to mental illness as: 1) displaying abnormal behavior more consistently than most people; 2) a psychopathology exhibiting frequent irresponsibility, the inability to cope, frequently being at odds with society, and an inaccurate perception of reality; and 3) the absolute absence or constant presence of a specific behavior that has a socially acceptable range of occurrences (Bailey and Dreyer, 1977).

CHARACTERISTICS OF MENTAL HEALTH

Maslow (1954), an eminent psychologist and writer, developed the following ideas about mentally healthy people:

1. They possess the ability to accept themselves, others, and nature. Stated another way, they have positive self-concepts and relate well to people and their environment.

2. They are able to form close relationships with others. Kindness, patience, and compassion are displayed for others.

3. They perceive the world as it really is and people as they really are. Problem solving occurs because these people are able to make decisions pertaining to reality rather than fantasy.

4. They are able to appreciate and enjoy life. Optimism prevails as they respond to people, places, and things in daily encounters.

5. They are independent or autonomous in thought and action and rely on personal standards of behavior and values. Such persons are able to face with relative serenity and happiness circumstances that would drive other people to self-destructive behavior.

6. They are creative, utilizing a variety of approaches as they perform tasks or solve problems.

7. Their behavior is consistent as they appreciate and respect the rights of others, display a willingness to listen and learn from others, and show reverence for the uniqueness and difference in others.

W. C. Menninger (of the Menninger Foundation, Topeka, Kansas) summarizes emotional maturity as the

1. Ability to deal constructively with reality

2. Capacity to adapt to change

3. Relative freedom from symptoms produced by tensions and anxieties

4. Capacity to find more satisfaction in giving than receiving

5. Ability to relate to other people in a consistent manner with mutual satisfaction and helpfulness

6. Capacity to redirect one's instinctive hostile energy into creative, constructive outlets

7. Capacity to love

The following is a comparison of some of the characteristics of mental health and mental illness:

MENTAL HEALTH	MENTAL ILLNESS
Accepts self and others	Feelings of inadequacy Poor self-concept
Ability to cope or tolerate stress. Can return to normal functioning if temporarily disturbed	Inability to cope Maladaptive behavior
Ability to form close and lasting relationships	Inability to establish a meaningful relationship
Uses sound judgment to make decisions	Displays poor judgment
Accepts responsibility for actions	Irresponsibility or inability to accept responsibility for actions
Optimistic	Pessimistic
Recognizes limitations (abilities and deficiencies)	Does not recognize limitations (abilities and deficiencies)
Can function effectively and independently	Exhibits dependency needs because of feelings of inadequacy
Able to perceive imagined circumstances from reality	Inability to perceive reality
Able to develop potential and talents to fullest extent	Does not reocgnize potential and talents due to a poor self-concept
Able to solve problems	Avoids problems rather than handling them or attempt to solve them
Can delay immediate gratification	Desires or demands immediate gratification
Mental health reflects a person's approach to life by communicating emotions, giving and receiving, working alone as well as with others, accepting authority, displaying a sense of humor, and coping successfully with emotional conflict.	Mental illness reflects a person's inability to cope with stress, resulting in disruption, disorganization, inappropriate reactions, unacceptable behavior and the inability to respond according to his expectations and the demands of society.

People who are mentally healthy do not necessarily possess all the characteristics listed. Under stress they may exhibit some of the traits of mental illness but are able to respond to the stress with automatic, unconscious behavior that serves to satisfy their basic needs in a socially acceptable way.

MISCONCEPTIONS ABOUT MENTAL ILLNESS

Altrocchi (1980) lists several misconceptions about abnormal behavior and mental illness. Summarized they are as follows:

1. *Abnormal behavior is different or odd, easily recognized.* We all are irrational at times and behave in an unusual or different manner. Such behavior may occur in the privacy of one's home, at work, or even in a public place, and still may go unnoticed by others. Maladaptive behavior can occur subtly; for example, the person who is suspicious of everyone and avoids contact with people. Unless he voices his concerns, his thoughts and behavior may go unnoticed. The depressed individual who is diagnosed as mentally ill may appear quiet, sullen, or distracted but doesn't necessarily exhibit abnormal or bizarre behavior.

2. *Abnormal behavior can be predicted and evaluated.* Newspaper articles prove otherwise. The following headline appeared in a local newspaper: "Snub starts 6 killings in Dallas Club." The article stated that a dancer pushed a man away after he apparently "got fresh" while they were dancing. Onlookers stated he blew her a kiss as he walked off, left the club, returned with a pistol and shot and killed her as she sat at the bar. He killed five other patrons and wounded a sixth. The man's employer was quoted as saying, "He was quiet, polite, was doing his job right." No motive was given for the man's sudden, unpredicted behavior.

3. *Internal forces are responsible for abnormal behavior.* Although internal forces may cause abnormal behavior, other factors (*e.g.,* people, culture, and environment) can influence one's behavior. Consider a couple who are having marital problems. Individually they may be mature, independent persons who are unable to live together owing to differences of opinion, values, or priorities. Stress and conflict from marital discord may result in abnormal or maladaptive behavior, such as regression, hostility, or even a suicide attempt.

4. *People who exhibit abnormal behavior are dangerous.* Coleman (1976) lists the following statistics about people in the United States with mental problems:

Six million children and teenagers are emotionally disturbed.

One million students withdraw from college yearly as a result of emotional problems.

Six million five hundred thousand individuals are mentally retarded.

Twelve million are alcoholic.

Twenty million are neurotic.

Two million are dependent on drugs.

Five million are antisocial personalities.

Three million are psychotic.

Two hundred fifty thousand attempt suicide each year.

Many of these people function to some extent in society and are not considered dangerous. They may turn to others for help in an attempt to cope with their problems.

5. *Maladaptive behavior is inherited.* Heredity may play a part in the development of some types of abnormal behavior; however, learning influences behavior. Children learn early in life how to satisfy their needs. They may cry excessively, become stubborn, have temper tantrums or manipulate a parent to achieve immediate gratification. Children as well as adults may observe specific behaviors used by others to meet their needs. As a result, they imitate behavior that they believe to be acceptable to others.

6. *Mental illness is incurable.* Much progress has occurred in the diagnosis and treatment of mental illness. Early detection and treatment may alleviate symptoms and allow the person to function normally in society. Persons with a chronic mental disorder may receive maintenance doses of medication, attend various therapies, or care for themselves with minimal supervision. The current trend toward deinstitutionalization emphasizes returning the patient to the community as a functioning person under the supervision of community mental health workers.

MAINTAINING MENTAL HEALTH

"A growing person is self-renewing . . . as new as each day. . . . Study his face and hands, listen to his voice . . . look for change . . . it is certain he has changed." (Powell, 1969, p. 28). *Emotional maturity, fully functioning, growing personally, fully human,* and *self-actualizing* are all terms used to describe the person who achieves and maintains mental health. Characteristics of mental health have already been discussed, but how does one maintain mental health? Harry Stack Sullivan, an eminent psychiatrist, states that people mistakenly believe that they can solve their own problems and maintain control of their lives without assistance from anyone or anything. The truth is that those who attempt to solve problems by themselves may become consumed by their problems and suffer some type of mental disorder or illness. Mental health is in part determined by relationships between those who either love or refuse to love one another.

Factors that influence the ability to achieve and maintain emotional maturity include interpersonal communication, dealing directly with one's emotions, and resorting to "human hiding places" or ego defense mechanisms (Powell, 1969).

INTERPERSONAL COMMUNICATION

Interpersonal communication is discussed at length in Chapter 3. A relationship is only as good as the interaction that occurs. Powell (1969) discusses five levels of communication that affect one's personal growth and maturity during interpersonal encounters. He refers to them as "the five degrees of willingness to go outside of himself, to communicate himself to others" (p. 50). A discussion of these levels of communication enables one to understand one method of maintaining mental health. They are presented in order from the least willingness to communicate with others to the most healthy response:

LEVEL 5: CLICHE CONVERSATION. No sharing of oneself occurs during this interaction. Comments such as "How are you doing?", "How's your new job?", or "Talk to you later" are empty, superficial statements in which no answers are expected. No personal growth can occur at this level.

LEVEL 4: REPORTING FACTS. The person who communicates at this level reveals very little about himself and expects minimal or no interaction from others. As the detective in a TV series said, "Just the facts, man." No personal interaction occurs at this level.

LEVEL 3: REVEALING IDEAS AND JUDGMENTS. Such communication occurs under strict censorship by the speaker who is watching the listener's response for an indication of acceptance or approval. If the speaker is unable to read the reactions of the listener, he may revert to safer topics or even say what he thinks the listener would like to hear rather than face disapproval or rejection.

LEVEL 2: SPONTANEOUS HERE-AND-NOW EMOTIONS. Revealing one's feelings or emotions takes courage since one faces the possibility of rejection by the listener. Powell (1969) states that if a person reveals the contents of his mind and heart, he may fear his emotional honesty will not be tolerated by another. As a result, the speaker may resort to dishonesty and superficial conversation to maintain contact with another person.

LEVEL 1: OPEN, HONEST COMMUNICATION. When this type of communication occurs, two people share emotions. They are "in tune" with each other, capable of experiencing or duplicating reactions of the other, as individual sopranos in a choir sing the same notes and sound as one voice. Such an interaction is termed complete emotional and personal communion and helps one to maintain emotional maturity. Open communication may not occur until persons relate to each other over a period, getting to know and trust each other.

As people respond to various stressors in their environment or within themselves, they may fluctuate from one level of communication to another in an attempt to alleviate tension or anxiety. Examine your own levels of communication. Which level do you use during most interactions? Do the levels differ with friends, families, co-workers, or patients?

FACING EMOTIONS

People handle their innermost thoughts and feelings in various ways. A comparison of healthy and unhealthy ways to deal directly with one's emotions during an interaction follows:

HEALTHY REACTIONS	UNHEALTHY REACTIONS
Be aware of any emotional response or feeling during an interaction with your environment or with another person. Try to identify what you are feeling.	Ignore any emotional response on your part. Bottle it up inside so that your mind is not aware of the response. Your body may feel the effects in the form of a headache or chest pain.
Admit that you are capable of experiencing various emotions, including anger, hostility, frustration, or disappointment.	Deny your true feelings by ignoring them or telling yourself they do not really exist. You are not the type of person who becomes angry or bitter.
Examine the intensity of each emotion you feel. What caused such a reaction? How is it impacting on your relationship with others?	Let the emotion rule you as you become defensive during an interaction. It's not you; it's the other guy who is at fault.
Share your emotional response. For example, saying "I need time to cool off. I'm too angry to think straight" is a healthy way of avoiding an unnecessary confrontation.	Allow yourself to lose control and become argumentative, incoherent, or disorganized. Blame your reaction on the other person or thing.
Let your mind tell you what is the correct approach to a specific interaction. Think before you act.	Let your emotions rule your actions. Act without thinking and be impulsive.

DEFENSE MECHANISMS

Mental mechanisms and *defense mechanisms* are terms used interchangeably to describe man's unconscious attempt to obtain relief from emotional conflict or anxiety. Coping mechanisms include both conscious and unconscious ways of adjusting to environmental stress.

Such mechanisms are supposedly in action by age 10 and are used as follows:

1. *To resolve a mental conflict.* For example, you are scheduled to work Friday night but have been invited to a concert you want to attend. How would you handle this mental conflict? Tell yourself you have a good work record so it is okay to miss one night of work? Convince

yourself that other people miss work for less significant reasons? Suddenly develop a headache Friday preventing you from going to work or attending the concert? These are just a few options available to resolve your conflict.

2. *To reduce anxiety or fear.* Anxiety is an unexplained feeling of apprehension, tension or uneasiness. The statement "I feel jittery, as if something terrible is about to happen" denotes anxiety. Fear is an emotional response to a recognizable object or threat that decreases when the danger or threat subsides. How do you think you would react if you were suddenly hospitalized to undergo tests to rule out the diagnosis of cancer? Would you deny the possibility, rationally discuss the possibility with your doctor, or elect not to think about the possibility? In any event your defense mechanisms would be called into action to reduce any anxiety or fear you experirence.

3. *Protect one's self-esteem.* You have worked for the same employer for 3 years when your immediate supervisor resigns to accept another position. Although you have received satisfactory periodic evaluations, yearly increases in salary, and have indicated an interest in the job, you are not offered the position. Such a decision would affect almost anyone's self-esteem. How would you protect yours? Would you believe that the incoming employee is much better qualified or would you blame your previous supervisor for showing favoritism toward the new employee? Perhaps you would elect not to talk about the situation because it upsets you too much. Your ego defenses are attempting to protect your self-esteem.

4. *Protect one's sense of security.* Webster defines security as safety or freedom from worry or uncertainty. Has your security ever been threatened? Suppose you were confronted by a robber while in a bank. How do you think you would react? Would you blame the security officer for allowing the robber to follow through with his intent? You might decide to comply with his demands, thinking no harm will come if you follow his directions. On the other hand, you may begin to hyperventilate and experience tachycardia as your emotions are expressed in physical symptoms.

Approximately 20 different mental mechanisms have been identified. Some are considered to be healthy defense mechanisms, whereas others are considered pathologic or characteristic of a mental disorder. The mechanisms are as follows:

1. *Suppression:* willfully or consciously putting a thought or feeling out of one's mind with the ability to recall the thought or feeling at will. A deliberate, intentional exclusion from the conscious mind is referred to as *voluntary forgetting.* "I'd rather not talk about it right now," "Let's talk about my accident later." or "I'm taking a vacation. My problems will still be here when I get back", are examples of

suppression. This mechanism generally is used to protect one's self-esteem.

2. *Repression:* one of the most common defense mechanisms, referred to as the "burying alive mechanism." The person is unable to recall painful or unpleasant thoughts or feelings because they are automatically and involuntarily pushed into one's unconsciousness. The inability to remember the reason for an argument or recall feelings of fear following an automobile accident are examples of repression.

3. *Rationalization:* the most common ego defense mechanism (referred to as self-deception at its subtle best). Rationalization is used to justify ideas, actions, or feelings with good, acceptable reasons or explanations. Generally it is used to maintain self-respect, prevent guilt feelings, and obtain social approval or acceptance. For example, a teen-aged girl who was not asked to the junior prom tells her friend, "John really wanted to date me but felt sorry for Sue and took her to the prom." A golfer overdrives the green by about 100 yards and states: "The wind really carried my golf ball. I didn't hit it that hard."

4. *Identification:* also referred to as "the imitator." People use it in an attempt to be like someone or to resemble the personality and traits of another. Such behavior preserves one's ego or self, the organized conscious mediator between person and reality.

5. *Compensation:* the act of "making up" for a real or imagined inability or deficiency with a specific behavior to maintain self-respect or self-esteem. The person overcomes an inability by becoming proficient in another area. For example, a short girl may become the manager of the girls' basketball team because she is not tall enough to qualify for the team. An unattractive man selects expensive, stylish clothes to draw attention to himself.

6. *Reaction–formation:* also referred to as overcompensation. The person exaggerates or overdevelops certain actions by displaying exactly the opposite behavior, attitude, or feeling from what he normally would show in a given situation. This mechanism is considered a protective drive by which the person prevents painful, undesirable, or unacceptable attitudes toward others from emerging. For example, a young man who dislikes his mother-in-law may act very polite and courteous toward her. A woman who hates children may talk very lovingly to a friend's young son (although privately she considers him a brat).

7. *Substitution:* the act of finding another goal when one is blocked. Also defined as the replacement of consciously unacceptable emotions, drives, attitudes, or needs by those that are more acceptable. A student nurse in a baccalaureate program who decides she is unable to master the clinical competencies and elects to become a respiratory technician is using the mechanism of substitution. This mechanism is used to reduce frustration and promote feelings of satisfaction or success.

8. *Displacement:* a mechanism that serves to transfer feelings such as frustration, hostility, or anxiety from one idea, person, or object to another. The substitute target is less threatening and allows the person to release emotional reactions. Have you ever slammed a door when you were angry or yelled at one person when you were angry at another? If so, you displaced your feelings toward the original person to another object (the door) and person. Parents often displace feelings of anger or frustration toward their children as they are more tolerant recipients of such displacement than other adults.

9. *Restitution or undoing:* the negation of a previous consciously intolerable action or experience to reduce or alleviate feelings of guilt. For example, a young man sends flowers to his fiancée after he embarrassed her at a cocktail party. A mother, who sent her son to his room because he broke an ashtray, decides to let him stay up an hour later to watch television.

10. *Projection:* often termed the "scapegoat" defense mechanism. The person rejects unwanted characteristics of self and assigns them to others. He may blame others for faults, feelings, or shortcomings that are unacceptable to self. A man who is late for work states, "My wife forgot to set the alarm last night so I overslept." After spilling a glass of milk while playing cards with a friend, a 10-year-old tells his mother, "Johnny made me spill the milk. He told me to hurry up and play." A common retort is "you made me do it!" or "see what you made me do!"

11. *Symbolization:* an object, idea, or act represents another through some common aspect and carries the emotional feeling associated with the other. External objects may become outward representations of internal ideas, attitudes, or feelings. The engagement ring symbolizes love and a commitment to another person. Wearing a white wedding gown generally symbolizes the bride's purity or chastity. Symbolization allows emotional self-expression.

12. *Regression:* retreating to past levels of behavior that reduce anxiety, allow one to feel more comfortable, and permit dependency. A 27-year-old woman acts like a 17-year-old on her first date with a fellow employee. A 5-year-old boy who is toilet trained becomes incontinent during his father's hospitalization. Both persons have regressed to earlier developmental levels to reduce feelings of anxiety.

13. *Sublimation:* the rechanneling of consciously intolerable or socially unacceptable impulses or behaviors into activities that are personally or socially acceptable. For example, a college student who has hostile feelings rechannels them by joining the debate team. An aggressive young woman volunteers to head the United Fund drive in her community.

14. *Denial:* the unconscious refusal to face thoughts, feelings, wishes, needs, or reality factors that are intolerable. Denial is also defined as

blocking the awareness of reality by refusing to acknowledge its existence. A person who is told he has terminal cancer denies the diagnosis by telling his family he had a little tumor on his lung and his doctor "removed all of it." A young woman denies that her marriage is failing by telling her estranged husband that all couples go through marital slumps and "things will be better tomorrow."

15. *Introjection:* attributing to oneself the good qualities of another; symbolically taking on the character traits of another person by "ingesting" his philosophy, ideas, knowledge, customs, mores, or attitudes. Psychiatric patients have claimed to be Mary Magdalene, Jesus Christ, Moses, and other biblical or well-known persons. They have been observed dressing and acting like the personage they profess to be. One patient who claimed to be Moses grew a beard and long hair, wore a blanket and sandals, and read his Bible daily. He refused to participate in activities unless he was called Moses.

16. *Conversion:* the transferring of a mental conflict into a physical symptom to release tension or anxiety. For example, an elderly woman experiences sudden blindness after witnessing a robbery. A middle-aged man develops paralysis of his lower extremities after he learns that his wife has terminal cancer.

17. *Fantasy:* imagined events or mental images (*e.g.,* daydreaming) to express unconscious conflicts, gratify unconscious wishes, or prepare for anticipated future events. Heather, a young woman on a popular television soap opera, fantasized that she had a child, as she sat in a rocking chair, held a baby doll, and sang lullabies.

18. *Isolation:* the process of separating an unacceptable feeling, idea, or impulse from one's thoughts (also referred to as emotional isolation). For example, an oncologist is able to care for a terminally ill cancer patient by separating or isolating his feelings or emotional reaction to the patient's inevitable death. He focuses on the treatment, not the prognosis.

19. *Dissociation:* the act of separating and *detaching* a strong, emotionally charged conflict from one's consciousness. This detached information is blocked from conscious awareness, which allows the person to defer or postpone experiencing an emotional impact or painful feelings. A woman who was raped was found wandering a busy highway in torn, disheveled clothing. When examined by the emergency room physician, the woman was exhibiting symptoms of traumatic amnesia. She separated and detached her emotional reaction to the rape from her consciousness.

20. *Intellectualization:* the act of transferring emotional concerns into the intellectual sphere. The person uses reasoning as a means of avoiding confrontation with unconscious conflicts and their stressful emotions. A young man shows no emotional response to the "dear John" letter he received from his fiancée; instead, he tells his roommate he is trying to figure out why she changed her mind about the upcoming

wedding. The young man is using intellectualization as a method of avoiding confrontation with his fiancée.

Defense mechanisms are categorized in various ways: healthy to unhealthy; sophisticated to primitive; most frequently to least frequently used. Such lists of defense mechanisms have been developed after extensive research of several psychological, sociological, and psychiatric nursing, texts and are based on the degree of personality disintegration and reality distortion that can occur when the mechanisms are used frequently. Although denial is listed as unhealthy, it can be a healthy mechanism if used for a short period during the grieving process. A woman who has just been informed of her husband's death may use denial as a temporary protective measure, postponing a confrontation with reality. If she is able to work through the denial stage and progress to the other stages of the grieving process, denial has not caused her personality to disintegrate. A middle-aged man who is told he has cirrhosis of the liver because of alcoholism ignores his doctor's recommendations and continues to drink. A few weeks later he is admitted to the hospital for portal hypertension and hemorrhaging esophageal varices. The use of denial has been detrimental to his health physically and emotionally and has distorted the reality of his prognosis, making it an unhealthy mechanism. (A defense mechanism exercise is included in the Learning Activities at the end of this chapter).

SIGNIFICANT OTHERS OR SUPPORT PERSONS

Although mental health can be maintained by means of positive interpersonal communication, facing one's emotions, and using ego defense mechanisms, people may reach out to other individuals or groups for support during periods of increased stress or anxiety. Such persons are referred to as *significant others* or *support persons*. For instance, labor and delivery is generally considered to be a normal, healthy biologic process; however, many women desire the presence and encouragement of a support person, one who assists the woman in coping with the stress and anxiety that may occur during the labor and delivery process as well as during the postpartum recovery period. As a student nurse, you are living in a dormitory for the first time in 18 years. You are required to abide by various rules and regulations that are much different from those set by your parents and therefore you are not certain you want to stay in the dormitory. How do you think you would cope with this stressful situation? Would you need to reach out to another person? If so, to whom?

Support persons or significant others can be anyone that the person feels comfortable with, trusts, and respects. A support person can act as a sounding board, simply listening while one vents various feelings or emotions, or he or she may interact as the need arises. Women who enjoy coffee breaks with neighbors may look on these neighbors as people to whom they can relate their troubled feelings. Nurses need to help people to identify support persons as well as suggesting people who might be supportive. A cancer patient who has just been told he has 6 months to live needs someone to help him work through the grieving process. A young mother hospitalized for emergency surgery would certainly benefit from the support of a significant other as she makes arrangements for the care of her children at home and prepares for emergency surgery. A teenager whose parents are contemplating divorce may need to explore feelings of guilt, anger, or resentment. A paraplegic just starting a new job may need a supportive person available 24 hours a day. These people could develop symptoms of mental illness if they are unable to cope with the various stressors they encounter. Crisis intervention, which generally occurs when someone is *unable to take action on his own* to solve a problem, will be discussed in a separate chapter.

SUMMARY

Various definitions of mental health and mental illness have been presented, as well as the factors that influence the development of mental health: 1) inherited characteristics; 2) nurturing during childhood; 3) and life circumstances. Agreed upon characteristics of mental health were summarized. A comparison of mental health and mental illness was explored. Methods of maintaining mental health, such as effective interpersonal communication, dealing directly with one's emotions, and utilizing ego defense mechanisms, were discussed. Five levels of communication were described to demonstrate one's willingness to communicate verbally with others. They include 1) cliche conversation; 2) reporting facts; 3) revealing ideas and judgments; 4) gut level emotions; and 5) open, honest communication. Healthy and unhealthy ways of dealing directly with one's emotions were compared, with the focus on: 1) awareness of one's emotional responses; 2) capability of experiencing negative emotions; 3) ability to examine the intensity of such emotions and sharing these emotional responses with others; and 4) ability to think through emotional reactions rather than letting the emotion rule one's actions. The dynamics of twenty defense mechanisms were discussed, including purpose, definitions, and examples. The importance of the presence of significant others or support persons was explained.

LEARNING ACTIVITIES

  I. Clinical Activities
    A. Evaluate your nurse–patient interactions:
      1. What communication level did you use during these interactions?

2. Identify defense mechanisms used by the patient and yourself. What purpose do you feel each served?

B. Evaluate the reports you received on each assigned patient:
  1. Identify the communication level used during this report.
  2. Discuss your emotional reactions to the report.
  3. State how you handled these emotional reactions.

C. Identify the support persons or significant others available to each assigned patient. If none are available, what would you do?

II. Independent Activities
  A. Complete the programmed instruction on "Understanding Defense Mechanisms" (Am J Nurs: Sept, 1972).
  B. Complete the following defense mechanism exercise.

DEFENSE MECHANISM EXERCISE

Identify the following examples of defense mechanisms.

1. Mary Jones has just been told her husband has cancer. She asks the doctor to repeat some laboratory work because she feels certain that the technician made a mistake.

2. When asked if she would care to talk about her husband's condition, Mary Jones says, "I'd rather not talk about it right now."

3. Mr. Jones died after a brief illness. When asked about the funeral, Mrs. Jones says, "I can't recall or remember anything about it except that there were a lot of people there."

4. Bill Smith imitates the characteristics and actions of one of the actors on his favorite television show.

5. Jane, a rather unattractive woman, dresses like a fashion plate to attract attention.

6. John, who has a strong desire to drink alcohol, condemns the use of alcohol by others.

7. A person who has just been admitted to a mental institution states, "I'm really not sick. I'm just in here to get a rest".

8. Charlet Green always wanted to be a registered nurse. When she realized that her grades were not good enough to stay in the nursing program, she decided to become a medical receptionist.

9. Jim Williams, an executive whose day did not go smoothly, immediately criticizes his wife when he arrives home for dinner.

10. Ted Rule, who has difficulty playing basketball, was cut from the basketball team during tryouts. He states, "I got cut because the coach doesn't like me".

(continued)

11. Carl White witnessed an accident while enroute to work. As he describes the accident to his secretary, she comments, "You're as cool as a cucumber. Didn't the accident upset you?"

12. A young prizefighter becomes very upset with his father and attempts to throw a right punch. His right arm becomes paralyzed as he tries to move it.

13. Hostile impulses are rechanneled into debating, sports, or business activities.

14. Kevin Martin, age 22, sulks and pouts after his fiancée refuses to go to a boxing bout with him.

15. A shy 15-year-old girl daydreams about being glamorous, beautiful, and rich.

C. Read one of the following for personal growth:

   1. Berne E: What Do You Say After You Say Hello?

   2. Edelson M: The Idea of a Mental Illness.

   3. Elis A: A Guide to Rational Living.

   4. Harris T: I'm O.K., You're O.K.

   5. James M, Jongeward D: Born to Win.

   6. Jourard S: Disclosing Man to Himself. The Transparent Self.

   7. Lair J: I Ain't Much Baby. I Ain't Well But I Sure Am Better.

   8. Powell J: Fully Human, Fully Alive.

SELF-TEST

1. List the factors that influence the development of mental health or mental illness.

2. Name a positive state in which the person is responsible, self-directive, and displays self-awareness.

3. Maternal deprivation and parental rejection are examples of:

4. List the characteristics of emotional maturity as described by Menninger.

5. State at least five comparisons of mental health and mental illness.

6. Explain the five levels of communication as discussed in this chapter.

7. List ways to handle one's emotions in a positive manner while interacting with others.

8. Explain how defense mechanisms promote or help one to maintain mental health.

Match the following.

9. Rationalization
10. Repression
11. Compensation
12. Undoing
13. Suppression
14. Displacement
15. Substitution
16. Symbolization
17. Regression
18. Denial
19. Conversion
20. Sublimation

a. "I'd rather not discuss my problems with you."
b. "Sorry I'm late. My car kept stalling."
c. A laboratory technician is unhappy with her work and elects to become a medical secretary.
d. An accountant is unable to recall the reason for his argument with his boss.
e. A paraplegic becomes a competitive arm wrestler.
f. Yelling at the dog after an argument with one's spouse
g. A doctor compliments the head nurse after criticizing her earlier.
h. A 41-year-old woman dresses like a teenager.
i. A hostile, aggressive young man becomes a boxer.
j. Reciting the Pledge of Allegiance or saluting the flag
k. A person living on the slope below a glacier disregards the danger it presents.
l. A young woman suddenly experiences chest pain after arguing with her husband.

21. Why are denial, projection, and introjection considered to be *unhealthy* ego defense mechanisms?

22. Explain the importance of a support person or significant other.

REFERENCES

Altrocchi J: Abnormal Behavior. New York, Harcourt Brace Jovanovich, 1980

American Psychiatric Association: A Psychiatric Glossary, 5th ed. Washington, American Psychiatric Press, 1980

Bailey D, Dreyer S: Therapeutic Approaches to the Care of the Mentally Ill. Philadelphia, FA Davis, 1977

Coleman C: Abnormal Psychology and Modern Life, 5th ed. Dallas, Scott, Foresman, 1976

Haber J, et al.: Comprehensive Psychiatric Nursing, 2nd ed. New York, McGraw–Hill, 1982

Haggerty BK: Denial isn't all bad. Nursing 80: Oct,

Halderly R, NcNulty E: Feelings, feelings. Nursing 79: Oct,

Hale B: Appearance can be deceiving. . . . Nursing 81: Feb,

Jahoda M: Current Concepts of Positive Mental Health. New York, Basic Books, 1958

Knowles R: Handling anger: Responding *vs.* reacting. Am J Nurs: Dec, 1981

Kreigh H, Perko J: Psychiatric and Mental Health Nursing, 2nd ed. Reston, Reston Publishing, 1983

Marmor J, Pumpion–Mundlin E: Toward an integrated conception of mental disorders. Journal of Nervous and Mental Disease: Jan, 1950

Maslow A: Motivation and Personality. New York, Harper & Row, 1954

Peterson M: Understading defense mechanisms: Programmed instruction. Am J Nurs: Sept, 1972

Powell J: Why Am I Afraid to Tell You Who I Am? Niles, Argus Communications, Allen, Texas, 1969

Reynolds B: Behavioral problems: Sudden blindness. Nursing 79: July,

Rogers C: On Becoming a Person. Boston, Houghton Mifflin, 1961

Walker JI: Everybody's Guide to Emotional Well-Being. San Francisco, Harbor Publishing, 1982

Wilson H, Kneisl C: Psychiatric Nursing, 2nd ed. Menlo Park, Addison–Wesley, 1983

2

HISTORY AND TRENDS

IN PSYCHIATRIC NURSING

... when psychiatric treatment is frightening, unjust, and humiliating, then the price of psychic survival demands that the patient become the deserving victim, not only in the minds of those providing treatment, but most importantly, in the minds of the patients themselves. The price of psychiatric treatment then becomes self-blame, self-hatred, loss of self-respect ... *Judith S. Banes, 1983*

LEARNING OBJECTIVES

1. Define psychiatric nursing.
2. Discuss the treatment of mentally ill people during the Middle Ages.
3. Describe how the following people contributed to the history and trends in psychiatric nursing:
   Philippe Pinel
   Benjamin Rush
   Dorothea Dix
   Clifford Beers
   Linda Richards
4. State the educational objectives of psychiatric nursing during the early 20th century as described by the National League for Nursing (NLN).
5. State the purpose of the "Standards of Psychiatric Mental Health Nursing Practice."
6. Describe the progress of psychiatric nursing during the 20th century.

PSYCHIATRIC nursing is "the branch of nursing concerned with the prevention and cure of mental disorders and their sequelae. It employes theories of human behavior as its scientific framework and requires the use of self as its art or expression in nursing practice" (Urdang, 1983, p. 1901). Activities involved in psychiatric nursing include 1) providing a therapeutic environment; 2) helping patients or clients learn positive coping skills concerning real problems that they face daily; 3) providing care for physical symptoms; 4) acting as a social agent; 5) participating in psychotherapy; 6) providing leadership for members of the health care team; 7) participating in patient education; and 8) participating in research.

EARLY CIVILIZATION

Psychiatric nursing came into being between 1770 and 1880 during a series of reform movements concerning the treatment of the mentally ill. Before that time, during the era of organic explanations, spirits were thought to possess the body and had to be driven away to effect a cure. The ancient Greeks, Romans, and Arabs believed emotional disorders were an organic dysfunction of the brain. They used a variety of treatment approaches such as sedation, good nutrition, good physical hygiene, music, and recreational activities.

During the fifth century B.C., Hippocrates described a variety of personalities or temperaments and proposed that mental illness was a disturbance of four body fluids or "humors," resulting alternately from heat, cold, dryness, and moisture. Aristotle concluded that the mind was associated with the heart, and a Greek physician, Galen, stated that the emotional or mental disorders were associated with the brain. The Greeks used temples as hospitals and provided an environment of fresh air, sunshine, and pure water to promote healing for the mentally ill. Riding, walking, and listening to the sounds of a waterfall were examples of therapeutic care.

MIDDLE AGES

During the Middle Ages, an era of alienation, social exclusion, and confinement, the humane treatment of mental illness suffered a setback while various theories pertaining to demon possession became evident. Persons who displayed abnormal behavior were considered to be lunatics, witches, or demons possessed with evil spirits. Superstition, mysticism, magic, and witchcraft prevailed as patients were locked in asylums, flogged, starved, tortured, or subjected to the procedure of bloodletting. Beheading, hanging, and burning at the stake were common occurrences. Exorcism was practiced in some monasteries. People who were considered to be mad were isolated by confinement to large houses and institutions for social order. They were beaten for disobedience, chained, and placed in cages or closets. The mentally ill were subjected to cruel forms of torture. Physicians described symptoms of a) depression, b) paranoia, c) delusions, d) hysteria, and e) nightmares. Such persons were thought to be incompetent and potentially dangerous. The first mental hospital, Bethlehem Royal Hospital, was opened in England. Pronounced "Bedlam," the name came to symbolize the animalistic treatment of patients who were exhibited for twopence a look. Harmless inmates sought charity on the streets.

During the eighteenth century or era of reason and observation, Philippe Pinel, a French physician, was placed in charge of La Bicêtre, a hospital for the insane in Paris. He began more humane treatment of the mentally ill by removing chains and advocating the humane treatment instead. Pinel classified the patients according to observable behaviors, developed a case history on each, and kept records of their conversations with him.

Weyer, a German physician, is considered to be the first psychiatrist because of his descriptions of several diagnostic categories.

EIGHTEENTH AND NINETEENTH CENTURIES

Benjamin Rush, often called "the father of American psychiatry," wrote the first American textbook on psychiatry and encouraged more humane treatment of the mentally ill. In 1783, during an era of moral treatment, he joined the staff of Pennsylvania Hospital and insisted that intelligent, kind attendants be hired to read to the patients, talk to them, and share in their activities.

In 1843 Thomas Kirkbride attempted to establish a training school for attendants at Pennsylvania Hospital to assist physicians in the care of mentally ill patients.

By 1872 New England Hospital for Women and Children and Womens' Hospital of Philadelphia had established schools of nursing, but no psychiatric services were available. During this period Dorothea Lynde Dix, a Boston teacher, spent much of her time working for improved conditions for the mentally ill. She devoted her life to the cause of building state mental hospitals to meet the needs of the mentally ill. The nurse's role was to oversee the care given and to ensure the smooth operation of the ward. Housekeeping duties, dietary management, and laundry care were considered nursing responsibilities.

As hospitals were established by the middle of the 19th century to provide long-term custodial care for the mentally ill, humane treatment became more prevalent. In 1882, the first psychiatric training school for nursing was established at McLean Hospital in Waverly, Massachusetts. It soon became a training school for nurses and was considered to be the first formally organized school for nurses in a hospital for the mentally ill.

In 1890, trained nurses were employed on nursing staffs of state mental hospitals. These nurses were relieved of menial tasks and were able to develop their skills to provide therapeutic nursing care. By the end of the 19th century there was a growing appreciation of the therapeutic role of the psychiatric nurse. Duties included 1) assisting the physician; 2) administering sedative drugs; and 3) providing hydrotherapeutic measures (*e.g.,* hot and cold douches, continuous baths, and wet-sheet packs).

TWENTIETH CENTURY

During the 20th century the mental health movement was strongly influenced by the publication of a book written by Clifford Beers, titled *A Mind That Found Itself* (1908). He spent approximately 3 years in mental institutions and described his observations and experiences. Beers used his influence to organize the National Society for Mental Hygiene in 1909, now known as the National Association for Mental Health. As a result of public awareness, large state mental hospitals were built in rural areas, where the patients could receive the benefits of fresh air, sunshine, and a rural environment.

In 1915, Linda Richards, the first graduate nurse in the United States and often referred to as "the first American psychiatric nurse," suggested that the mentally ill receive the same quality of care as do the physically ill. She stated that caring for the mentally ill required a degree of patience and tact that the average student did not possess. Clinical experience in state mental hospitals provided students with a chance to cultivate these qualities. Several advancements occurred as the National Committee on Mental Hygience and the American Nurses' Association promoted study of the insane by publishing journal articles. Textbooks focusing on psychiatric nursing practice were written, and the National League for Nursing conventions discussed undergraduate psychiatric nursing education (1915–1935). These educational objectives included

1. Teaching the student nurse the relationship between physical and mental illness and the application of nursing principles to mental health nursing

2. Teaching the student nurse the causes of mental disease or illness and modern methods of treatment

3. Teaching the student nurse how to assess behaviors of patients who are mentally ill, so that they may recognize early signs or symptoms.

4. Teaching the student nurse the relationship of environmental conditions and mental disorders

5. Teaching the student to be resourceful, versatile, and adaptable while giving individualized care (Smoyak, 1982).

Clinical experiences in psychiatric hospitals were considered an essential part of the student nurses' basic experience and were standardized in 1937. Students were given the opportunity to care for patients with varying degrees of mental disorders, including organic diseases. Experiences focused on hydrotherapy; physical, occupational, recreational, and diversional therapy; and patient education. Nursing interventions included emphasis on cleanliness, proper elimination and adequate nutrition, as well as supervising continuous baths to promote relaxation.

By 1939 approximately one half of all nursing schools provided psychiatric nursing courses for students, but participation in such courses did not become a requirement for nursing licensure until 1955.

Phenothiazines and other major tranquilizers were discovered in the treatment of major symptoms of psychoses, enabling patients to be more responsive to therapeutic care. Open-door policies were implemented in large mental institutions, allowing patients to leave the units or wards under supervision.

In 1963, the Community Mental Health Act authorized funding for the establishment of community health centers to provide the following services to the public: 1) emergency mental health care, such as crisis centers and telephone hot-lines; 2) inpatient care or hospitalization; 3) partial hospitalization such as daycare centers and therapeutic communities; 4) aftercare, including halfway houses and foster homes; and 5) consultation services, as provided in counseling centers. This act played an important part in the specialization of psychiatric nursing services.

During the present century psychiatric nursing also began to evolve as a clinical specialty. Nurses were previously involved as managers and coordinators of activities as they provided therapeutic care based on the medical model. By advanced study and clinical practice, experienced in a master's program in psychiatric nursing, clinical specialists and nurse practitioners are able to gain expert knowledge in the care and prevention of psychiatric disorders.

STANDARDS OF PSYCHIATRIC–MENTAL HEALTH NURSING PRACTICE

In 1973 the American Nurses' Association developed 14 standards of psychiatric mental health nursing practice. These follow:

STANDARDS OF PSYCHIATRIC–MENTAL HEALTH NURSING PRACTICE

Standard I	Data are collected through pertinent clinical observations based on knowledge of the arts and sciences, with particular emphasis on psychosocial and biophysical sciences.
Standard II	Clients are involved in the assessment, planning, implementation, and evaluation of their nursing care program to the fullest extent of their capabilities.
Standard III	The problem-solving approach is used in developing nursing care plans.
Standard IV	Individuals, families, and community groups are assisted to achieve satisfying and productive patterns of living through health teaching.
Standard V	The activities of daily living (ADL) are used in a goal-directed way in work with clients.
Standard VI	Knowledge of somatic therapies and related clinical skills are used in working with clients.
Standard VII	The environment is structured to establish and maintain a therapeutic milieu.
Standard VIII	Nursing participates with interdisciplinary teams in assessing, planning, implementing and evaluating programs and other mental health activities.
Standard IX	Psychotherapeutic interventions are used to assist clients to achieve their maximal development.
Standard X	The practice of individual, group, or family psychotherapy requires appropriate preparation and recognition of accountability for the practice.
Standard XI	Nursing participates with other members of the community in planning and implementing mental health services that include the broad continuum of promotion of mental health, prevention of mental illness, treatment, and rehabilitation.
Standard XII	Learning experiences are provided for other nursing care personnel through leadership, supervision, and teaching.

(continued)

| Standard XIII | Responsibility is assumed for continuing educational and professional development, and contributions are made to the professional growth of others. |
| Standard XIV | Contributions to nursing and the mental health field are made through innovations in theory and practice and participation in research. |

OTHER EVENTS INFLUENCING PSYCHIATRIC NURSING

The following is a chronological listing of other important events influencing psychiatric nursing:

DATES	EVENTS
1856 to 1929	Emil Kraeplin differentiated manic–depressive psychosis from schizophrenia and stated that schizophrenia was incurable.
1856 to 1939	Sigmund Freud introduced psychoanalytic theory and therapy. He explained human behavior in psychological terms and proved that behavior can be changed in certain situations.
1857 to 1939	Engene Bleuler described the psychotic disorder of schizophrenia (formerly referred to as *dementia praecox*).
1870 to 1937	Alfred Adler focused on the area of psychosomatic medicine, referring to organ inferiority as the causative factor.
1875 to 1961	Carl Jung described the human psyche as consisting of a social mask (persona), hidden personal characteristics (shadow), feminine identification in man (anima), masculine identification in women (animus), and the innermost center of the personality (self).
1920	First textbook on psychiatric nursing, *Nursing Mental Diseases*, by Harriet Bailey.
1930s	Introduction of insulin shock therapy, pentylenetetrazol (Metrazol) therapy, electroconvulsive therapy, and prefrontal lobotomy, to treat mentally ill patients with psychotic disorders.
	International Committee for Mental Hygiene
	The Hill–Burton Act funded the building of psychiatric units.
1940s	Funding of graduate nursing programs to prepare clinical specialists by the Mental Health Act of 1946

DATES	EVENTS
1946 to 1971	Care of the mentally ill is brought into the mainstream of health care.
	National Mental Health Act provided funds for professional training programs.
	World Federation for Mental Health provided funds for research and education.
1947	Helen Render wrote *Nurse–Patient Relationships in Psychiatry.*
1949	Establishment of the National Institute of Mental Health to 1) provide grant-in-aides; 2) fund training programs and demonstration projects; and 3) provide support for research.
1952	Hildegarde Peplau wrote *Interpersonal Relations in Nursing,* a text that provided the basis for the development of therapeutic roles in nurse–patient relationships. This book was of paramount importance in the development of psychiatric nursing as a profession.
1955	Development of Joint Commission on Mental Illness and Health to study and evaluate needs and resources
1961	World Psychiatric Association examined the social consequences of mental illness.
1961	Economic Opportunity Act stressed improvement of social environments to prevent the development of mental illness.
1963 to 1975	The Mental Retardation Facilities and Community Mental Health Centers Construction Act provided federal funds to help state and local agencies to decentralize mental health care; provided community services and facilities to treat substance abusers such as drug addicts and alcoholics; and proposed that community mental health programs include special programs to treat children and the elderly.
1970s	Fifty graduate psychiatric nursing programs are established in the United States.
	Establishment of private psychiatric hospitals and psychiatric units in general hospitals.
	Insurance companies provided coverage for psychiatric care.
	Emphasis on deinstitutionalization and community living for mental patients, focusing on teaching them ADLs and self-care.

PSYCHIATRIC NURSING IN THE TWENTIETH CENTURY

Schools of nursing offer a variety of programs in psychiatric nursing. Licensed practical nursing schools generally address the topics of human behavior or mental health and mental illness, and may integrate mental health concepts into various classes such as pediatrics, obstetrics and the aging process. Psychiatric nursing clinical experience usually is not offered in such one-year programs, although state board examinations do include questions pertaining to basic mental health concepts. If a licensed practical nurse elects to continue and become a registered nurse, psychiatric nursing experience needs to be obtained in a ladder program.

Associate degree programs may offer a 5- to 10-week course in psychiatric nursing with or without clinical rotation to psychiatric or mental health settings. Some schools integrate psychiatric nursing concepts throughout the 2-year program, after core courses in developmental psychology or abnormal psychology. Psychiatric nursing experience may occur in a medical–psychiatric unit, private psychiatric hospital, state psychiatric facility, or in a community mental health setting. Emphasis is on nursing intervention under the direction of a more experienced registered nurse.

Baccalaureate schools generally provide more time for psychiatric nursing and clinical experiences, and place a heavier emphasis on theoretical foundations, the assessment process, statistics, group dynamics, patient or client education and the nurse's role in preventive care.

Graduate schools offering a master's degree in psychiatric or mental health nursing generally require 48 to 50 hours of core courses, clinical experience, research, electives, and a practicum. Courses available may focus on leadership, life cycle, conceptual bases, physiological bases, and client assessment. The graduate student may elect to become a clinical nurse specialist or a nurse practitioner, depending on the courses available.

Psychiatric nursing experience as a student provides a valuable foundation for a variety of career opportunities after graduation. The following is a list of such positions and examples of how psychiatric nursing experience can be an asset.

CAREER OPPORTUNITIES	EXAMPLES
Obstetric nursing	Helping the mother in labor and/or support person cope with anxiety or stress during labor and delivery
	Providing support to bereaved parents in the event of fetal demise, inevitable abortion, or the birth of an infant with congenital anomalies

CAREER OPPORTUNITIES	EXAMPLES
	Providing support to an unwed mother who must decide whether to keep her child or give it up for adoption
Oncologic nursing	Helping cancer patients or other terminally ill individuals on oncology units to work through the grieving process
	Providing support groups for families of terminally ill patients
Industrial (occupational health) nursing	Implementing or participating in industrial substance abuse programs for employees and/or their families
	Providing crisis intervention during an industrial accident or the acute onset of a physical or mental illness (*e.g.,* heart attack, or anxiety attack)
	Teaching stress management
Public health nursing	Assessing the person both physically and psychologically (*e.g.,* The newly diagnosed diabetic may develop a low self-concept, or the recovering stroke patient may exhibit symptoms of depression due to a slow recovery.)
Office nursing	Assisting the patient in explaining somatic or emotional concerns during the assessment process
	Providing support with the problem-solving process when people call the office and the physician is unavailable. Acting as a community resource person
Emergency room nursing	Providing crisis intervention as the need arises (*e.g.,* during natural disasters, accidents, or unexpected illnesses causing increased anxiety, stress, or immobilization)

SUMMARY

Psychiatric nursing began to emerge as a nursing subspecialty between 1770 and 1880, when reform movements occurred concerning the treatment of mentally ill people. This chapter focuses on the history and trends in psychiatry and psychiatric nursing by discussing the treatment of mentally ill persons during the periods of early civilization, the Middle Ages, and the 18th, 19th and 20th centuries, mentioning the contributions of Hippocrates, Aristotle, Galen, Pinel, Weyer, Rush, Kirkbride, Dix, Beers, and Richards. "The Standards of Psychiatric Mental Health Nursing Practice" are included, as well as a chronological listing of important acts and events influencing psychiatric nursing. An overview of student psychiatric nursing experiences for licensed practical nurses, associate degree nurses, baccalaureate nurses and graduate students was presented. Examples of how a psychiatric nursing experience can be an asset for graduate nurses working in obstetric, oncologic, industrial, public health, office, and emergency room settings were given.

SELF-TEST

1. Define psychiatric nursing:
2. State how the following pertain to the history of psychiatric nursing:
   a. Era of organic explanations
   b. Era of alienation, social exclusion and confinement

   Match the following:

3. Hippocrates
4. Philippe Pinel
5. Benjamin Rush
6. Dorothea Dix
7. Linda Richards

    a. Devoted time to the cause of building state mental hospitals
    b. Removed chains from the mentally ill and advocated the use of kindness
    c. First graduate nurse and first American psychiatric nurse
    d. Wrote the first American textbook on psychiatry
    e. Proposed that mental illness was a disturbance of four fluids or "humors"

8. State the origin of the word "Bedlam".
9. Compare psychiatric nursing duties during the time Dorothea Dix worked for improved conditions for the mentally ill and 1890, when trained nurses were employed in state mental institutions.
10. Discuss how Clifford Beers influenced psychiatry and psychiatric nursing.
11. List the educational objectives of psychiatric nursing as stated by the National League for Nursing conventions (1915–1935).
12. Discuss the function of the Community Mental Health Act of 1963.
13. Review the "Standards of Psychiatric Mental Health Nursing Practices" and summarize the role of the psychiatric nurse.
14. State the contributions of the following people to psychiatric nursing:
    a. Harriet Bailey
    b. Helen Render
    c. Hildegarde Peplau

15. Discuss the application of psychiatric nursing concepts in other fields of nursing, such as
   a. emergency room
   b. public health nursing
   c. oncologic nursing
   d. obstetric nursing

REFERENCES

Banes JS: An ex-patient's perspective of psychiatric treatment. J Psychosoc Nurs: Mar, 1983

Haber J et al: Comprehensive Psychiatric Nursing, 2nd ed. New York, McGraw–Hill, 1982

Horwitz E: Madness, Magic and Medicine. Philadelphia, JB Lippincott, 1977

Kahlman N, Waughfield CG: Mental Health Concepts. Albany, Delmar Publishers, 1983

Kreigh HZ, Perko JE: Psychiatric and Mental Nursing: A Commitment to Care and concern, 2nd ed. Reston VA, Reston Publishing, 1983

Mereness D, Taylor C: *Essentials of Psychiatric Nursing,* 10th ed. St. Louis, CV Mosby, 1978.

Murray RB, Huelskoetter MM: Psychiatric Mental Health Nursing: Giving Emotional Care. Englewood Cliffs, Prentice–Hall, 1983

Pasquali E et al: Mental Health Nursing: A Bio-Psycho-Cultural Approach. St. Louis, CV Mosby, 1981

Smoyak S, Rouslin S (eds): A Collection of Classics in Psychiatric Nursing Literature. Thorofare, NJ, Charles B Slack, 1982

Stuart G, Sundeen S: Principles and Practice of Psychiatric Nursing, 2nd ed. St. Louis, CV Mosby, 1983

Urdang L (ed): Mosby's Medical and Nursing Dictionary. St. Louis, CV Mosby, 1983

Wilson H, Kneisl C: Psychiatric Nursing, 2nd ed. Menlo Park, Addison–Wesley, 1983.

3

T H E R A P E U T I C

I N T E R A C T I O N S

LISTEN

When I ask you to listen to me
   and you start giving advice
   you have not done what I asked.

When I ask you to listen to me
   and you begin to tell me why I shouldn't feel that way,
   you are trampling on my *feelings*.

When I ask you listen to me
   and you feel you have to *do* something to solve my problem,
   you have failed me, strange as that may seem.

Listen! All I asked, was that you listen.
   not talk or do—just hear me.
Advice is cheap: 10 cents will get you both Dear Abby and
   Billy Graham in the same newspaper.
And I can do for myself; I'm not helpless.
   Maybe discouraged and faltering, but not helpless.

When you do something for me *that I can and need to do
   for myself,* you contribute to my fear and weakness.

But, when you accept as a simple fact that I do feel what I feel,
   no matter how irrational, then I can quit trying to convince
   you and can get about the business of understanding what's
   behind this irrational feeling.
   And when that's clear, the answers are obvious and I don't need
   advice.

Irrational feelings make sense when we understand what's
    behind them.

Perhaps that's why prayer works, sometimes, for some people
    because God is mute, and he doesn't give advice or
    try to fix things. "They" just listen and let you work it out for
    yourself.

So, please listen and just hear me. And, if you want to
    talk, wait a minute for your turn; and I'll listen to you.

Anonymous

"The greatest gift I can give is to understand and to touch another
person. When this is done, I feel contact has been made."

Satir (1976)

LEARNING OBJECTIVES

1. Describe a therapeutic interaction.
2. Define the process of communication.
3. State the factors that influence communication.
4. Explain how one may develop good communication skills.
5. Discuss how communication blocks can occur.
6. Compare social and therapeutic interactions.
7. List essential conditions for a therapeutic relationship to occur as described by Carl Rogers.
8. Describe the elements of nonverbal communication.
9. Explain the phases of a therapeutic relationship.
10. Cite examples of interpersonal therapeutic techniques.
11. Discuss the interaction or process recording.

ACCORDING to Webster, an interaction is a mutual or reciprocal action that can occur between or among people. Interaction that facilitates growth, development, maturity, improved functioning, and improved coping is considered therapeutic (Rogers, 1961).

Therapeutic communication, relationship, intervention, environment, and milieu all are terms that refer to nurse–patient interactions. The focus of this chapter is to discuss the nurse's ability to establish a therapeutic relationship through communication and interaction.

COMMUNICATION

The process of communication includes three elements: the sender, the message, and the receiver. Communication is the giving and receiving of information. The sender prepares or creates a message when a need occurs and sends the message to a receiver or listener, who then decodes it. The receiver may then return a message or feedback to the initiator of the message. Communication is a learned process influenced by attitudes, one's sociocultural or ethnic background, past experiences, knowledge of subject matter, and the ability to relate to others. Interpersonal perceptions also affect one's ability to communicate because they influence the initiation and response of communication. Such perception occurs through the senses of sight, sound, touch, and smell. Environmental factors that influence communication include time, place and the presence of one or several persons.

The factors influencing communication follow:

1. *Attitude.* Attitudes are developed in various ways and may be the result of interacting with the environment, assimilating the attitudes

of others, life experiences, intellectual processes, or a traumatic experience. Descriptive terms include accepting, caring, prejudiced, judgmental, and open or closed minded.

2. *Sociocultural or ethnic background.* People of French or Italian heritage often are referred to as gregarious and talkative, willing to share thoughts and feelings. People from East Asian countries such as Thailand or Laos, who are quiet and reserved, may appear stoic and reluctant to discuss personal feelings with persons outside their families.

3. *Past experiences.* Previous positive or negative experiences influence one's ability to communicate. For example, a child who has been told continually to be quiet or to speak only when spoken to, may become withdrawn and noncommunicative. A teenager who has been "put-down" by parents or teachers whenever attempting to express any feelings may develop a poor self-image and feel his opinions are not worthwhile. As a result, the teenager avoids interacting with others.

4. *Knowledge of subject matter.* A person who is well-educated or knowledgeable about certain topics may feel more secure when discussing these topics with others. A word of caution: knowledgeable people need to communicate with others at their level of understanding. The receiver of the message may neglect to ask questions because he doesn't want to appear ignorant. As a result he may not receive the correct information.

5. *Ability to relate to others.* Some people are "natural-born talkers" who claim to have "never met a stranger." Others may possess an intuitive trait that enables them to say the right thing at the right time and relate well to persons. "I feel so comfortable talking with her", "She's so easy to relate to", and "I could talk to him for hours" are just a few comments made about people who have the ability to relate to others. Such an ability can also be a learned process, the result of practicing communicative skills over a period of time.

6. *Interpersonal perceptions.* Satir (1976) warns the reader to beware of looking without seeing, listening without hearing, touching without feeling, moving without awareness, and speaking without meaning. The following passage reinforces the importance of perception: "I know that you believe you understand what you think I said, but I'm not sure you realize that what you heard is not what I said" (Lore 1981). Adler and Towne (1978) list seven types of listening that can impair communication. They include:

Pseudolistening: "Counterfeit communication" in which the listener appears interested but ignores the speaker. Such inattention may be the result of preoccupation or boredom.

Stage hogging: Such a person is not interested in listening to others, but wants only to express his own ideas while others listen.

Selective listening: This person selectively screens out information he does not want to hear.

Insulated listening: Responding to a comment and then forgetting the conversation, or failure to hear in the first place, generally occurs as a result of lack of interest or preoccupied thinking.

Defensive listening: One who becomes defensive during a conversation may feel a personal attack is about to occur. Such a person may be suspicious of conversation around or near him, accusing people of talking about him.

Ambushing: Have you ever felt as if you were being asked "twenty questions" or cross-examined during a conversation? One student nurse noted on an interaction recording (process recording) that she didn't realize her anxiety level was so high as she attempted to relate to a patient until she counted the number of questions she asked, merely to "keep the conversation going."

Insensitive listening: A person who is insensitive takes comments at face value and doesn't recognize any hidden meanings that may occur during a conversation.

7. *Environmental factors such as time, place, and the presence of people.* Timing is quite important during a conversation. Consider the child who has misbehaved and is told by his mother, "Just wait 'til your father gets home." By the time father does arrive home, the child may not be able to relate to him regarding the incident that occurred earlier. Some people prefer to "buy time" to handle a situation involving a personal confrontation. They want time to think things over or "a cooling-off period." The place in which communication occurs, as well as the number of people present, have a definite influence on interactions. A subway, crowded restaurant, or grocery store would not be a desirable place to conduct a disclosing, serious, or philosophic conversation.

NONVERBAL COMMUNICATION

As mentioned earlier, communication can be verbal, written, or nonverbal. The latter is considered a more accurate description of true feelings because one has less control over nonverbal reactions. Nonverbal communication includes position or posture, gestures, touch, physical appearance, facial expressions, vocal cues, and distance or spatial territory.

1. *Position or posture.* The position one assumes can designate authority, cowardice, boredom, or indifference. For example, a nurse standing at the foot of a patient's bed with her arms folded across her chest gives the impression that she is in charge of any interaction that may occur. A student nurse slumped in her chair, doodling on a pad gives the appearance of boredom.

2. *Gestures.* Pointing, finger tapping, winking, hand clapping, eyebrow raising, palm rubbing, hand wringing, and beard stroking are examples of nonverbal gestures that communicate various thoughts and

feelings. Reflect on these gestures and your reactions to them. What gestures are common in your nonverbal communication? Do they betray feelings of insecurity, anxiety, or apprehension or do they express feelings of power, enthusiasm, eagerness, or genuine interest?

3. *Touch.* Hand shaking, hugging, holding hands, and kissing all denote positive feelings for another person. Reactions to touch depend on one's age, sex, cultural background, interpretation of the gesture, and appropriateness of the touch. The nurse should exercise caution when touching people. The depressed or grieving patient may respond to touch as a gesture of concern, whereas the sexually promiscuous person may consider touching an invitation to sexual advances. An abused child may recoil from the nurse's attempt to comfort him, whereas the dying patient may be comforted by the presence of a nurse sitting by the bedside silently holding his hand.

4. *Physical appearance.* People who are depressed may pay little attention to their appearance. They may appear unkempt and unconsciously don dark-colored clothing, reflecting their depressed feelings. Confused or disoriented persons may forget to put on items of clothing, put them on inside out, or dress inappropriately. Weight gain or weight loss also may be a form of nonverbal communication. People who exhibit either may be experiencing feelings of anxiety, depression, loneliness, or a low self-concept. The manic patient may dress in brightly colored clothes with several items of jewelry and excessive make-up. People with a positive self-concept may communicate such feelings by appearing neat, clean, and well-dressed.

5. *Facial expressions.* A blank stare, startled expression, sneer, grimace, and broad smile are examples of facial expression denoting one's innermost feelings. Clowns use facial expressions to convey feelings of sadness, happiness, surprise, disgust, and other emotional reactions. Commercials on television and billboard advertisements make use of facial expressions to sell various products.

6. *Vocal cues.* Pausing or hesitating while conversing, talking in a tense or flat tone, or speaking tremulously are vocal cues that can agree with or contradict one's verbalization. Speaking softly may indicate a concern for another whereas speaking loudly may be the result of feelings of anger or hostility. For example, a person who is admitted to the hospital for emergency surgery may speak softly but tremulously stating, "I'm okay. I just want to get better and go home as soon as possible." The nonverbal cues should indicate to the nurse that the patient is not okay and the patient's feelings should be explored.

7. *Distance or spatial territory.* Hall (1966) describes four zones of distance awareness utilized by adult, middle-class Americans. They include the intimate, personal, social, and public zones. Intimate distance includes love-making, wrestling, and other actions that involve touching another body. The personal zone refers to an arm's length distance of approximately 1½ ft to 4 ft. Physical contact, such as hand

holding, still can occur. This is the zone in which therapeutic communication occurs. The social zone, in which formal business and social discourse occurs, occupies a space of 4 ft to 12 ft. The public zone, in which no physical contact and little eye contact occurs, ranges from 12 ft to 25 ft. People who maintain communication in this zone remain strangers.

COMMUNICATION SKILLS

The following suggestions are given to enable one to develop good communication skills for effective therapeutic interactions.

Know Yourself: What motivates your interest in helping others? Identify your emotional needs so that they don't interfere with the ability to relate to others. Be aware of any mood swings that you may exhibit. Patients are very sensitive to the emotions and reactions of helping persons. One student stated at the beginning of a therapeutic interaction, "Mr. Williams asked me what was wrong today. I tried not to show that I had a headache. He said I wasn't my usual cheery self. I'm surprised he realized I wasn't feeling up to par."

Be Honest With Your Feelings: Don't wear a mask to protect yourself or avoid contact with others. Your body language, gestures, and tone of voice can reveal your true feelings or reactions to patient behavior. Your non-verbal communication may contradict your spoken word if you are not honest with the patient. Nurses who work with cancer patients often find it hard to relate to terminally ill persons. They may avoid contact as much as possible, so that their emotions are not revealed to the patients when they are asked questions such as, "Will I be getting better?", "Is it cancer?", or "Am I going to die?". It is okay to cry with a terminally ill patient who is emotionally upset or depressed. A student nurse told a 17-year-old cancer patient who used vulgar language, "I like you, but I don't like to hear you use profanity when you speak to me."

Be Secure in Your Ability to Relate to People: Don't allow the behavior of others to threaten or intimidate you. Remember that all behavior has meaning. Ask yourself, "What is the patient trying to communicate?"

Be Sensitive to the Needs of Others: Listen attentively by utilizing eye-to-eye contact, focusing your attention on the speaker and assuming a personal distance of 1½ ft to 4 ft. Use tact and diplomacy while conversing with others.

Be Consistent: Consistency in what you say and do encourages the development of trust.

Recognize Symptoms of Anxiety: Knowing anxiety when it appears in yourself and those you relate to is important. Anxiety impairs communication if the person is unable to concentrate or express feelings.

Watch Your Nonverbal Reactions: Be aware of your body language because it punctuates and modifies verbal messages. Use gestures cautiously to emphasize meanings, reactions, or emotions.

Use Words Carefully: When relating to others these words should be used cautiously: I, you, they, it, but, yes, no, always, never, should, and ought. Satir (1976) refers to these words as "powerful words" that may be used thoughtlessly, appear to be accusations, be easily misunderstood, cause confusion or ambivalence, or imply stupidity.

Recognize Differences: The fact that people may have personality or age differences, or may have conflicting loyalties can impair communication.

Recognize and Evaluate Your Own Actions and Responses: Are you open or close minded, cooperative or uncooperative, and supportive or nonsupportive, when you converse with someone? Are you available when needed or do you tend to put someone on hold if you are busy? Never cut a conversation short by hanging up in the middle of a self-disclosing interaction. Refer the person to someone whom you feel can be supportive regarding the issues at hand.

INEFFECTIVE COMMUNICATION

Stalls can occur during the process of communication. The nurse needs to be aware of the various reasons for ineffective communication. These reasons include

1. Ineffective communication skills used by the helping person. He may not send the message he intended to send. A list of effective interpersonal communication skills and examples of each are presented later in this chapter.

2. Failure to listen on the part of the helping person. Some individuals are doers rather than listeners. They focus on task-oriented nursing instead of therapeutic communication. The patient also may not hear the message sent because of a variety of reasons, such as stress, anxiety, fear, denial, or anger.

3. Conflicting verbal and nonverbal messages. Ambivalence on the part of the sender may confuse the receiver since he senses conflicting signals and doubts the helping person's interest in him.

4. A judgmental attitude. Someone who displays prejudice or a judgmental attitude when relating to others may never really get to know the

person. A sensitive person may pick up on a judgmental attitude and refuse to relate to others, thinking that all people are judgmental. A student nurse shared in postclinical conference that her assigned patient was quite defensive as she attempted to relate to him. She later learned that he was labeled a juvenile delinquent because he had lived in a low socioeconomic part of town. His parents were migrant workers and left the children to care for each other while they worked in the fields. The patient related experiences that he had had with teachers as he attended various schools. He was shunned by the middle-class students and stereotyped as a member of the street gangs.

5. Misunderstanding because of multiple meanings of English words. Consider the word "cup." It may mean a drinking receptacle, a hole on a golf green, or a winner's cup (trophy). The sender should select words that are not confusing in meaning.

6. False reassurance. Clichés such as "Everything will be okay" or "Don't worry, the doctor will make you well" are considered examples of false reassurance. No one can always predict or guarantee the outcome of a situation. There are too many variables, such as a person who desires to maintain a sick role, nonsupportive families, or an illness that is irreversible (e.g., cancer or multiple sclerosis). Patients who receive false reassurance quickly learn not to trust people if they do not respond to treatment as predicted.

7. Giving advice rather than encouraging the person to make decisions, however small they may be, may facilitate dependency. It may also cause the patient to feel inadequate because he is not given the opportunity to make choices pertaining to personal care. The patient will accept advice only when wanted. Feelings of dependency and inadequacy may occur and impair therapeutic communication if the patient receives no positive feedback during nurse–patient interactions. It is much more constructive to encourage problem solving by the patient.

8. Disagreeing with or criticizing a person who is seeking support. Belittling a person may result in the development of a low self-concept and incapability of coping with stressors. Thoughts and feelings are not important, or so the patient thinks.

9. The inability to receive information because of a preoccupied or impaired thought process. The receiver may be prepared to hear a different message from the one sent. Someone who is preoccupied with thoughts is not as receptive to messages as a person with a clear mind. Impaired thought processes, such as delusions or hallucinations also interfere with communication. A person who hears voices telling him that he is being poisoned is not receptive to a nurse's request that he take his medication.

10. Changing the subject if one becomes uncomfortable with the topic being discussed

INTERACTIONS

Two types of interactions may occur when the nurse is working with patients or families who seek help for physical or emotional needs. They are referred to as social and therapeutic interactions. Social interactions occur daily as the nurse greets the patient and passes the time of day, so to speak, with what is referred to as small talk. Comments such as "Good morning. It's a beautiful day out", "How are your children?", and "Have you heard any good jokes lately?" are examples of socializing. During a therapeutic interaction the nurse helps or encourages the patient to communicate feelings of perceptions, fears, anxieties, frustrations, expectations, and increased dependency needs. "You look upset. Would you like to share your feelings with someone?", "I'll sit with you until the pain medication takes effect," and "No, its true that I don't know what it is like to lose a husband, but I would think it would be one of the most painful experiences one might have," are just a few examples of therapeutic communication.

The following is a comparison of social helping and therapeutic helping as discussed by Purtilo (1978):

SOCIAL HELPING	THERAPEUTIC HELPING
A personal or intimate relationship occurs.	A personal, but not intimate relationship occurs.
Not necessarily concerned with the identification of needs	Needs are identified by the person with the help of the nurse if necessary.
Personal goals may or may not be discussed.	Personal goals are set by the patient.
May create constructive or destructive dependency	Promotes constructive dependency, interdependency, and independency
May use a variety of resources during socialization	Uses specialized professional skills while employing nursing interventions
Social helping may be referred to as doing a favor for another person, such as lending someone money, taking food to a houseridden elderly couple, or giving advice to a young girl who has just broken her engagement.	Therapeutic helping promotes the functional use of one's latent inner resources. Encouraging verbalization of feelings following the death of one's child or exploring ways to cope with increased stress are examples of therapeutic helping.

Purtilo (1978) also recommends the following approaches when communicating in a therapeutic manner:

1. Translate any technical information into layman's terms.

2. Clarify and restate any instructions or information given. Patients usually do not ask doctors or nurses to repeat themselves.

3. Display a caring attitude.

4. Exercise effective listening.

5. Do not overload the listener with information.

Rogers (1961) lists eight conditions essential for a therapeutic relationship to occur. They include

1. *Empathy.* The helper is able to zero in on the feelings of another person. To "walk in another's shoes" describes emphathetic understanding because such action enables one to experience the feelings of another and respond to them. A person seeking help feels understood and accepted. He is then able to relate to another, to explore feelings, and to try new behaviors.

2. *Respect.* The helper considers the person to be deserving of high regard and cares deeply for the person as a human being. Consistency on the part of the helper conveys respect.

3. *Genuineness.* The helper is sincere, honest, and authentic in responses. He becomes a role model as he meets the patient's needs rather than his wants.

4. *Self-disclosure.* Exposing a view of one's attitudes, feelings, and beliefs is self-disclosure. It can occur on the part of the helper as well as the patient. Appropriate self-disclosure by the helper provides a role for the other person to model, thus becoming more open, revealing more about himself, and feeling more secure.

5. *Concreteness and specificity.* The ability to identify feelings by skillful listening requires the helper to be realistic, not theoretical, while assisting the person in expressing specific feelings. He should not expect a patient to be a textbook picture of an illness and stereotype or label symptoms.

6. *Confrontation.* Discussing discrepancies in the person's behavior must be done in an acceptant manner after the helper has established a good rapport with the person. Those with emotional problems may perceive themselves differently than they think others regard them. Such feelings may result in anxiety and inappropriate behavior in an attempt to reconcile these perceived discrepancies.

7. *Immediacy of relationship.* Recognizing one's own feelings and sharing them with the patient is essential to a therapeutic relationship. The helper needs to be able to share spontaneous feelings but not necessarily all of them. The sharing of too many negative expressions can be detrimental during the beginning of a relationship. Once a relationship exists the helper shares spontaneous feelings when he feels the patient will profit from such a discussion.

8. *Self-exploration.* If the patient is to make progress, he needs to engage in self-exploration. Feelings of discomfort or fear may initially emerge; however, the more the patient investigates his feelings, the more he learns to cope and adapt.

CONFIDENTIALITY

Confidentiality is important during a nurse–patient interaction. The patient has a right to privacy. All information concerning the patient is considered personal property and is not to be discussed with other patients or outside the hospital setting. When discussing a patient, as in preclinical or postclinical conference, the patient's name and descriptive information that might identify him should not be mentioned. It may be necessary for a student nurse to reassure a patient that confidentiality will be maintained except when: 1) the information may be harmful to the patient or others; 2) the patient does not intend to comply with the treatment plan; and 3) the patient threatens self-harm. One way to convey this is simply to state "Only information that will be helpful in assisting you toward recovery will be provided to others on the staff." The student nurse has an obligation to share such information with the nursing staff or with the patient's doctor. Family members should be told that permission must be obtained from patients 18 years old and older before the attending physician, social worker, or other members of the health care team can discuss the patient's progress with them.

THERAPEUTIC RELATIONSHIP: PHASES

Initiating Phase

The first step of the threapeutic relationship is called the initiating or orienting phase. During this phase the nurse sets the stage for a one-to-one relationship by becoming acquainted with the patient. Both the nurse and the patient may experience anxiety when they first meet. A comment such as "Sometimes it's hard to talk to a stranger" is a good way to begin a discussion on initiating a relationship. Assessment of the patient occurs as the nurse and patient agree on the time, place, and duration of each meeting. Communication styles of the nurse and patient are explored to facilitate rapport and open communication as the patient begins to share innermost feelings and conflicts. The patient must feel accepted as he develops a feeling of trust toward the nurse. Allow the patient to set the pace of the relationship. He is a unique person who is ill and may be experiencing feelings of loneliness, fear, anger, disgust, despair, or rejection. As a patient, he seeks comfort and help to handle various stressors. In doing so the patient accepts another's assistance in problem solving or goal setting. The following tasks are to be accomplished during the initiating phase:

1. Building trust and rapport
2. Establishing a therapeutic environment

3. Establishing a mode of communication acceptable to both the patient and nurse

4. Initiating a therapeutic contract by establishing a time, place, and duration for each meeting, as well as the length of time the relationship will be in effect

5. Assessing the patient's strengths and weaknesses

Working Phase

The second phase of the therapeutic relationship is known as the working or middle phase. The patient begins to relax, trusts the nurse, and is able to discuss mutually decided on goals with the nurse as the assessment process continues and a plan of care develops. Perceptions of reality, coping mechanisms, and support systems are identified at this time. Alternative behaviors and techniques are explored to replace those that are maladaptive. The nurse and patient discuss the meaning behind such behavior, as well as any reactions by the nurse such as fear, intimidation, embarrassment, or anger. During the working phase, the patient is able to focus on unpleasant, painful aspects of life with the nurse's supportive help. Therapeutic tasks accomplished during the working phase include

1. Exploring perception of reality

2. Developing positive coping behaviors

3. Identifying available support systems

4. Promoting a positive self-concept

5. Encouraging verbalization of feelings

6. Developing a realistic plan of action

7. Implementing the plan of action

8. Evaluating the results of the plan of action

9. Promoting independence

Terminating Phase

The final step of the therapeutic relationship is the terminating phase. The nurse terminates the relationship when the mutually agreed on goals are reached, the patient is transferred or discharged, or the nurse has finished her clinical rotation. At this time it is not uncommon for the patient to show regressive behavior, hostility, or attempt to prolong the relationship as he experiences symptoms of separation anxiety. The nurse must realize that

1. Termination needs to occur if a therapeutic relationship is to be a complete process. Preparation for termination begins during the initiating phase.

2. The nurse and patient will experience a variety of feelings that need to be recognized and shared. By this process the patient learns that it is acceptable to feel sadness or loss when separation occurs.

3. The patient has a right to see the nurse's reactions during the termination of a relationship. The nurse also may experience feelings of sadness when separation occurs and may unconsciously prolong the terminating phase.

4. This may be the first successful termination experience for the patient.

5. This may be the first time that the patient feels important to another person.

6. The longer the relationship, the longer the preparation for termination occurs.

Some mutually accepted goals resulting in the termination of a therapeutic relationship include the ability to

1. Provide self-care and maintain one's environment

2. Demonstrate independence and work interdependently with others

3. Recognize signs of increased stress or anxiety

4. Cope positively when experiencing feelings of anxiety, anger, or hostility

5. Demonstrate emotional stability

INTERPERSONAL TECHNIQUES

The following is a list of therapeutic interpersonal communication techniques and examples of each.

THERAPEUTIC TECHNIQUES	EXAMPLES
Using silence	
Accepting	"Yes." "That must have been difficult for you."
Giving recognition or acknowledging	I noticed that you've made your bed.
Offering self	I'll walk with you.
Giving broad openings or asking open-ended questions	Is there something you'd like to do?
Offering general leads or door-openers	Go on. You were saying . . .

THERAPEUTIC TECHNIQUES	EXAMPLES
Placing the event in time or in sequence	When did your nervousness begin?
Making observations	I notice that you're trembling. You appear to be angry.
Encouraging description of perceptions	What does the voice seem to be saying? How do you feel when you take your medication?
Encouraging comparison	Has this ever happened before? What does this resemble?
Restating	*Patient:* I can't sleep. I stay awake all night. *Nurse:* You can't sleep at night.
Reflecting	*Patient:* I think I should take my medication. *Nurse: You* think you should take your medication?
Focusing on specifics	This topic seems worth discussing more in depth. Give me an example of what you mean.
Exploring	Tell me more about your job. Would you describe your responsibilities?
Giving information or informing	His name is . . . I'm going with you to the beauty shop.
Seeking clarification or clarifying	I'm not sure that I understand what you are trying to say. Please give me more information.
Presenting reality or confrontation	I see no elephant in the room. This is a hospital, not a hotel.
Voicing doubt	I find that hard to believe. Did it happen just as you said?
Encouraging evaluation or evaluating	Describe how you feel about taking your medication. Does participating in group therapy enable you to discuss your feelings?
Attempting to translate into feelings or verbalizing the implied	*Patient:* I'm empty. *Nurse:* Are you suggesting that you feel useless?
Suggesting collaboration	Perhaps you and your doctor can discuss your home visits and discover what produces your anxiety.
Summarizing	During the past hour we talked about your plans for the future. They include . . .
Encouraging formulation of a plan of action	If this situation occurs again, what options would you have?
Asking direct questions	How does your wife feel about your hospitalization?

INTERACTION OR PROCESS RECORDING

Interaction is a tool used to analyze nurse–patient interactions and is seen in various formats. It is used to teach communication skills to student nurses in the clinical setting, focusing on verbal and nonverbal communication. The following format has been used successfully in an associate degree program:

Patient's initials:

Age:

Diagnosis:

Goal of interaction: State your goal.

Description of environment: Give a visual description of the setting in which the conversation took place, including noise level, odors, as well as the patient's physical appearance and posture.

Verbal communication: State the communication verbatim, including what the patient states and your responses. List in sequential order and identify therapeutic and nontherapeutic techniques used during the conversation. Identify any defense mechanisms used by the patient.

Nonverbal communication: Include your thoughts and feelings, as well as any facial expressions, gestures, position changes, or changes in eye contact, voice quality, and tone by the patient or yourself.

Evaluation of this interaction: Discuss whether the goal was met. What changes would you make, if any, after evaluating this interaction?

Excerpts of an interaction recording by a second-year associate degree student during her clinical rotation on a medical floor in a general hospital are given. Although the patient was diagnosed as acute low back pain, the staff had observed symptoms of anxiety and suggested that the student and patient would both benefit from the assignment.

Patient's initials: JW

Age: 33

Diagnosis: Acute low back pain

Goal of interaction: To identify the cause of his low back pain and explore methods of alleviating pain

Description of environment: A private room at the end of the corridor with no offensive odors or disturbing noises. The room is rather bare, with no evidence of get-well cards, pictures, or plants.

The patient was dressed in a hospital gown and was found lying with his back to the door as I entered the room. The lights were turned off and the curtains were drawn.

STUDENT	PATIENT

1. "Good morning. My name is . . . I will be your nurse for this morning." (Smiling; speaking softly; gazing directly at JW while walking to the side of the bed.)
  a. Giving recognition
  b. Giving information
  c. Offering self
	2. "Oh. How long will you be here?" (Turns over in bed and briefly gazes at me with a blank facial expression; speaks in a low voice.)

3. I'll be here until 1:30. I understand you are having back pain. Could you describe the pain to me?"
  a. Giving information
  b. Encouraging description of perception
	4. "It started when I was moving a chair in my living room after my son spilled some spaghetti on the rug." (Maintains eye contact and grimaces as he sits up in bed.)

5. "Tell me more about the pain." (Maintained eye contact while sitting in the chair beside his bed.) a. Exploring	6. "It's a sharp, stabbing pain that occurs whenever I move from side to side or try to get up and walk."

The patient confided in the student that he experienced episodes of low back pain since he was 25 years old. He stated that although he had no history of injury to his back, the pain occurred whenever he was working and either had an argument with his boss or worried about financial problems at home. This was his third hospitalization within 1 year, and the family doctor suggested that he talk with a counselor because his history and physical were negative. The interaction resumed as follows:

STUDENT	PATIENT
7. "How do you feel about your doctor's recommendation?" (Maintaining eye contact; sitting) a. Encouraging description of perceptions	8. "I guess he knows what he is doing." (Serious expression; breaks eye contact; fingers sheets nervously.)
9. "Perhaps you and the counselor can discover the cause of your back pain? Then you'll be able to prevent future hospitalizations." a. Suggesting collaboration	10. "I hope so. I can't afford to miss any more work."

Evaluation of interaction: JW was quite receptive to any questions or comments I made and readily discussed his hospitalization for lower back pain. He is willing to undergo counseling at the suggestion of his family doctor to identify the cause of his recurrent pain. I feel this interaction was effective because it showed JW I cared about him as a person and showed an active interest in his physical condition.

SUMMARY

The process of communication and the three elements necessary to interact with another person were discussed. They include sender, message, and receiver. Influencing factors that determine the outcome of communication include attitudes, socioeconomic or ethnic background, past experiences, knowledge of subject matter, the ability to relate to others, interpersonal perceptions, and environmental factors. Seven types of ineffective listening were presented: pseudolistening, stage hogging, selective listening, insulated listening, defensive listening, ambushing, and insensitive listening. Ten suggestions for developing good communication skills were listed, focusing on honesty, consistency, sensitivity, security, and careful selection of words relating to others. Eight communication blocks or stalls such as a judgmental attitude, ambivalence, false reassurance, failure to listen, giving advice, disagreeing with or criticizing the patient, the inability to receive information, and the use of ineffective communication skills were discussed. Two types of interactions, social and therapeutic, were compared. Rogers' eight essential conditions for a therapeutic relationship were summarized: empathy, respect, genuineness, self-disclosure, concreteness or specificity, confrontation, immediacy of relationship, and self-exploration. Confidentiality was explained, with focus on the nurse's responsibility to the patient. The effect of nonverbal communication behaviors or reactions such as the posture or position one assumes, gestures, touch, physical appearance, facial expressions, vocal clues, and distance or spatial territory were explored. Three phases of the therapeutic relationship were described, these are the orienting or initiating, working, and terminating phases. Therapeutic tasks of each phase were stated. A list of therapeutic interpersonal communication techniques and examples of each were included for reference. An example of the interaction or process recording was given, with an explanation of its purpose.

LEARNING ACTIVITIES

    I. Clinical Objectives
        A. Establish a therapeutic relationship with a patient. Identify therapeutic and nontherapeutic techniques during your interactions.
        B. Observe various nonverbal gestures and facial expressions of

patients and personnel in the clinical setting. List those nonverbal reactions used most frequently. Discuss your reactions to each individual observed.

II. Independent Activities

   A. The following are questions pertaining to therapeutic interactions. Share your responses in postclinical conference.

      1. Explain why a nurse's personality is considered by some to be the most effective tool in establishing a therapeutic interaction.

      2. State how one's personality could be detrimental to a therapeutic relationship.

      3. Describe how you would handle feelings of anger or annoyance generated by a patient's behavior.

   B. Role play the following:

      1. A social interaction with a 19-year-old, newly admitted male patient.

      2. The orienting phase of a therapeutic interaction with a 23-year-old female patient exhibiting symptoms of depression.

      3. The terminating phase of a therapeutic relationship with an alcoholic 33-year-old man.

   C. Describe possible reactions or behaviors of patients during the following phases of the nurse–patient relationship:

      1. Initial or orienting phase

      2. Working phase

      3. Terminating phase

   D. After reviewing the list of therapeutic communication techniques listed in the chapter, state those techniques you commonly use and explain why.

SELF-TEST

1. Describe the purpose of each phase of the therapeutic relationship.
2. Explain the communication process.
3. List the factors influencing communication.
4. Explain a stall or communication block and why it may occur.
5. List four types of listening that can impair communication.
6. Explain the importance of honesty, sensitivity, and consistency when developing communication skills.
7. Differentiate between social and therapeutic communication.
8. Explain the difference between sympathy and empathy.
9. What purpose does confrontation serve in a therapeutic interaction?
10. Why is confidentiality important in nursing?

11. Explain the statement "Don't invade his spatial territory."

12. State the purpose of a process or interaction recording.

REFERENCES

Adler R, Towne N: Looking Out/Looking In: Interpersonal Communication. New York, Holt, Rinehart, and Winston, 1978

Amacher NJ: Touch is a way of caring. Am J Nurs: May, 1973

Arnold H: A guide to one-to-one relationships. Am J Nurs: June, 1976

Barry P: Psychosocial Nursing Assessment and Intervention. Philadelphia, JB Lippincott, 1984

Brill N: Working With People: The Helping Process, 2nd ed. Philadelphia, JB Lippincott, 1978

Coltrene F, Pugh C: Danger signals in staff/patient relationships in the therapeutic milieu. J Psych Nurs: June, 1978

Duldt B et al.: Interpersonal Communication in Nursing. Philadelphia, FA Davis, 1984

Elliot E: My name is Mrs. Simon. Ladies Home Journal, August, 1984.

English M: Ordeal. Nursing 83: Oct, 1983

Fagin C: Psychotherapeutic nursing. In: Psychiatric/Mental Health Nursing: Contemporary Readings. New York, D. Van Nostrand, 1978

Ferszi G, Taylor P: The patient's right to cry. Nursing 84: Mar, 1984

Forsyth D: Looking good to communicate better with patients. Nursing 83: July, 1983

Gearratona C: Reach out, reach out and touch . . . Henry. Nursing 84: Febr, 1984

Haber J et al: Comprehensive Psychiatric Nursing, 2nd ed. New York, McGraw–Hill, 1982

Hall E: The Hidden Dimension. New York, Doubleday and Co, 1966

Hannan J: Talking is treatment, too. Am J Nurs: Nov, 1974

Horney K. Our Inner Conflicts. New York, Norton Press, 1945

Knowles RD: Dealing with feelings: Affirmations. Am J Nurs: Apr, 1982

Lego S: Psychotherapeutic Interview (film). Am J Nurs:

Littlefield N: Therapeutic relationship: A brief encounter. Am J Nurs: Sept, 1982

Lore A: Effective Therapeutic Communication. Bowie, Robert J Brady, 1981

McAuliffe K, McAuliffe D: I Care. Nursing 84. April, 1984

Murray R, Zenter J: Nursing Concepts for Health Promotion. Englewood Cliffs, Prentice–Hall, 1975

Nurse–patient interactions: Techniques of therapeutic communication (filmstrip). Trainex

Nurse–patient interactions: Blocks to therapeutic communication (filmstrip). Trainex

Osterlund B: Humor: A Serious approach to patient care. Nursing 83: Dec,1983

Peplau H: Interpersonal Relations in Nursing. New York, Putnam, 1952

Poole K: Breaking the ice. Nursing 81: Febr, 1981

Purtilo R: Health Professionals/Patient Interaction, 2nd ed. Philadelphia, WB Saunders, 1978

Rogers C: Characteristics of a helping relationship. Personnel Guidance Journal: Sept, 1958

Rogers C: On Becoming A Person. Boston, Houghton, Mifflin & Co, 1961

Ruditis S: Developing trust in nursing interpersonal relationships. J Psych Nurs: Apr, 1979

Satir V: Making Contact. Berkley, CA, Celestial Arts, 1976

Searight R: Being honest with Gary was the least and the most we could do. Nursing 80: Febr, 1980

Sene B: Termination in the student–patient relationship. Backer B, Dubbert P, Eisenman E (eds): Psychiatric/Mental Health Nursing: Contemporary Readings. New York, D. Van Nostrand, 1978

Shanken WJ, Shanken P: How to be a helping person. J Psych Nurs: Febr, 1976

Strauch B et al: Caring enough to give your patient control. Nursing 80: August, 1980

Suprina R: Curing with kindness. Nursing 81: May, 1981

Williams JC: Why did Annie hate us so? Nursing 78: May, 1978

Wilson H, Kneisl C: Psychiatric Nursing, 2nd ed. Menlo Park, Addison–Wesley, 1983.

4

NURSING DIAGNOSIS AND

NURSING PROCESS

1982 ANA STANDARDS OF PSYCHIATRIC–MENTAL HEALTH NURSING

Standard 1: Theory. The nurse applies appropriate theory that is scientifically sound as a basis for decisions regarding nursing practice.

Standard 2: Data Collection. The nurse continuously collects data that is comprehensive, accurate, and systematic.

Standard 3: Diagnosis. The nurse uses nursing diagnoses and standard psychiatric diagnoses to express conclusions supported by recorded assessment data and current scientific premises.

Standard 4: Planning. The nurse develops a nursing care plan with specific goals and interventions delineating nursing actions unique to each client's needs.

Standard 5: Intervention. The nurse intervenes as guided by the nursing care plan to implement nursing actions that promote, maintain, or restore physical and mental health, prevent illness, and rehabilitate.

Standard 6: Evaluation. The nurse evaluates client responses to nursing actions to revise the data base, nursing diagnoses, and nursing care plan.

Nursing is "the diagnosis and treatment of human responses to actual or potential health problems."

American Nurses' Association

Psychiatric nursing is a specialized area of nursing practice employing theories of human behavior as its scientific aspect and purposeful use of self as its art. It is directed toward both preventive and corrective impacts upon mental illness and is concerned with the promotion of optimum health for society.

Congress for Nursing Practice, 1973

LEARNING OBJECTIVES

1. Define psychiatric nursing.
2. State the purpose of the nursing process in the psychiatric setting.
3. Describe the five steps of the nursing process.
4. Differentiate between objective and subjective data.
5. State the benefits of using the nursing diagnosis.
6. Apply the steps of the nursing process while caring for a patient in a psychiatric setting.

THE nursing process is a problem-solving approach that serves as an organizational framework for the practice of nursing. It consists of 1) an assessment of the patient; 2) a statement of the nursing diagnosis; 3) a formulation of a plan of nursing care; 4) nursing actions or interventions; and 5) an evaluation of the patient's response. Murray states that "the nursing process is an ongoing systematic series of actions, interactions, and transactions with a person(s) in need of health care, using the problem-solving method, so that empathic and intellectual processes and scientific knowledge form the basis for your outward actions observable to others" (1980, p. 19).

ASSESSMENT

This phase of the nursing process includes data collection about the person, family, or a group by the methods of observation, examination, and interviewing. Two types of data are collected: objective and subjective. Objective data include information obtained verbally from the patient, as well as the results of inspection, palpation, percussion, and auscultation during an examination. Subjective data are obtained as the patient, family members, or significant others provide information spontaneously, during direct questioning, or during the health history.

A nursing history guide or form generally is used as an assessment tool to process information obtained about 1) previous illnesses and hospitalizations, 2) understanding of or insight into health problems, 3) educational level, 4) intellectual capacity, 5) communication patterns, 6) religious practices, 7) coping patterns, 8) activities of daily living (ADLs), and 9) expectations of health care. A detailed nursing history guide pertaining to the patient in a psychiatric setting is described in several texts (e.g., Barry's *Psychosocial Nursing Assessment and Intervention*, JB Lippincott, 1983).

Murray (1980) lists obstacles to avoid while assessing patients.

1. Stereotyping the patient

2. Perceiving the patient as an object or thing instead of a person

3. Viewing the person as someone to meet your needs rather than as someone whose needs must be met

4. Considering the assessment tool as a task instead of a basis to plan individualized patient care.

NURSING DIAGNOSIS

The nursing diagnosis is a statement of an existing problem or of a potential health problem or need that a nurse is both licensed and competent to treat. It is not "a diagnostic test, a piece of equipment, a nursing problem, a nursing need, a sign or symptom, or a healthy response" (Price, 1980, p. 668). "To make a nursing diagnosis is to come to a conclusion based on a scientific determination of a person's nursing needs. It is the result of a systematic assessment of the patient's behavior, the nature of the illness, and numerous other factors. It should be based on a scientific body of knowledge and should then serve as a guide for nursing care" (Lengel, 1982, p. 4). Lengel discusses the following benefits of using a nursing diagnosis. It facilitates:

1. A clearer definition of areas of nursing practice, providing guidelines for independent practitioners

2. Better direction in the formulation of nursing care plans, focusing on the care of the whole patient or the patient's biopsychosocial needs

3. A clearer view of the need for nursing care or intervention as a description of nursing care rendered, problems encountered, and nursing actions taken

4. Better individualized, meaningful nursing care due to a holistic approach

5. Effective discharge planning due to the setting of short- and long-term goals

6. Continuity of care due to effective communication that identifies patient problems and needs

7. Nursing care standards and desired quality of care for an institution, thus facilitating quality assurance

8. Closure of the gap between theory and practice in nursing education, reducing the "reality shock" experienced by newly graduated nurses

9. Encouragement for research

Clough (Haber, 1983) states that the formulation of a nursing diagnoses is the result of assessment, problem identification, determining the cause of a problem, labeling the problem, and classification of the problem.

The following nursing diagnoses were identified and accepted by the National Group on Classification of Nursing Diagnoses at the Fourth and Fifth National Conferences:

Nursing Diagnoses Accepted for Clinical Testing*

Airway clearance, ineffective

Bowel elimination, alterations in: Constipation

Bowel elimination, alterations in: Diarrhea

Bowel elimination, alterations in: Incontinence

Breathing patterns, ineffective

Cardiac output, alterations in: Decreased

Comfort, alterations in: Pain

Communication, impaired verbal

Coping, ineffective individual

Coping, ineffective family: Compromised

Coping, ineffective family: Disabling

Coping, family: Potential for growth

Diversional activity, deficit

Fear (specify)

Fluid volume deficit, actual

Fluid volume deficit, potential

Gas exchange, impaired

Grieving, anticipatory

Grieving, dysfunctional

Home maintenance management, impaired

Injury, potential for

Knowledge deficit (specify)

Mobility, impaired physical

Noncompliance (specify)

Nutrition, alterations in: Less than body requirements

Nutrition, alterations in: More than body requirements

Nutrition, alterations in: Potential for more than body requirements

*These diagnoses are published in Kim M, Moritz D (eds): Classification of Nursing Diagnoses. Proceedings of the 3rd and 4th National Conferences. New York, McGraw–Hill, 1982.

Parenting, alterations in: Actual

Parenting, alterations in: Potential

Rape trauma syndrome

Self-care deficit (specify level: feeding, bathing and hygiene, dressing and grooming, toileting)

Self-concept, disturbance in

Sensory perceptual alterations

Sexual dysfunction

Skin integrity, impairment of: Actual

Skin integrity, impairment of: Potential

Sleep pattern disturbance

Spiritual distress (distress of the human spirit)

Thought processes, alterations in

Tissue perfusion, alterations in

Urinary elimination, alterations in patterns

Violence, potential for

Nursing Diagnoses Accepted for Clinical Testing at the Fifth National Conference†

Activity intolerance

Anxiety

Family processes, alterations in

Fluid volume, alterations in: Excess

Health maintenance alteration

Oral mucous membrane, alterations in

Powerlessness

Social isolation

Gebbie (1975) lists the following nursing diagnoses commonly seen in psychiatric settings and includes descriptions of each:

1. *Anxiety, mild*

Increased questioning

Restlessness

---

†From the North American Nursing Diagnosis Association, St. Louis University, Dept. of Nursing, 3525 Caroline St., St. Louis, MO, 63104

Increased awareness

Increased attending

2. *Anxiety, moderate*

Voice tremors

Voice pitch changes

Rate of verbalization

Shakiness

Pacing

Increased muscle tension

Narrowing focus of attention

Diaphoresis

Increased heart rate

Increased respiratory rate

Increase in verbalization

3. *Anxiety, severe*

Inappropriate verbalization

Purposelessness

Perceptual focus fixed

Perceptual focus scattered

Tachycardia

Hyperventilation

4. *Anxiety, panic*

Difficulty in verbalization

Immobilization

Inability to focus on reality

Dilated pupils

Pallor

5. *Confusion*

Disoriented to person (or time, place, object, purpose)

Inappropriate verbal or nonverbal behavior

Statements reflecting recognition of confusion

Other possible defining characteristics

Impaired attention span

Restlessness

Purposeless responses (activity)

Inappropriate activity (responses or affect)

Anxiety

Agitation

Apprehension

Fright

Verbosity

Confabulation

Rambling speech

Dependent and demanding attention-getting behavior

Withdrawal

Belligerence

Combativeness

Facial expression specific to confusion

Hyperactive

6. *Grieving, acute*

Loss of significant object

Expansion of distress at loss

Denial of loss

Guilt

Anger

Sorrow

Choked feelings

Changes in eating habits

Alterations in sleep patterns

Alterations in activity level

Altered libido

Altered communication patterns

7. *Grieving, anticipatory*

Potential loss of significant object

Expression of distress at potential loss

Denial of loss

Guilt

Anger

Sorrow

Choked feelings

Changes in eating habits

Alterations in sleep patterns

Alterations in activity level

Altered libido

Altered communication patterns

8. *Grieving, delayed*

Loss of significant object at least 1 year in past

Express of distress at loss

Denial of loss

Guilt

Anger

Sorrow

Choked feelings

Changes in eating habits

Alterations in sleep patterns

Alteration in activity level

Altered libido

Altered communication patterns

9. *Manipulation*

Lack of empathy

Self-centered

Covert use of others to meet own goals

Avoidance of open communication

Conscious attempt to influence others

Unconscious attempt to influence others

Attempt to "play" people against each other

10. *Self-concept: Alterations in body image*

Alterations in verbalization regarding body

Alterations in response to body change

Self-motivation and self-destruction

Denial of altered body state

Alteration in perceived focus of control

Expressed feelings of hopelessness

Expressed feelings of helplessness

Expressed feelings of powerlessness

Other possible defining characteristics:

    Alteration in ability to accept positive reinforcement

    Alteration in ability to make change, grow, adapt

    Alteration in ability to adapt redependency and independence

11. *Sensory/perceptual alterations*

Disoriention in time

Disoriention to place

Disoriention to persons

Altered abstraction

Altered conceptualization

Change in problem-solving abilities

Report of change in sensory acuity

Measured change in sensory acuity

Change in behavior pattern

Anxiety

Apathy

Change in usual response to stimuli

Indication of body image alteration

12. *Sleep–rest activity, dysrhythmia*

Restless when asleep

Restless when awake

Change in activity level

Dozing

Insomnia

Difficulty in arousing

Delayed response to stimuli

Increased response to stimuli

Irritability

Verbalization of sleep disturbances

Verbalization of fatigue

Lethargy

13. *Thought processes impaired*

Impaired attention span

Discrepancy between chronological age and development level

Inappropriate behavior

Impaired recall ability

Decreased ability to grasp ideas

Decreased ability to order ideas

Impaired ability to reason

Impaired ability to conceptualize

Impaired judgment

Impaired perception

Impaired decision-making

EXAMPLES OF NURSING DIAGNOSES

The following are examples of nursing diagnoses focusing on the psychological needs of hospitalized patients identified by student nurses in a medical–psychiatric setting.

1. Fifty-two-year-old male with congestive heart and metabolic acidosis. This man's chief complaint was shortness of breath. History revealed two heart attacks, chronic constipation, and kyphosis. The student nurse noted the following nursing diagnoses pertaining to psychological needs:

Moderate anxiety exhibited by voice tremors, increased verbalization, increased muscle tension, and diaphoresis owing to illness and hospitalization

Ineffective individual coping, demonstrated by the increased use of withdrawal, isolation, and suppression

Sleep pattern disturbance of insomnia because of anxiety and physical condition

Sexual dysfunction or impotence owing to anxiety and fear

Fear of disability because of congestive heart failure

2. Forty-five-year-old female with chronic congestive heart failure and lymphoma, admitted for chemotherapy. Chief complaints included shortness of breath, rapid weight loss, and fatigue. The following nursing diagnoses were made pertaining to the patient's psychological needs:

Acute grief exhibited by denial and anger related to terminal condition of lymphoma

Possible disturbance in self-concept due to alterations in body image such as hair loss, weight loss, and dry skin

Ineffective individual coping, demonstrated by the increased use of suppression, projection, dissociation, and denial

Acute anxiety related to illness, hospitalization, and separation from spouse; evidenced by increased restlessness, rapid pulse, and increased questioning about illness

Sexual dysfunction of decreased libido owing to anxiety, physical condition, and poor self-concept

3. Twenty-eight-year-old female with partial bowel obstruction and recurring cancer with metastasis to the liver. Her chief complaint during the admission assessment was "My cancer is spreading and intertwining in my bowels. I feel like a raw apple being sliced into pieces". The student nurse discussed the following nursing diagnoses during clinical post conference:

Anticipatory grief, bargaining stage, related to terminal illness as noted in her statements "I wish we could go to Florida for one more Christmas" and "I wish I could live long enough to raise my kids."

Moderate anxiety due to impending death, exhibited by increased questioning, tremors, and voice trauma

Ineffective individual coping from increased anxiety and lack of support systems, demonstrated by the use of fantasy and symbolization

Alteration in self-concept due to terminal illness and change in physical appearance

Alterations in comfort due to abdominal pain

Fear of death and of children's getting cancer

Sexual dysfunction from weakened physical condition

Sleep pattern disturbance of insomnia and restlessness because of anxiety, fear, and abdominal pain

Social isolation due to physical condition and low self-concept

The nursing diagnosis should not describe nursing actions, list medical diagnosis, list diagnostic tests, contain vague information about the need or problem, list symptoms, or list equipment.

FORMULATION OF PLAN OF NURSING CARE

The next phase of the nursing process includes priority setting, goal setting, and planning interventions. Priority setting considers the urgency or seriousness of the problem or need and its impact on the person. Is there a threat to the person's life, dignity, or integrity? Are there problems or needs that negatively affect the patient? Do problems exist that affect normal growth and development? Maslow's hierarchy of needs generally is used as a guide for problem solving during the formulation of a plan of care. These needs include physical needs, safety, love and belonging, self-esteem, and self-actualization.

Goal setting occurs as the nurse and patient mutually discuss and state expected outcomes. Such goals should be short-term as well as long-term to evaluate the patient's progress. Short-term goals are individualized, derived from the diagnoses, and can be met in a short amount of time. They should be realistic and achievable; measurable, observable, and behavioral; patient centered; and time designated. Long-term goals are future oriented and considered the desired result of nursing intervention (Murray, 1980).

Four purposes of a care plan are to

1. Communicate information and appropriate actions or interventions about the patient to all care-givers.
2. Provide individualized, comprehensive care, focusing on short- and long-term goals.
3. Provide continuity of care by all care-givers 24 hours a day by stating what needs to be done, when, and how.
4. Facilitate an ongoing, accurate evaluation of care. These purposes must be considered since the nurse uses available resources while planning appropriate nursing interventions. Resources include the patient who can describe measures that have helped or failed in the past, the family, other nurses and health care providers sharing common goals, literature, and research.

General principles to be considered in writing a plan of care include

1. Individualize or personalize the plan of care according to the nursing diagnoses or problem list. Ask yourself, "If a person who knew nothing about the patient read the care plan, what would be learned about the patient's needs?"

The following is a brief sample plan of nursing care for a patient with the diagnosis of depression:

Assessment Data	Nursing Diagnoses	Goals	Nursing Interventions
Weight loss of 10 lb in 2 wks Retardation of speech	Ineffective individual coping: Depression	Learn effective coping skills to decrease depression	Encourage ventilation of feelings.
Numerous bodily complaints (i.e., headache, back and abdominal pain) Insomnia Fatigue Restlessness	Sleep pattern disturbance: Insomnia	Establish a positive sleep pattern to ensure adequate rest	Administer antidepressant medication as ordered. Limit naps during the day. Encourage exercising and participation in daily activities. Offer warm milk, back rub, etc. at h.s. Limit noise and other distraction in the patients's room
		Explore support systems	Explore coping mechanisms.
Feelings of worthlessness and low self-esteem, evidenced by the statement "I'm no good. No one needs me anymore." Divorced 2 wks ago	Disturbance in self-concept	Establish a positive self-concept	Treat the patient with respect. Reinforce any positive action taken by the patient. Help the patient to identify positive traits. Give the patient honest praise for accomplishments.

2. Use simple, understandable language to communicate information about the patient's care.

3. Be specific when stating nursing actions.

4. Prioritize nursing care (i.e., list nursing actions for ineffective airway clearance before those for impaired physical mobility or sexual dysfunction).

5. State short- and long-term goals.

NURSING ACTIONS OR INTERVENTIONS

Also referred to as implementation of care, this phase occurs as the nurse or member of the health care team performs assigned nursing interventions. It includes verbal and nonverbal communication; individual approaches to promote or maintain health, stability or recovery; and promotion of independent functions, such as self-care when appropriate. The care-giver continually assesses the patient during this phase of the nursing process because of changing responses that may occur. Kozier (1983) lists seven activities required during intervention. They include

1. A review and update of data as the need arises
2. Revision of the nursing care plan to meet potential and existing needs or problems
3. Establishing a helping relationship with the patient
4. Determining the need for nursing care
5. Implementing nursing orders (*e.g.,* measure abdominal girth, monitor intake and output, or spend 30 minutes every shift talking with the patient)
6. Continual assessment of the patient's responses to nursing interventions, including both negative or positive responses.
7. Communication of action taken as well as the patient's response to provide continuity of care.

EVALUATION

The evaluation phase of the nursing process is referred to as the ongoing assessment of the patient's problems, needs, and nursing diagnosis when one is making rounds, during consultation with other health team members; or while one is giving patient care. Evaluation includes predicting outcomes through short- and long-term goals. Care-givers must evaluate current, new, or resolved problems or needs, as well as the recurrence of a problem or need. Kozier (1983) lists four possible outcomes of the evaluation process: 1) the patient has responded favorably or as expected to care; 2) short-term goals were met but long-term goals have not been met; 3) the patient was unable to meet or achieve any goals; and 4) new problems or needs have been identified. As a result of the evaluation process, the care plan is maintained, modified, or totally revised.

SUMMARY

The nursing process is a problem-solving approach that consists of patient assessment, statement of the nursing diagnosis, formulation of a plan of nursing care, nursing actions or interventions, and evaluation of the patient's response. It serves as an organizational framework for the practice of nursing. Each of the five steps of the nursing process were defined and discussed, including collection of objective and subjective data; the use of a nursing history guide as an assessment tool; obstacles to avoid while assessing patients; benefits of the nursing diagnoses; goal setting; principles to consider in writing a plan of care; activities required during nursing intervention; and possible outcomes of the evaluation process. Nursing diagnoses accepted for clinical testing as well as nursing diagnoses commonly seen in psychiatric settings were listed. Examples of nursing diagnoses focusing on the psychological needs of hospitalized patients in a medical–psychiatric setting were given, in addition to a sample plan of nursing care for a patient with the diagnosis of depression.

LEARNING ACTIVITIES

I. Clinical activities
   A. Using the steps of the nursing process, develop a care plan for an assigned patient in the psychiatric setting focusing on psychological or emotional needs.
   B. Evaluate the care plan daily and modify or revise it when necessary.
II. Independent activities
   A. Read one or more of the following articles listed in the references:
      1. Dossey H, Guzzetta C: Nursing diagnoses. Nursing 81: June, 1981
      2. Wolff M, Erikson R: The assessment man: Nurs Outlook: Feb, 1977
      3. Price: Nursing Diagnoses: Making a concept come alive. Am J Nurs: Apr, 1980
   B. Develop a care plan for the patient described in the following paragraph. Focus on emotional or psychological needs.

      This 50-year-old man complains of chronic low back pain from degenerative disk disease and various somatic symptoms. He alleges that he is disabled and cannot work or pursue his hobbies owing to his back pain. This person was divorced approximately 6 years ago at age 44 and described the divorce in great detail during his initial assessment. He refers to himself as a failure, stating "I never could do anything well enough to please my father and then my marriage ended in a divorce. Things never did go right for me. I don't have any friends." He alleges having difficulty falling asleep at night, that he has lost 18 pounds the past year, and that he "does not feel like" eating. He has no social or civic involvements and alleges financial problems because he is receiving social security disability benefits of $637.00 per month. During the interview his voice became tremulous as he discussed his divorce. He rubbed the arm of the chair incessantly, chain smoked four cigarettes, and complained of headaches, dizziness, restlessness in his legs, and back pain.

SELF-TEST

1. Name the five steps of the nursing process.
2. List the information obtained during the assessment phase of the nursing process.
3. According to Murray (1980), during the assessment process, the nurse should avoid:
4. Benefits of using a nursing diagnosis include:
5. Four nursing diagnoses accepted for clinical testing that identify psychological or emotional needs or problems include:
6. The phase of the nursing process that includes priority setting and goal setting is termed what?
7. Three purposes of a nursing care plan are:
8. Principles to consider when writing a plan of care include:
9. State several activities that occur during the phase of nursing intervention
10. Describe the evaluation phase of the nursing process.

REFERENCES

American Nurses' Association: Standards of Psychiatric and Mental Health Nursing Practice. Kansas City, American Nurses' Association, 1982

Barry PD: Psychosocial Nursing Assessment and Intervention. Philadelphia, JB Lippincott, 1984

Bower F: The Process of Planning Nursing Care, 2nd ed. St. Louis, CV Mosby, 1977

Carpenito LJ: Nursing Diagnoses: Applications to Clinical Practice. Philadelphia, JB Lippincott, 1983

Dossey H, Guzzetta C: Nursing diagnosis. Nursing 81: June, 1981

Gebbie KM, Lavin MA (eds): Classification of Nursing Diagnoses. St. Louis, CV Mosby, 1975

Kozier B, Erb G: Fundamentals of Nursing: Concepts and Procedures, 2nd ed. Menlo Park, Addison–Wesley, 1983

Lamonica E: The Nursing Process: A Humanistic Approach. Menlo Park, Addison–Wesley, 1979

Lancaster J: Adult Psychiatric Nursing. Garden City, NJ, Medical Examination Publishing, 1980

Lengel NL: Handbook of Nursing Diagnosis. Bowie, Robert J. Brady, 1982

Lewis S, Collier I: Medical–Surgical Nursing: Assessment and Management of Clinical Problems. New York, McGraw–Hill, 1982

Mayers MG: A Systematic Approach to the Nursing Care Plan. New York, Appleton Century Crofts, 1972

Monken SS: After assessment–What then? Nurs Clin North Am: Mar, 1975

Murray R, Zentner J: Nursing Assessment and Health Promotion through the Life Span, 2nd ed. Englewood Cliffs, Prentice–Hall, 1979

Murray R, Zentner J: Nursing Concepts for Health Promotion, 2nd ed. Englewood Cliffs, Prentice–Hall, 1979

Murray R et al.: The Nursing Process in Later Maturity. Englewood Cliffs, Prentice–Hall, 1980

Price M: Nursing diagnosis: Making a concept come alive. Am J Nurs: Apr, 1980

Rich P: Making the most of your charting time. Nursing 83: Mar, 1983

Schmeltzer C: Teaching the nursing process: Practical method. J Nurs Ed: Nov, 1980

Urdang L (ed): Mosby's Medical and Nursing Dictionary. St. Louis, CV Mosby, 1983

Wilson H, Kneisl, C: Psychiatric Nursing, 2nd ed. Menlo Park, Addison–Wesley, 1983

Wolff H, Erikson R: The assessment man. Nurs Outlook: Febr, 1977

Yura H, Walsh M: The Nursing Process: Assessing, Planning, Implementing, Evaluating, 2nd edition. New York, Appleton Century Crofts, 1973.

5

THE THERAPEUTIC

ENVIRONMENT

TAKE TIME

Take time to work—
  It is the pride of success.

Take time to think—
  It is the source of power.

Take time to play—
  It is the secret of perpetual youth.

Take time to read—
  It is the fountain of wisdom.

Take time to be friendly—
  It is the road to happiness.

Take time to dream—
  It is hitching your wagon to a star.

Take time to look around—
  It is too short a day to be selfish.

Take time to laugh—
  It is the music of the soul.

Anonymous

LEARNING OBJECTIVES

1. Differentiate between therapeutic environment and therapeutic community.
2. List criteria for a therapeutic environment.
3. Define psychiatric mental health team.
4. List the disciplines that participate in the promotion of a therapeutic environment.
5. Explain the nurse's role in the following conceptual models of patient care:
   Biological
   Psychological
   Behavioral
   Social
   Interpersonal
   Existential
   Communication
   Nursing
6. State the goals of psychotherapy.
7. List the purposes of group therapy.
8. Explain the purpose of family therapy.
9. State the mechanisms common to all therapy groups.
10. Differentiate between operant conditioning and systematic desensitization.
11. Discuss nursing interventions during electroconvulsive therapy.
12. Explain the importance of assessing a patient's spiritual needs.

MORAL, *milieu, environmental, interpersonal* or *situational therapy,* as well as *therapeutic environment,* are terms that refer to a specially structured setting that encourages people to function within the range of social norms through modification of the person's life circumstances and immediate environment. Moral therapy is a term that was used in the 1800s, emphasizing "friendly interactions, discussion of problems and daily pursuit of purposeful activity . . . based on the assumption that the insane were basically normal people who had lost their reason as a result of severe psychological and social problems" (Altrocchi, 1980, p. 23). Altrocchi refers to moral therapy as a revolution before its time, with a 70% to 90% recovery rate.

Therapeutic community is a special type of milieu or environmental therapy using the social and interpersonal interactions in the hospital as therapeutic tools to bring about change in the patient by encouraging active participation in treatment. A therapeutic community is democratic, rehabilitative, permissive, and communal (Stuart and Sundeen, 1983).

Therapeutic environments can occur in a variety of settings, such as the hospital, community home, or in the private practice of a counselor or therapist. Regardless of the setting, certain criteria must be met to help patients to develop a sense of self-esteem and personal worth, to feel secure, to establish trust, to improve their ability to relate to others, and to return to the community. The environment should

1. Be purposeful and planned to provide safety from physical danger and emotional trauma. It also should have furniture to facilitate a home-like atmosphere, privacy, provisions for physical needs, and opportunities for interaction and communication among patients and personnel.

2. Provide a testing ground for new patterns of behavior while the patient takes responsibility for his actions. Behavioral expectations should be explained to the patient, including the existing rules, regulations, and policies.

3. Be consistent when setting limits. This reflects aspects of a democratic society. All patients are treated as equally as possible, with respect to restrictions, rules, and policies.

4. Encourage participation in group activities and free-flowing communication in which the patient has the freedom to express himself in a socially acceptable manner.

5. Respect the person and treat him with dignity. Adult–adult interactions should prevail, when appropriate, promoting equal status of interactors, exchange of interpersonal information, and avoiding any "power plays." The person should be encouraged to use personal resources to resolve problems or conflicts.

6. Convey an attitude of overall acceptance and optimism. Conflict between staff members must be handled and resolved in some manner to maintain a therapeutic environment. Patients are perceptive of such reactions and may feel that they are the cause of conflicts among personnel.

7. Continually assess and evaluate the patient's progress, modifying treatment and nursing interventions as needed.

MENTAL HEALTH TEAM

Members of several disciplines participate in the promotion of a therapeutic environment. Referred to as the psychiatric mental health team, they include psychiatrists; clinical psychologists; psychiatric social workers; psychiatric nurses, nurse assistants or technicians; occupational, education, art, musical, psychodrama, recreational, play, and speech therapists; chaplains; dietitians; and auxiliary personnel. A summarized description of these disciplines follows.

DISCIPLINE	DESCRIPTION
Psychiatrist	Licensed physician with at least 3 years of residency training in psychiatry, including 2 years of clinical psychiatric practice Specializes in the diagnoses, treatment, and prevention of mental and emotional disorders Conducts therapy sessions and serves as leader of the mental health team. Prescribes medication and somatic treatment
Clinical psychologist	Has a doctoral degree in clinical psychology, is licensed by state law, and has completed a psychology internship (supervised work experience) Provides a wide range of services from diagnostic testing, interpretation, evaluation, consultation to research. May treat patients individually or in a group therapy setting.
Psychiatric social worker	Possesses a baccalaureate, master's or doctoral degree. Uses community resources and adaptive capacities of individuals and groups to facilitate positive interactions with the environment. Conducts the intake interview; family assessment; individual, family and group therapy; discharge planning; and community referrals
Psychiatric nurse	A registered nurse who specializes in mental health nursing by employing theories of human behavior and the therapeutic use of self. Gives holistic nursing care by assessing the patient's mental, psychological, and social status. Provides a safe environment, works with patients dealing with everyday problems, provides leadership, and assumes the role of patient advocate. A master's degree is required for the clinical nurse specialist who does family, group, and individual therapy.
Psychiatric technician or nurse assistant	High school graduate who receives in-service education pertaining to the job description. Assists the mental health team in maintaining a therapeutic environment, providing care, and supervising patient activities
Occupational therapist	Possesses a baccalaureate or master's degree in occupational therapy. Uses creative techniques and purposeful activities, as well as a therapeutic relationship, to alter the course of an illness. Assists with discharge planning and rehabilitation, focusing on *(continued)*

DISCIPLINE	DESCRIPTION
	vocational skills and activities of daily living (ADL) to raise self-esteem and promote independence.
Educational therapist	College graduate who specializes in the field of educational therapy. Determines effective instructional methods, assessing the person's capabilities and selecting specialized programs to promote these capabilities. May include remedial classes, special education for "maladjusted" children, or continuing education for hospitalized students with emotional or behavioral problems (e.g., anorexia nervosa, depression, or substance abuse)
Art therapist	College graduate with a master's degree and specialized training in art therapy. Encourages spontaneous creative art work to express feelings or emotional conflicts. Assists the patient in analyzing expressive work. Uses basic child psychiatry to diagnose and treat emotional or behavioral problems. Attention is paid to the use of colors as well as symbolic or real-life figures and settings. (e.g., One dying child drew a series of sailboats on the ocean, beginning with colorful sails and ending with drab grey just before his death. He had interpreted the sailboats as his body sailing the sea of life and death.)
Musical therapist	College graduate with a master's degree and training in music therapy. Focuses on the expression of self through music such as singing, dancing, playing an instrument or composing songs and writing lyrics. Deanna Edwards, a musical therapist who originally worked with Kübler-Ross, uses music to relate to the elderly, dying, and emotionally disturbed. (She has written such songs as "Teach Me To Die," "Put My Memory in Your Pocket," and "Catch A Little Sunshine.") Music therapy promotes improvement in memory, attention span and concentration and provides an opportunity for the individual to take pride in his achievement.
Psychodrama therapist	College graduate with advanced degree and training in group therapy. This therapy is also referred to as role-playing therapy. People are encouraged to act out their emotional problems through dramatization and role playing. This type of therapy is excellent for children, adolescents, and people with marital or family problems. The therapist helps

DISCIPLINE	DESCRIPTION
	the people to explore past, present, and potential experiences through role play and assists group members in developing spontaneity and successful interactional tools (Lancaster, 1980, p. 497). The audience may participate by making comments about and interpretations of the persons acting.
Recreational or activity therapist	College graduate with a baccalaureate or master's degree and training in recreational or activity therapy. Focuses on remotivation of patients by directing their attention outside themselves rather than preoccupation with personal thoughts, feelings, and attitudes. Patients learn to cope with stress through activity. Activities are planned to meet specific needs and encourage the development of leisure-time activities or hobbies. Recreational therapy is especially useful with those people who have difficulty relating to others (*e.g.*, the regressed, withdrawn, or immobilized person). Examples of recreational activity include group bowling, picnics, sing-alongs, and bingo. One group of student nurses presented a puppet show during a sing-along for patients with organic brain syndrome. The people related well to the puppets who visited them individually because they encouraged singing. The students also dressed like clowns as they recruited sedentary patients to participate in activities. CVA patients responded to the clowns who tossed balloons at them by hitting the balloons with their affected limbs (exercise that is considered active range-of-motion activity) and tossing bean bags into baskets. A volunteer, under the direction of the recreational therapist, visited the patients daily with her pet poodle as she delivered mail. The patients responded positively to the poodle.
Play therapist	A psychiatrist, licensed psychologist, psychiatric nurse, psychiatric social worker, or other person trained in counseling. A play therapist observes the behavior, affect, and conversation of a child who plays in a protected environment with minimal distractions, using games or toys provided by the therapist. The therapist tries to gain insight into the child's thoughts, feelings, or fantasies and helps the child to understand and work through emotional conflicts. One child

(continued)

DISCIPLINE	DESCRIPTION
	was observed hitting the boy doll and calling him stupid. The therapist explored the child's behavior and discovered that he was a victim of child abuse.
Speech therapist	College graduate with a master's degree and training in speech therapy. Speech therapists assess and treat disturbed children or people who have developmental language disorders involving nonverbal comprehension, verbal comprehension, and verbal expression. Failure to develop language may occur as a result of deafness, severe mental handicap, gross sensory deprivation, institutionalization (*e.g.*, an orphanage), or an abnormality of the central nervous system (CNS). The speech therapist may work with a neurologist or otologist in such cases.
Chaplain	College graduate with theological or seminary education. Identifies the spiritual needs of the person and support persons and provides spiritual comfort as needed. May act as a counselor if such education has been obtained. The chaplain may attend the intake interview and staff meetings to provide input about the patient as well as to plan holistic health care.
Dietitian or clinical nutritionist	Person with graduate level education in the field of nutrition. The dietitian serves as a resource person to the psychiatric mental health team as well as a nutritional counselor for clients with eating disorders, such as anorexia nervosa, bulimia, pica, and rumination.
Auxiliary personnel	Refers to volunteers, housekeepers, or clerical help who come in contact with patients. Such persons receive in-service training on how to deal with psychiatric emergencies as well as how to interact therapeutically with patients.

Mental health teams consist of a variety of disciplines, depending on the needs of the patients and the therapeutic environment. Because of budgetary constraints, it is not uncommon for the occupational or activities therapist to serve as the recreational, occupational, music and art therapist, especially in smaller, privately owned or community hospitals.

CONCEPTUAL MODELS OF PATIENT CARE

Various models of care exist within the therapeutic environment. Each model considers aspects of human behavior, methods of assessment and treatment, and implications for nursing interventions. Originally four models of care existed: biologic (Kraeplin); psychological (Freud, Sullivan, and Erikson); behavioral (Pavlov, Watson, and Skinner); and social (Meyer and Sullivan). Present models also include the interpersonal (Horney, Fromm, Reich, and Sullivan); existential (Sartre, Heidegger and Kierkegaard); communication (Berne and Watzlawick); and nursing models (Peplau, King, Orem, Rogers, and Roy).

Biologic Model

The biologic or medical model states that mental illness is a disease that is the result of a specific etiology affecting the brain and emphasizes physical, chemical, genetic, environmental, and neurologic causes. As a result, signs and symptoms or syndromes provide the basis for a differential diagnosis, which then determines the treatment. The psychiatrist or attending physician may prescribe antipsychotic or antidepressant drugs, while at the same time utilizing interpersonal treatment approaches that vary from intensive to brief, superficial therapy sessions and avoids placing the blame for deviant behavior on the patient. The nurse who functions under the biologic model deals with the patient's somatic complaints as well as responses to psychopharmacology, electroconvulsive therapy, insulin therapy, psychosurgery, and hydrotherapy. This model is considered particularly useful in treating acute schizophrenic and depressed patients. It is used frequently in modern psychiatric care and encourages research pertaining to the causes of mental illness. *The Diagnostic and Statistical Manual of Mental Disorders* (DSM-III) is used to evaluate clinicl syndromes, personality disorders, and physical disorders.

Psychological Model

The psychological or psychoanalytical model states that the personality is pathologic or defective owing to developmental conflicts such as childhood deprivation, confused communication between parent and child, or poor family relationships. Negative experiences due to the inability to cope can result in adult neurosis as well as other pathologic disorders. This model uses psychotherapy or psychoanalysis to bring the person's unconscious problems to the awareness level. Free association (the verbalization of thoughts as they occur without censorship), and the interpretation of dreams are techniques used, to help the patient recognize intrapsychic conflict. Emphasis is placed on learning appropriate responses. Nurses who work in an environment that uses the psychological model help the patient to handle here-and-now problems by developing more positive coping skills. A surrogate parent role may be necessary temporarily while the nurse encourages the patient to explore and interpret feelings and behavior.

Behavioral Model

Proponents of the behavioral model believe that learned abnormal behavior is used to avoid uncomfortable experiences or because it leads to positive reinforcement. Such behavior becomes habitual and needs to be modified or unlearned through treatment approaches such as desensitization, aversive control, extinction, shaping, assertiveness training, relaxation therapy, or operant conditioning. The patient is not encouraged to explore the past or underlying conflicts. Behavioral approaches are useful for some personality disturbances, adjustment disorders, and behavioral disorders, and are considered complete when the symptoms disappear. The nurse participates in the treatment regimen by setting limits, teaching the patient relaxation techniques, promoting assertiveness, and focusing on the characteristics of mental health. She also works closely with the clinician and patient, for example during the desensitization process of anxiety disorders such as agoraphobia.

Social Model

The social model focuses on how the patient functions in society and society's impact on his personality and life experiences. Symptoms occur as a result of the inability to function or cope positively with society or one's environment. Some theorists believe that culture itself defines what is socially acceptable or normal. What is considered normal by one culture may be considered deviant behavior by another and therefore is labeled mental illness. The social model is considered useful with various disorders and focuses on altering the patient's relationship with society or reorganizing the system the patient lives in, not his personality. Treatment approaches include group or family therapy, day hospitals, outpatient or walk-in clinics, and group homes. Crisis intervention may be necessary. The nurse working in the social model establishes a therapeutic milieu by focusing on recreational, occupational, and social competencies of the patient. She is a member of the interdisciplinary team and takes part in discharge planning by identifying community and social support systems as well as peer support. Some clinicians feel that patients should not be hospitalized involuntarily but rather should be allowed to select their own treatment regimen and therapist.

Interpersonal Model

The interpersonal model stresses that behavior is the result of interpersonal relationships and early life experiences including infancy. Anxiety can occur during a disturbed mother–child relationship and is a "major factor in personality development as well as the development of all emotional illnesses and psychopathology" (Rowe, 1980, p. 19). Intrapsychic conflicts or conflicts within one's personality are derived from interpersonal conflicts. Treatment approaches focus on exploration of the patient's progress through the stages of personality development and ability to relate to others. As the person communicates with the clinician or nurse, he experiences a closeness that enables him to develop trust, enhance self-esteem, and demonstrate healthy behavior. The nurse functions in various roles: 1) resource person, 2) teacher, 3) leader, 4) surrogate, and 5) counselor. Therapy terminates when the patient is able to establish satisfying interpersonal relationships.

Existential Model

The existential approach stresses the here-and-now in the evaluation of a personality disorder by focusing on three aspects of the person's ability to relate: the person and himself, the person and others, and the person and the world in which he lives. The person develops deviant behavior when he is out of touch with himself or his environment. Such behavior is the result of inhibitions or restrictions that are self-imposed and prevent the person from choosing possible alternative behaviors. The person feels helpless, sad, and lonely, and is unable to engage in rewarding interpersonal relationships. Such people tend to allow tradition and the demands of others to dominate behavior or reactions. Encounter approaches (meeting of two or more persons who appreciate each other's existence) include confrontation about one's behavior and responsibility for it, searching for the meaning of one's life, exploring one's life goals and intent to accomplish them, and enhancing one's self-awareness (Stuart and Sundeen, 1983).

Communication Model

All behavior has meaning and communicates feelings, thoughts, or attitudes. Maladaptive or disruptive behavior can be the result of faulty communication. Conversely, poor or faulty communication can cause feelings of anxiety or frustration to occur. For example, a young child is admonished frequently by her mother and told she is a "bad girl." She is never permitted to tell her mother how she feels. In response to these pent-up feelings, the young girl begins to act out by disobeying her parents and hitting other children. Such behavior is the result of faulty communication with her mother. Have you ever argued with someone and felt frustrated or upset afterwards? The argument was a poor or faulty communicative process resulting in such feelings.

Berne (1964) founded transactional analysis (TA), a communication model that combines psychoanalytic and interpersonal insights with a communication approach. The focus is on here-and-now interactions that occur between or among people. These transactions or communication patterns are analyzed as parent–adult–child interactions and feedback is given to clarify any problems. Family therapy, behavior therapy, role playing, or reality therapy may be used to facilitate good communication skills.

Nursing Model

In the past, psychiatric–mental health nursing followed the medical model. Nurses were taught and supervised by psychiatrists. Peplau and Muller were responsible in part for the emergence of theory-based mental health nursing practice, in which the nurse serves as therapist. Although there is no one universally accepted model, various models focus on the holistic approach to biopsychosocial needs. The plan of care is based on the nursing process (see Chapter 4) and various psychotherapeutic modalities. The nurse collaborates with the patient as well as other care-givers in formulating the nursing care plan and setting short- and long-term goals. Fitzpatrick (1982) and Chinn (1983) discuss specific nursing models and their applications in the mental health setting.

Eclectic Approach

An individualized style or approach that incorporates one's own resources as a unique person and theoretical knowledge best suited to one's use is referred to as eclectic. Therapists may specialize in one particular conceptual model or combine aspects of different ones. The therapist realizes there is no one way to deal with all of life's stresses or problems of living and is open to new ideas and approaches as the need arises.

TREATMENT MODALITIES IN THE THERAPEUTIC ENVIRONMENT

There are as many treatment modalities as there are books written about the care of psychiatric patients. Chapters include information on relationship therapies, alternative therapies, somatic therapies, psychosocial intervention, intervention modes, helping relationships, and crises intervention.

Some of the more common categories of treatment modalities that will be discussed include psychotherapy, group therapy, family or systems therapy, behavior therapy, management therapy, and somatic therapy.

Crisis intervention is discussed in the following chapter.

Psychotherapy

A *Psychiatric Glossary* (1980) defines *psychotherapy* as "a process in which a person who wishes to relieve symptoms or resolve problems in living or is seeking personal growth enters into an implicit or explicit contract to interact in a prescribed way with a psychotherapist" (p. 116). Walker (1983) states that psychotherapy helps a person to learn and possibly to adopt better ways of coping with problems.

The goals of psychotherapy include reducing patient discomfort or pain, improving the patient's social functioning, and improving the patient's ability to perform or act appropriately. These goals are achieved by

1. Establishing a therapeutic therapist–patient relationship
2. Providing an opportunity for the patient to release tension as problems are discussed
3. Assisting the patient in gaining insight about the problem
4. Providing the opportunity to practice new skills
5. Reinforcing appropriate behavior as it occurs
6. Providing consistent emotional support

Types of individual psychotherapy include: psychoanalysis, uncovering therapy, hypnotherapy, reality therapy, and supportive therapy.

PSYCHOANALYSIS. The term *psychoanalysis,* introduced by Freud, is used to describe a lengthy method of psychotherapy in which the patient talks in an uncontrolled, spontaneous manner termed free association. The therapist assists the patient in exploring repressed anxieties, fears, and images of childhood by interpreting dreams, emotions, and behaviors. A reliving experience is encouraged by the therapist to enable the patient to deal with once harmful emotions. Sessions last approximately 45 minutes, 4 to 5 days a week for approximately 3 to 5 years. It is an expensive form of therapy.

UNCOVERING THERAPY. Uncovering therapy, also referred to as intensive, insight, or investigative psychotherapy, assists the person in gaining insight by uncovering conflicts, mainly unconscious, so that they can be treated openly and effectively. The patient then "works through" the conflict through repeated exploration of the newly gained insight.

HYPNOTHERAPY. Hypnotherapy is an adjunct to psychotherapy used to help people learn to relax, effect behavioral change, uncover repressed feelings and thoughts, and control attitudes. The therapist places the person in a trance and encourages discussion of emotional conflicts. A person who undergoes hypnosis is generally submissive, abandons control, and responds with a high degree of mental and physical suggestibility. Hypnosis is considered effective in the treatment of overeating, smoking, and other addictive disorders. A hypnotized person can not be forced to perform actions that conflict with his values and beliefs.

REALITY THERAPY. Reality therapy is based on the premise that persons who are mentally unhealthy are irresponsible. They cannot meet all of their basic needs, and they refuse to face reality. Responsibility either was never learned or was abandoned at some point in life. The therapist helps the person to overcome denial of the real world and meet his needs by assuming responsibility for his actions. This is done as the therapist becomes involved in an active relationship with the patient, rejects unrealistic behavior displayed by the patient, and teaches the patient better ways to meet his needs in the real world. Reality therapy stresses the present because the past cannot be changed. It also forces the patient to make a value judgment by facing issues of right and wrong, assuming responsibility for his actions.

SUPPORTIVE THERAPY. Supportive psychotherapy is used to handle conscious conflicts or current problems. The therapist utilizes techniques such as reassurance, unburdening, environmental modification, persuasion, and clarification. Reassurance helps the patient to restore self-confidence and decrease feelings of fear and anxiety. Psychological reassurance occurs when parents are told it is normal to experience occasional feelings of hostility and aggressiveness toward one's children.

Ventilating one's feelings through conscious, free expression is referred to as unburdening. Two purposes are served by unburdening: 1) sharing one's feelings, which makes them appear less intense; and 2) revealing oneself, resulting in a form of self-punishment. Recently, a middle-aged man placed an apology in a local newspaper to a childhood classmate he had accused of stealing a sandwich. The article stated that he had felt guilty for several years and had to unburden himself even if the classmate did not see the apology.

Environmental modification or manipulation is done to relieve a patient's symptoms and distress. Advising a young mother to hire a babysitter so that she can have time to herself, placing a child in a foster home because of a poor interpersonal relationship with his parents, who are undergoing a divorce, or suggesting that a middle-aged man take a vacation to overcome feelings of prolonged or unresolved grief are examples of environmental modification or manipulation.

Persuasion is used to give direct suggestions to influence behavior and may include an element of environmental modification. For example, a teenager who smokes and drinks excessively when stressed is told to try jogging, swimming, or other physical exercise to release tension, anxiety, or frustration.

Clarification is a process by which the therapist helps the patient to gain a clearer picture of reality by understanding his feelings and behavior. Explaining to an alcoholic that his illness is a result of a poor self-image or a woman that she needs to be hospitalized because of self-destructive behavior are both examples of clarification of reality.

Group Therapy

Group therapy provides the opportunity for a person to examine his interactions, learn and practice successful interpersonal communication skills, explore emotional conflicts, realize that others experience feelings of fear, anger, and frustration, and effect personality change. Selection of group members depends on the primary goal of the group. Some therapists prefer a heterogenous or well-diversified group to provide stimulation among members rather than a homogenous group (*e.g.,* all adolescent alcoholics) that may dwell on common problems and support each other's defense systems (Haber, 1983).

Members of a group meet at least once or twice a week, exchange information, provide support for each other, and work together to meet a primary goal. Morgan (1973) lists the following mechanisms common to all therapy groups (pp. 101–102):

1. Group acceptance: Individuals feel they are respected, accepted, and belong to the group.

2. Reality testing: Group members can monitor each person's reactions and behaviors, providing feedback in an open and nonthreatening manner.

3. Universalization: Group members feel secure when they realize that they do not have unique problems and are not so different from other persons.

4. Ventilation: Group therapy provides an opportunity for ventilation of various emotions that otherwise would be "bottled-up" inside.

5. Intellectualization: The member gains insight into his problems as he learns to examine or explore symptoms in himself as well as other group members.

6. Altruism: " . . . the phenomenon of group members giving support, advice, encouragement, and love to one another" (Haber, 1983, p. 101).

7. Transference: The individual develops an emotional attachment to another person, such as the therapist or members of the group.

8. Interaction: Group therapy provides the person with the opportunity to assert himself and improve communication skills with others outside the group.

Groups are available to children, adolescents, couples, parents, alcoholics, substance abusers, and other people with various problems. Examples of specific groups include: psychodrama, activity therapy, didactic therapy, repressive–inspirational groups (AA), and free-interaction groups such as encounter or sensitivity groups. Group members may be encouraged to attend individual therapy sessions regularly as well as group sessions.

Family or Systems Therapy

Morgan (1973) gives an excellent presentation on "different" family members who do not conform to predictable "family patterns," thus causing difficulty in interpersonal family relationships. He states that an adjustment in the family relationship must be made by treating the family in a type of modified group therapy referred to as family or systems therapy. One change in a system or family necessitates that all parts must change. Walker (1983) states that such therapy attempts to establish open communication and healthy interactions within the family. (Duvall's theory is discussed in Chapter 8.) Family or systems therapy is recommended when turmoil and hostility occurs within the family unit as a result of one member's illness or emotional conflicts. For example, a 45-year-old mother of three teenage children is hospitalized with terminal cancer. The husband is unable to accept his wife's illness and displaces his anger toward the children. Role changes occur as the oldest daughter assumes her mother's duties. She is unable to participate in school activities or date her steady boyfriend because of her responsibilities. The oldest daughter becomes hostile and aggressive toward her younger siblings and resentful of her mother's illness. Family or systems therapy would encourage acting out these role changes to show family members the behavioral changes occurring. This approach would show the members how they relate to each other and teach them positive ways to get along.

Morgan lists nine basic theoretical concepts of family therapy (1973, pp. 117–118). They are summarized as follows:

1. There is no single-patient concept in family therapy.

2. The identified patient is symptomatic of family psychopathology or disorder. In other words, the patient's symptoms are only part of a wider, family problem.

3. Social environment and pressures impact on a family's interpersonal relationships and may disrupt the family unit.

4. "Scapegoating" is a characteristic feature of pathogenic or disordered families. One member of the family is "chosen" or unconsciously allows family members to displace feelings of anger or hostility to him.

5. Pathologic double-bind situations that occur in families are particularly disruptive to children and adolescents. Such situations can lead to feelings of insecurity as well as hostile, aggressive behavior.

6. A symbiotic relationship may exist between the mother and child. Such a relationship is pathogenic because it sustains dependency on the part of the child to fulfill needs of the mother.

7. One parent may be aggressive, domineering, overprotective, insecure, or rejecting of children. Such behavior indicates a disordered interaction in a seriously disturbed family.

8. Both sick and healthy family systems attempt to preserve their unity and function. Personality changes in one person affect the other family members.

9. Consistent contradictions are typical of disordered family communication, resulting in distrust, confusion, and meaningless or no communication.

Family therapists use various techniques or methods to help the family solve individual as well as family problems. One of the goals of family therapy is to help the family develop healthy ways to maintain a balance as members change and grow. Conflicts and anxiety are resolved within the unit. In one approach the therapist joins the family by participating in conversations and nonverbal communication. The therapist is then able to form a family diagnosis and to plan appropriate intervention to bring about change in the system. Change occurs as a result of the therapist's directives and tasks assigned to family members.

Behavior Therapy

Behavior therapy is "a mode of treatment that focuses on modifying observable and, at least in principle, quantifiable behavior by means of systematic manipulation of the environment and behavioral variables thought to be functionally related to the behavior" (American Psychiatric Association, 1980, p. 13). It aims to eliminate symptoms such as temper tantrums or bedwetting or to develop desirable behavior. Behaviorists believe that problem behaviors are learned and therefore can be eliminated or replaced by desirable behaviors through new learning experiences.

Rowe (1980) lists the following general principles about behavior therapy:

1. Faulty learning can result in psychiatric disorders.

2. Behavior is modified through the application of principles of learning.

3. Maladaptive behavior is considered to be excessive or deficient; thus, behavior therapy seeks to promote appropriate behavior and decrease or eliminate the frequency, duration, or place of occurrence of inappropriate behavior.

4. One's social environment is a source of stimuli that support symptoms; therefore, it also can support changes in behavior through appropriate treatment measures.

Behavior techniques include: behavior modification, systematic desensitization, aversion therapy, cognitive behavior therapy, assertiveness training, and implosive therapy.

BEHAVIOR MODIFICATION AND SYSTEMATIC DESENSITIZATION. Two models of learning theory are used in behavior modification: Pavlov's theory of conditioning, which states that a stimulis elicits a response (a red Delicious apple stimulates one's salivary glands); and Skinner's operant conditioning theory, which states that the results of a person's behavior determine whether the behavior will recur in the future (a child is given a spanking when he breaks an ashtray while playing with it). In operant conditioning, rewards are given for good behavior, such as physical reinforcers (food) or social reinforcers (approval, tokens of exchange), and are withheld if maladaptive behavior occurs. Such rewards generally encourage positive or good behavior, bringing about a change in attitudes and feelings. Operant conditioning has been successful with language training of autistic children, teaching ADL and social skills to intellectually retarded children and adults, and teaching social skills to regressed psychotic patients.

Systematic desensitization is useful with Pavlov's theory of conditioning. This approach of behavior therapy eliminates a patient's fears or anxieties by stressing relaxation techniques that inhibit anxious responses. The patient is taught various ways to relax as he vividly imagines a fear. For example, a postman is intensely afraid of dogs because he was bitten by one. He is taught relaxation techniques and then is asked to visualize a dog several yards away. He is instructed to imagine himself walking toward the dog, and whenever he becomes anxious he is instructed to divert his attention by using a relaxation technique. This imagined role-playing situation continues until the man no longer experiences anxiety. The next step would be to approach a live dog slowly while using relaxation techniques to decrease anxiety. Therapy is successful if the patient loses his intense fear of dogs.

AVERSION THERAPY. This type of therapy uses unpleasant or noxious stimuli to change inappropriate behavior. The stimulus may be a chemical, such as Antabuse or apormorphine, used to treat alcoholics; electrical, such as the using of a pad and buzzer apparatus to treat a child who has urinary

incontinence while sleeping, or visual, such as the films of an auto accident shown to drivers who are arrested for speeding or for driving while
under the influence of alcohol or drugs. Aversion therapy has been used
in the treatment of alcoholism and compulsive unacceptable or criminal
social behavior.

COGNITIVE BEHAVIOR THERAPY. This behavioral approach utilizes confrontation as a means of helping patients restructure irrational beliefs and
behavior. In other words, the therapist confronts the patient with a specific irrational thought process and helps to rearrange maladaptive thinking, perceptions, or attitudes. Thus, by changing thoughts, one can change
feelings and behavior. Cognitive behavior therapy is considered a choice
of treatment for depression and adjustment difficulties. Rational emotive
therapy is a type of cognitive therapy that is effective with groups whose
members have similar problems.

ASSERTIVENESS TRAINING. During assertiveness training, patients are taught
how to relate appropriately to others using frank, honest, and direct
expressions whether these are positive or negative in nature. In other
words, one voices opinions openly and honestly without feeling guilty.
One is encouraged not to be afraid to show an appropriate response, negative or positive, to an idea or suggestion. Many people are unable to say
how they feel and hold back their feelings. Others may show inconsiderate
aggression and disrespect for the rights of others. Assertiveness training
teaches one to ask for what is wanted, take a position on various issues,
and take specific actions to obtain what one wants while respecting the
rights of others. Such training is beneficial to mentally ill as well as mentally healthy persons.

IMPLOSIVE THERAPY OR FLOODING. Implosive therapy is the opposite of systematic desensitization. Persons are exposed to intense forms of anxiety pro-
ducers, either in imagination or in real life. Such flooding is continued
until the stimuli no longer produce disabling anxiety. It is used in the
treatment of phobias and other problems causing maladaptive anxiety.

Management Therapy

Occupational, educational, art, music, and recreational activities all have
psychotherapeutic value and are called management therapy.

Occupational therapy uses purposeful activities as a way of meeting a
person's needs and provides for personal change and growth. Creative
media such as clay, woodburning, or painting are used to express creative
needs or feelings and conflicts that a person is unable to express verbally.
Activities such as rug weaving or sanding provide outlets for the release

of anger, hostility, and frustration. The therapist also may focus on activities that improve living skills, such as grocery shopping, cooking, and self-care.

Somatic Therapy

The biologic treatment of mental disorders is referred to as somatic therapy. It includes: clinical psychopharmacology (use of psychotropic drugs); electroconvulsive therapy (ECT); insulin shock or coma therapy; psychosurgery; and physiotherapy. Such approaches are used to treat the patient by improving physical and psychological well-being.

CLINICAL PSYCHOPHARMACOLOGY. Also referred to as pharmacotherapy, chemotherapy, psychotropic drug therapy, psychoactive drug therapy, and the use of psychotherapeutic drugs, this somatic regimen has changed psychiatric treatment more than any other single development. Modern psychopharmacology is responsible for deinstitutionalization of state mental hospitals and the success of community-based treatment centers. For the most part, acute psychotic patients, who were once on locked wards and restrained, are able to function with moderate to minimal supervision without restraints, hydrotherapy, or ECT. Hyperactive and depressed patients can be medicated so that they do not harm themselves or others while receiving psychiatric treatment. (Antipsychotic drugs, antidepressant drugs, lithium, antianxiety agents, sedative–hypnotics, and antiparkinson agents are discussed in Chapter 7.)

ELECTROCONVULSIVE THERAPY. Introduced by Cerletti and Bini in 1937, ECT uses electric current to induce convulsive seizures (electroshock or ECT). Electronarcosis is a type of ECT that produces a sleeplike state; electrostimulation avoids producing convulsions by using anesthetics and muscle relaxants. ECT is indicated in the treatment of severe depressions, psychosis, catatonia or mania; in situations in which the patient shows no response to drug therapy; or when rapid results are necessary. The following is a step-by-step description of the ECT procedure:

1. A thorough physical including heart, lung, and bone examination should precede any treatment.
2. The patient should be NPO at least 4 hours before treatment.
3. Vital signs are taken 30 minutes before treatment.
4. Instruct the patient to empty the bladder just before or after vital signs are taken.
5. Remove dentures, contact lenses, or any prosthesis that may injure the patient during treatment.

6. A sedative may be given to decrease anxiety.

7. An atropinelike drug is given to dry up body secretions and prevent aspiration.

8. The patient is given a quick-acting anesthetic such as Brevital after being placed on a padded mat or table.

9. Medication such as Anectine is given to produce muscle paralysis or relaxation and prevent severe muscle contractions.

10. Oxygen may be administered by way of an Ambu bag if spontaneous respirations are decreased.

11. A tongue depressor is generally in place to prevent biting of the tongue or obstruction of the airway.

12. Two electrodes are applied to the temples to deliver electrical shock.

13. The limbs are restrained gently to prevent fractures in the event of a severe clonic seizure. Usually the seizure is barely noticeable; slight toe twitching, finger twitching, or goose bumps may occur.

14. The patient awakens approximately 20 to 30 minutes after treatment and appears groggy and confused.

15. Vital signs are taken during the recovery stage and the nurse stays with the patient until he is oriented and able to care for himself.

Six to twelve treatments (one treatment 2 to 3 times a week) are generally required to be effective. During ECT, memories gradually come back over a period of 2 to 3 weeks, although the patient may not recall events immediately surrounding treatment.

Contraindications for ECT are rare but cardiac patients are considered poor risks as are patients with brain tumors or abdominal aneurysms. Side-effects include memory disturbances and rare skeletal complications such as vertebral compressions or fractures.

INSULIN SHOCK OR COMA THERAPY. Insulin shock therapy was first used in 1933 to treat schizophrenia. An injection of a large dose of insulin was given to the patient to produce a profound state of hypoglycemia (low blood sugar level). The true coma generally occurs about 3 hours after the insulin is given. A glucagon injection is then given and the patient awakens within 10 to 20 minutes. Insulin shock has been replaced by psychotherapy, psychotropic drugs, and ECT.

PSYCHOSURGERY (LOBOTOMY). Originating in 1936, psychosurgery is a surgical intervention to sever fibers connecting one part of the brain with another or to remove or destroy brain tissue. It is designed to affect the patient's psychological state, including modification of disturbed behavior, thought content, or mood. Prefrontal lobotomy and transorbital lobotomy are the two types of psychosurgery still used in research and treatment centers for chronic patients and those who are nonresponsive to all other recommended approaches.

PHYSIOTHERAPY. Hydrotherapy and massages are used for their relaxing effects in the treatment of psychiatric patients. They are short-lasting and produce few side-effects if any. In the past, hydrotherapy was used to treat agitated and depressed patients by the application of wet packs and cold sheets. Tubs also were used to contain restrained patients in hot or cold water for a period of time. Present-day hydrotherapy includes hot baths, whirlpool baths, showers, and swimming pools.

LIMIT SETTING. Limit setting is an important aspect of the therapeutic milieu. Limits reduce anxiety, minimize manipulation, provide a framework for the patient to function, and enable a patient to learn to make requests. Eventually the patient learns to control his own behavior. The first step in limit setting is to give advanced warning of the limit and the consequences that will follow if the patient does not adhere to the limits. Choices should be provided whenever possible, this allows the patient a chance to participate in the limit setting. For example, a 17-year-old substance abuse patient is informed that he is to keep his room orderly, practice good personal hygiene, and attend therapy sessions twice a week. If he does not follow these rules or regulations, he is to forfeit one or more of his privileges. He will be allowed to state his feelings about the limits and to decide which of his privileges will be discontinued temporarily.

The consequence of limit setting should not provide a secondary gain (*e.g.,* individual attention) nor should it lower self-esteem. The consequence should occur immediately after the patient has exceeded the limit. Consistency must occur with all personnel on all shifts to contribute to a person's security and to convey to the patient that someone cares.

SPIRITUAL CARE OF THE PSYCHIATRIC PATIENT

> "When a person enters a hospital, he brings along his spiritual beliefs—possibly intensified by his illness. These beliefs can effect both his recovery rate and his attitude toward treatment . . . "
>
> *Pumphrey, 1977, p. 64*

> "Respecting the faith is but one small aspect of our total concern for clients, and is, perhaps, also a much overlooked aspect of tender loving care."
>
> *Peck, 1981, p. 158*

The first statement was made by a chaplain; the second by a nurse. Both are attuned to the spiritual needs of hospitalized patients, whether they have physical or emotional problems. If the nurse is to establish a therapeutic relationship with a patient, she first needs to establish trust which is in turn built on faith.

The initial interview should include a cultural assessment, focusing on the patient's existing support system. Who are trusted persons? What religious practices are part of the cultural background? Does he exhibit any spiritual needs? Does he indicate a belief in home remedies or cultural practices as part of his treatment?

Some religious groups condemn modern scientific practice, whereas others support medicine in general. The nurse needs to be familiar with the attitudes and requirements of various religious groups if she is to be effective while giving care.

Once the nurse has established a therapeutic relationship with a patient, she should inform the mental health care team of the patient's spiritual needs. As a plan of care is developed, the help of the chaplain or other personnel the patient feels should be involved in his treatment may be elicited. This should be done in conjunction with the members of the mental health team, who must consider the patient's spiritual as well as physical and psychological needs.

Meeting the spiritual needs of hospitalized patients is discussed more in depth in Chapter 9.

PROTECTIVE CARE OF THE PSYCHIATRIC PATIENT

Protective care of the psychiatric patient focuses on providing observation and care so that the patient does not injure himself, injure others, or become injured when around other patients. He must be supervised so that he does not use poor judgment, lose self-respect, destroy property, embarrass others, or leave the hospital without permission. Specific nursing interventions are given in various chapters focusing on suicide, disorientation, confusion, sadism, etc.

SUMMARY

The terms *therapeutic environment* and *community* are defined in this chapter. A therapeutic environment 1) is purposeful and planned; 2) provides a testing ground; 3) reflects a democratic atmosphere; 4) encourages social interaction; 5) respects the individual; 6) conveys an attitude of acceptance and optimism; and 7) continually assesses and evaluates the patient's progress, modifying treatment and nursing interventions as the need arises. A summarized description of each of the following members of the mental health team was given: psychiatrist, clinical psychologist, psychiatric nurse, nurse assistant or technician, various therapists (including occupational, educational, art, music, psychodrama, recreational, play and speech therapists), chaplain, and dietitian. The following conceptual models of patient care, including the role of the psychiatric nurse, were discussed: biological, psychological, behavioral, social, interpersonal, existential, communication, and nursing. The term *eclectic approach* was explained. Treatment modalities in the therapeutic environment were presented according to the following categories: psychotherapy, group therapy, family or systems therapy, behavior therapy, management therapy, and somatic therapy. The purpose and goals of psychotherapy were listed as were the mechanisms common to all therapy groups, including: group acceptance, reality testing, universalization, ventilation, intellectualization, transference, and interaction. Basic theoretical concepts of family therapy were explained, as well as general principles regarding behavior therapy. The following behavior techniques were presented: 1) behavior modification, 2) systematic desensitization, 3) aversion therapy, 4) cognitive behavior therapy, 5) assertiveness training, and 6) implosive therapy. Somatic therapy, the biologic treatment of mental disorders, focused on: clinical psychopharmacology, electroconvulsive therapy (ECT), insulin shock therapy, psychosurgery, and physiotherapy. A step-by-step description of ECT, and nursing intervention, was discussed. Also explained were limit setting, spiritual care, and protective care of the psychiatric patient.

LEARNING ACTIVITIES

I. Clinical activities
  A. Evaluate the psychiatric setting in which you receive your clinical experience. Does it meet the criteria of a therapeutic environment? If not, list changes necessary to establish a therapeutic milieu.
  B. List the members of the mental health team.
  C. Identify conceptual models of patient care being used.
  D. Are the following identifiable as part of the therapeutic environment:
    1. Limit setting
    2. Protective care
    3. Management therapy
II. Independent activities
  A. Interview a member of the mental health team. Ask the following questions:
    1. How do you view your role as a member of the psychiatric mental health team?

    2. What are your goals for the unit?

    3. What are your goals for a specific patient? On which model of therapeutic intervention are these goals based?

B. Read one or more of the references on:

    1. Musical therapy

    2. Spiritual needs of hospitalized patients

C. Develop a nursing care plan for a patient receiving ECT.

SELF-TEST

1. State three purposes of a therapeutic environment:

2. Explain the rationale for protective care of the psychiatric patient.

3. Describe the purpose of limit setting.

4. List functions of each of the following in the mental health setting:
    Psychiatrist
    Clinical psychologist
    Psychiatric social worker
    Psychiatric nurse
    Chaplain

5. State the purpose of psychodrama:

Match the following models of care and their descriptions

6. Psychological

7. Social

8. Biologic

9. Existential

10. Behavioral

    a. Mental illness is the result of a specific factor affecting the brain.

    b. Focuses on recreational, occupational, and social competencies of the patient.

    c. The personality is defective owing to a developmental conflict.

    d. Learned abnormal behavior needs to be modified or unlearned.

    e. Stresses the present in evaluating a personality disorder.

Complete the following:

11. Name the adjunctive therapy used to help people uncover repressed feelings or thoughts or to effect behavioral change (*e.g.*, to stop smoking).

12. Intensive, insight therapy is also referred to as:

13. Psychological reassurance, unburdening, and clarification are examples of:

14. The elimination or replacement of desirable behaviors by means of new learning experiences is known as:

15. Token economy or rewarding a person for good behavior is called:

16. The use of noxious stimuli to change appropriate behavior is called:

17. Contraindications for ECT include:

18. Side-effects of ECT are:

REFERENCES

American Psychiatric Association: A Psychiatric Glossary, 5th ed. Washington, American Psychiatric Press, 1980

Babcock D: Transactional Analysis. In Backer B, Dubbert P, Eisenman E (eds): Psychiatric/Mental Health Nursing: Contemporary Readings. New York, D Van Nostrand, 1978

Barker P: Basic Child Psychiatry, 4th ed. Baltimore, University Park Press, 1983

Beavers S: Music therapy. Am J Nurs: Jan, 1969

Berne E: Games People Play. New York, Grove Press, 1964

Brill N: Working With People: The Helping Process, 2nd ed. Philadelphia, JB Lippincott, 1978

Burgess A: Psychiatric Nursing in the Hospital and the Community, 3rd ed. Englewood Cliffs, Prentice–Hall, 1981

Burley EJ, Steiger TB: Behavior modification: Two nurses tell it like it is. In Backer B, Dubbert P, Eisenman E (eds): Psychiatric/Mental Health Nursing: Contemporary Readings. New York, D Van Nostrand, 1978

Carser D: Primary nursing in the milieu. J Psych Nurs: Feb, 1981

Chinn P, Jacobs M: Theory and Nursing: A Systematic Approach. St. Louis, CV Mosby, 1983

Devine B: Therapeutic milieu/milieu therapy: An overview. J Psych Nurs: Mar, 1981

Faro B: By losing control of herself, Linda controlled her parents and us. Nursing 80: Apr, 1980

Fitzpatrick J, et al: Nursing Models and Their Psychiatric Mental Health Applications. Bowie, Robert J Brady, 1982

Fowler RS, Fordyce WE, Berni R: Operant conditioning in chronic illness. In Backer B, Dubbert P, Eisenman E (eds): Psychiatric/Mental Health Nursing: Contemporary Readings. New York, Van Nostrand, 1978

Gasten E: Music in Therapy. New York, Macmillan, 1968

Haber J et al: Comprehensive Psychiatric Nursing. New York, McGraw–Hill, 1982

Hinds P: Music: A milieu factor with implications for the nurse–therapist. J Psych Nurs: June, 1980

Kornfield D, Finkel J: Psychiatric Management for Medical Practitioners. New York, Grune & Stratton, 1982

Lancaster J: Adult Psychiatric Nursing. Garden City, NJ, Medical Examination Publishing, 1980

Morgan AJ, Moreno JW: The Practice of Mental Health Nursing: A Community Approach. Philadelphia, JB Lippincott, 1973

Murray R, Huelskoetter MM: Psychiatric Mental Health Nursing. Englewood Cliffs, Prentice–Hall, 1983

Parriott S: Music as therapy. Am J Nurs: Aug, 1969

Payne D, Clunn P: Psychiatric Mental Health Nursing. Garden City NJ, Medical Examination Publishing, 1977

Peck ML: The therapeutic effect of faith. Nurs Forum: Feb, 1981

Pumphrey J: Recognizing your patient's spiritual needs. Nursing 77: Dec, 1977

Rowe C: An Outline of Psychiatry, 7th ed. Dubuque, Wm C Brown, 1980

Stuart G, Sundeen S: Principles and Practice of Psychiatric Nursing, 2nd ed. St. Louis, CV Mosby, 1983

Walker JI: Everybody's Guide to Emotional Well-Being. San Francisco, Harbor Publishing, 1982

Wheelright J: Treating the emotions: Part II: Trouble in the Family. Life Magazine: Mar, 1982

Yalom, ID: The Theory and Practice of Group Psychotherapy, 2nd ed. New York, Basic Books, 1975

6

CRISIS INTERVENTION

LEARNING OBJECTIVES

1. Define the term *crisis.*
2. List the characteristics of a crisis.
3. Describe the following phases of a crisis:
   Precrisis
   Impact or shock
   Crisis or defensive retreat
   Recoil, acknowledgment, or the beginning of resolution
   Resolution, adaptation, or change
   Postcrisis
4. Discuss how the following balancing factors can influence the development of a crisis:
   Realistic perception of the event
   Adequate situational support
   Adequate coping mechanisms
5. Define crisis intervention.
6. State the goals of crisis intervention.
7. Describe the steps of crisis intervention.
8. Discuss the importance of legal immunity for the crisis worker.
9. Differentiate between voluntary and involuntary admission to a psychiatric facility.
10. Discuss the legal rights of patients hospitalized in psychiatric facilities.
11. Using crisis intervention, plan therapeutic care for a young couple experiencing a crisis situation.

MOST people exist in a state of equilibrium; that is, their everyday lives contain some degree of harmony in their thoughts, wishes, feelings, and physical needs. Such an existence generally remains intact unless there is a serious interruption or disturbance of one's biologic, psychological, or social integrity. As undue stress occurs, one's equilibrium can be affected and the person may lose control of feelings and thoughts, thus experiencing an extreme state of emotional turmoil. When this occurs a person may be experiencing a crisis.

A crisis may be maturational or situational. A maturational crisis is an experience such as puberty, adolescence, young adulthood, marriage, or the aging process, in which one's life-style is continually subject to change. These are the normal processes of growth and development that evolve over an extended period and require the person to make some type of change. An example of a maturational crisis is retirement, in which a person faces the loss of a peer group as well as a status identity. A situational crisis refers to an extraordinary stressful event that could affect an individual or family regardless of age group, or socioeconomic or socio-cultural status. Examples include economic difficulty, illness, accident, divorce, or death.

CHARACTERISTICS OF A CRISIS

A crisis generally occurs suddenly, when a person, family, or group of individuals is inadequately prepared to handle the event or situation. Normal coping methods fail, tension rises, and feelings of anxiety, fear, guilt, anger, shame, and helplessness may occur. Most crises are generally short in duration, lasting 24 to 36 hours; rarely do they last longer than 4 to 6 weeks. They can cause increased psychological vulnerability, resulting in potentially dangerous, self-destructive, or socially unacceptable behavior, or they can provide an opportunity for personal growth. The outcome of a crisis depends upon the availability of appropriate help (Mitchell, 1981).

PHASES OF A CRISIS

The following phases of a crisis are generally described by theorists: 1) precrisis; 2) impact; 3) crisis; 4) resolution; and 5) postcrisis. The general state of equilibrium in which a person is able to cope with everyday stress is called the *precrisis phase*. When a stressful event occurs, the person is said to be experiencing the *impact phase*. For example, a young couple is told by their pediatrician that their 5-year-old son has inoperable cancer. Once the shock is over, the young parents become acutely aware of their son's critical illness and poor prognosis. This is an extraordinarily stressful event and a threat to their chid's life as well as to their integrity as a family. They are in the *crisis phase* and may experience much confusion and disorganization because they feel helpless and are unable to cope with the son's physical condition. When the young parents are able, with or without intervention of others, to regain control of their emotions, handle the situation, and work toward a solution concerning their son's illness, they are in the *resolution phase* of a crisis. If they are able to resume normal activities while living their son's hospitalization and illness, they are in the *postcrisis phase*. Such an experience may produce permanent emotional injury or may make the young parents feel a stronger bond with each other and their son, depending on their ability to cope.

Murray (1979) lists the four phases of crisis as 1) initial, impact, or shock phase; 2) defensive retreat; 3) phase of recoil or acknowledgment; and the 4) phase of resolution or adaptation and change. These phases are similar to the five phases just described. They are outlined here.

PHASES	DESCRIPTION
Precrisis	State of equilibrium or well-being
Initial, impact or shock	High level of stress Inability to reason logically Inability to apply problem solving behavior Inability to function socially Helplessness Anxiety Confusion Chaos Disorganization Possible panic May last a few hours to a few days
Crisis or defensive retreat	Inability to cope results in attempts to redefine the problem, avoid the problem, or withdraw from reality Ineffective, disorganized behavior interferes with daily living. Denial of problem Rationalization about cause of the situation Projection of feelings of inadequacy onto others May last a brief or prolonged period of time
Recoil, acknowledgment, or beginning of resolution	Acknowledges reality of the situation Attempts to use problem-solving approach by trial and error Tension and anxiety resurface as reality is faced. Feelings of depression, self-hate, and low self-esteem may occur.
Resolution, adaptation, and change	Occurs when the person perceives the crisis situation in a positive way Successful problem solving occurs Anxiety lessens. Self-esteem rises. Social role resumed
Postcrisis	May be at a higher level of maturity and adaptation owing to acquisition of new positive coping skills, or may function at a restricted level in one or all spheres of the personality due to denial, repression, or ineffective mastery of coping and problem-solving skills. Persons who cope ineffectively may express open hostility, exhibit signs of depression, or abuse alcohol, drugs, or food. Symptoms of neurosis, psychosis, chronic physical disability, or socially maladjusted behavior may occur.

PARADIGM OF BALANCING FACTORS

Aguilera (1982) illustrates a paradigm of balancing factors that determine whether a crisis occurs as the result of a stressful event. These factors, which can affect a return to equilibrium, are 1) a realistic perception of an event; 2) adequate situational support; and 3) adequate coping mechanisms to help resolve a problem.

A realistic perception occurs when a person is able to distinguish the relationship between an event and feelings of stress. For example, a 45-year-old executive recognizes the fact that his company is on the verge of bankruptcy because of inefficient projected financial planning by the board of trustees. He does not place the blame on himself and view himself as a failure, although he realizes the seriousness of the situation and feels stressed. His *perception* rather than the actual event will determine his reaction to the situation.

The executive may discuss the situation with a financial consultant, lawyer, or the firm's accountant. Such persons available in the environment are considered to be situational supports because they reflect appraisals of one's intrinsic and extrinsic values. Support by these people may prevent a state of disequilibrium and crisis from occurring. The less readily available emotional or environmental support systems are (*i.e.,* family or friends), the more overwhelming or hazardous will the person define the event, thus increasing vulnerability to crisis.

Coping mechanisms are those methods one usually employs to cope with anxiety or stress and reduce tension in difficult situations. They may be conscious or unconscious, revealing themselves in behavioral responses, for example, denial, intellectualization, productive worrying, grieving, crying, aggression, regression, withdrawal, or repression. The executive may cope by burying himself in his work, calling an emergency meeting of the board of trustees to discuss the situation, or withdrawing from the situation. Coping mechanisms are used during early developmental stages, and, if found effective in maintaining emotional stability, will become a part of one's life-style in dealing with daily stress. The person who has met developmental tasks and achieved a level of personal maturity generally will adapt more readily in a crisis.

Murray (1979) lists additional factors that may influence the development of a crisis. They include the physical and emotional status of a person, previous experience with similar situations, and cultural influences.

Using the crisis theory paradigm (Aguilera, 1982) a comparison of what could happen in the presence or absence of adequate balancing factors during a stressful situation, that of the young parents whose son has cancer, is presented.

STRESSFUL EVENT. A young couple is told that their son has inoperable cancer.

STATE OF DISEQUILIBRIUM OCCURS. The impact of their son's illness results in feelings of increased anxiety, tension, and helplessness. They experience a threatened loss: their son's life.

NEED TO RESTORE EQUILIBRIUM. Parents recognize the need to decrease feelings of anxiety, tension, and helplessness so that they can handle their own feelings and their son's illness.

Balancing Factors

REALISTIC PERCEPTION OF THE EVENT:

Prognosis of illness is poor because the cancer is inoperable.

PERCEPTION DISTORTED:

Question seriousness of illness

ADEQUATE SITUATIONAL SUPPORT:

Receive support of pastor, parents, and close friends

INADEQUATE SITUATIONAL SUPPORT:

No religious affiliation. Decline help from the hospital chaplain. Poor interpersonal relationship with both sets of parents. No close friends to turn to for help.

ADEQUATE COPING SKILLS:

Able to discuss their feelings and thoughts with each other, family members, and friends.

INADEQUATE COPING SKILLS:

Inability to communicate openly with each other. Each blame the other for not recognizing signs of their son's illness earlier.

RESOLUTION OF PROBLEM:

Able to apply problem-solving process. Decide to
  Stay with their son and make the most of their time together as a family.
  Provide the best medical care possible to keep their son comfortable.
Anxiety lessens after the problem-solving process applied
Able to carry on with routine daily activities while son is hospitalized.

PROBLEM UNRESOLVED:

Uncertain what to do about son's illness. Confusion, anxiety, and feelings of helplessness persist. Usual copying mechanisms do not alleviate the fear of a threatened loss. They avoid reality with overactivity.

NO CRISIS:

CRISIS:

Presence of severe or extraordinary stress that is time limited and precipitated by the son's illness.

DEFINITION AND GOALS OF CRISIS INTERVENTION

"Crisis intervention is an active but temporary entry into the life situation of an individual, a family, or a group during a period of stress" (Mitchell,

1981, p. 11). It is an attempt to resolve an immediate crisis when a person's life goals are obstructed and usual problem-solving methods fail. The patient or client is called on to be active in all steps of the crisis intervention process, including clarifying the problem, verbalizing feelings, identifying goals and options for reaching goals, and deciding on a plan.

Crisis intervention can occur in a variety of settings, for example, as the emergency room, industrial dispensary, classroom, surgical intensive care unit, or psychiatric unit. The generic approach focuses on a particular kind of crisis, with direct encouragement of adaptive behavior, general support, environmental manipulation, and anticipatory guidance. The individual approach stresses the present, shows little or no concern for the developmental past, and places an emphasis on the immediate causes of disequilibrium. It can be used as secondary or tertiary prevention and can be effective in preventing future crisis.

The goals of crisis intervention are

1. To decrease emotional stress and protect the crisis victim from additional stress

2. To assist the victim in organizing and mobilizing resources or support systems to meet unique needs and reach a solution for the particular situation or circumstances that precipitated the crisis. It is hoped that this action will prevent hospitalization, reduce the risk of chronic maladaptation, and promote adaptive family dynamics.

3. Returning the crisis victim to a precrisis or higher level of functioning.

STEPS IN CRISIS INTERVENTION

Aguilera (1982) lists four steps in the process of crisis intervention. They include: 1) assessment; 2) planning therapeutic intervention; 3) implementing techniques of intervention; and 4) resolution of the crisis and anticipatory planning.

When working with developmental crisis (also referred to as maturational or internal crisis) or a situational crisis (also referred to as accidental or external crisis), the crisis worker should be aware of the following usual occurrences (Lego, 1984):

1. Most crises occur suddenly, without warning; therefore, there is inadequate prior preparation to handle such a situation.

2. The person in crisis perceives it to be life threatening.

3. There is a decrease or loss of communication with significant others.

4. Some displacement from familiar surroundings or significant others occurs.

5. All crises have an aspect of an actual or perceived loss, involving a person, object, idea, or hope.

Assessment

The assessment process attempts to answer questions such as "What has happened?", "Who is involved?", "What is the cause?", and "How serious is the problem?" The crisis worker determines the following during the assessment process:

1. The onset of the crisis.

2. The precipitating factor (including who, what, when, and where) of the situation.

3. The person's perception of the event. Does it pose a threat to self-esteem, dependency needs, sexual role mastery, or biologic function?

4. The degree of disruption to the person and others, for example, anxiety level, presence of symptoms, and nonverbal behavior. How distressed is the individual? Has it disrupted the person's social life? If so, outside support may not be available.

5. The person's strengths, past methods used in coping, and usual support systems. Who are the person's friends? With whom does he live? Does he have a supportive clergyman?

6. Whether the individual is suicidal or homicidal. (The reader is referred to the chapter on suicidal behavior for additional information.)

7. Whether there are complicating dangers present, such as an acute physical disorder, health hazards, fire, or some other natural disaster.

8. Should the patient be involved in an outpatient crisis therapy group, or is hospitalization necessary?

The final step during the assessment process is the formulation of one or more nursing diagnoses, such as anxiety; ineffective individual coping; impaired verbal communication; and alterations in family processes.

Planning Therapeutic Intervention

With information gained through the assessment process, and the formulation of one or more nursing diagnoses, several specific interventions are proposed. The person should be involved in the choice of alternative coping methods. The needs and reactions of significant others must be considered, as well as the strengths and resources of all persons providing support. Doing something positive, even if the assessment is incomplete, is helpful in a crisis and is better than no help at all.

Therapeutic Intervention

Therapeutic intervention depends on preexisting skills, creativity and flexibility of the crisis worker, and the rapidity of the person's response.

The crisis worker helps the person to establish an intellectual understanding of the crisis by noting the relationship between the precipitating factor and the crisis. He also helps the crisis victim to explore coping mechanisms, remember or recreate successful coping devices used in the past, or devise new coping skills. Reducing immobility caused by anxiety and encouraging verbalization of feelings is an immediate goal of the crisis worker. An attempt also is made to establish new supportive and meaningful relationships and experiences, reopening the person's social world.

Murray (1979) recommends the following therapeutic techniques while performing crisis intervention:

1. Display acceptance and concern, and attempt to establish a positive relationship.

2. Encourage the person to discuss present feelings, such as denial, guilt, grief, or anger.

3. Help the person to confront the reality of the crisis by gaining an intellectual as well as an emotional understanding of the situation. Do not encourage the person to focus on *all* the implications of the crisis at once.

4. Explain that the person's emotions are a normal reaction to the crisis.

5. Avoid giving false reassurance.

6. Clarify fantasies, contrasting them with facts.

7. Do not encourage the person to place the blame for the crisis on others because such encouragement prevents the person from facing the truth, reduces the person's motivation to take responsibility for behavior, and impedes or discourages adaptation during the crisis.

8. Set limits on destructive behavior.

9. Emphasize the person's responsibility for behavior and decisions.

10. Assist the person in seeking help with everyday activities of daily living (ADL) until resolution occurs.

11. Nursing intervention is evaluated and modified as necessary.

Resolution and Anticipatory Planning

During the evaluation phase or step of crisis intervention, reassessment must occur to ascertain that the intervention is reducing tension and anxiety successfully rather than producing negative effects. Reinforcement is provided whenever necessary while the crisis work is reviewed and accomplishments of the crisis victim are emphasized. Assistance is given to formulate realistic plans for the future, and the person is given the opportunity to discuss how present experiences may help in coping with future crises.

CRISIS INTERVENTION MODES

The steps in crisis intervention just presented generally are evident during individual crisis counseling. Persons may elect to participate in a crisis group that resolve various crises through use of the group process (seen in self-awareness groups, personal growth groups, or short-term group therapy). Such groups generally meet for 4 to 6 sessions. They provide support and encouragement to persons who depend on others for much of their sense of personal fulfillment and achievement.

Family crisis counseling includes the entire family during sessions lasting approximately 6 weeks. This type of counseling is considered the preferred method of crisis intervention for children and adolescents.

Telephone hot-lines such as CONTACT and ADAPT serve suicide prevention and crisis intervention telephone counseling centers on a 24-hour basis. They are generally staffed by volunteers who have had intensive training in telephone interviewing and counseling and can give the person in crisis immediate help.

Home crisis visits are available in some situations; for example, if additional information needs to be obtained following a telephone interview; if a caller is assessed as being highly suicidal; or if concerned persons notify a crisis center of potential patients or clients in crisis.

LEGAL ASPECTS OF CRISIS INTERVENTION*

Most people are not required by law to help a person in crisis; however, there are some exceptions such as police officers, firefighters, and emergency medical personnel. In certain states doctors and nurses also are expected to provide help during an emergency or crisis situation. They generally have legal immunity while providing reasonable and prudent care according to a set of previously established criteria and should not hesitate to aid people who need their help.

The criteria or standard of care for a person providing crisis intervention states that the person who begins to intervene in a crisis is obligated to continue the intervention unless a more qualified person relieves him. Discontinuing care constitutes "abandonment," and the care-giver is liable for any damages suffered as a result of the abandonment. Unauthorized or unnecessary discussion of the crisis incident is considered a breach of confidentiality. Touching a crisis victim without his permission could result in a charge of battery. Permission can be obtained verbally or by nonverbal actions that express a desire for help. Implied consent is permission to care for an unconscious crisis victim to preserve life or prevent

*The following information is a summary of simple, broad statements regarding the legal aspects of crisis intervention and in no way is intended to provide legal counsel. The intent of the author is to inform the crisis worker of the potential for legal liabilities.

further injury. "Failure to act in a crisis carries a greater legal liability than acting in favor of the treatment" (Mitchell, 1981, p. 34). Negligence may be charged if a person is injured by the actions of a crisis worker; however, the victim must prove that the worker acted with a blatant disregard for standard care. Usually the charge is dropped if the care-giver can prove he acted in a prudent and reasonable manner.

EMERGENCY ADMISSION TO A PSYCHIATRIC FACILITY

Admission to a psychiatric facility during a crisis can generally occur in one of two ways: 1) voluntary admission and 2) involuntary admission or commitment. During a voluntary admission, the person retains all civil rights while he presents himself for psychiatric evaluation. Admission for psychiatric treatment generally is based on verification by one or two physicians that the person is emotionally disturbed. If the person so chooses, he may sign himself out of the psychiatric facility after a reasonable period of time by giving written notice, unless he is found to be harmful to himself or others.

An involuntary admission or commitment occurs when, after examination by one or two physicians or a qualified mental health professional, the person is found to be mentally disturbed and likely to cause harm to himself or others. A legal hearing may be held before the involuntary admission occurs, and the patient is then detained for a longer period for treatment. Reevaluation of the person's condition must occur before release. A patient's advocate generally meets with the patient within 24 hours and explains his rights during involuntary admission.

The following are examples of patient or client rights during hospitalization in a psychiatric facility according to modern mental health status. They include the rights to

1. Treatment, including a) a humane psychological and physical environment; b) adequate treatment in a least restrictive environment; c) a current, written, individualized treatment plan; and d) informed consent concerning one's condition, progress, explanations of procedures, risks involved, alternative treatments, consequences of alternative treatments, and any other information that may help the patient to make an intelligent, informed choice

2. Refuse treatment, unless such action endangers others, or withdraw from treatment if risks outweigh benefits

3. A probable cause hearing within 3 court days of admission to secure a speedy recovery from involuntary detention if found sane in a court of law (writ of habeas corpus)

4. Communicate freely with others by letter, telephone, or visits, unless such activities are specifically restricted in one's treatment plan

5. Personal privileges: a) wearing one's own clothing; b) maintaining personal appearance to individual taste; and c) receiving the basic necessities of life

6. Maintain one's civil rights, including a) legal representation; b) employment; c) hold public office; d) vote; e) execute a will; f) drive; g) marry; h) divorce; i) hold public office; or j) enter into a contract

7. Religious freedom and education

8. Privacy and confidentiality: Information, records, and correspondence may be disclosed only with the patient's written consent. The exception occurs when the public becomes endangered; namely the patient is transferred to another facility; the patient's attorney, law enforcement officers, or a court request information; the patient participates in research; or insurance companies require information to complete insurance claims.

9. Aftercare: Individuals discharged from mental health facilities have the right to adequate housing and aftercare planned by professional staff.

SUMMARY

This chapter focused on the theory of crisis intervention by defining a crisis; listing the characteristics of a crisis, and describing the phases or stages of a crisis. The paradigm of balancing factors used to determine whether a crisis occurs during an exceptionally stressful situation was presented. A definition and the goals of crisis intervention were stated. The four steps of crisis intervention were summarized, including 1) assessment, 2) planning therapeutic intervention, 3) therapeutic intervention, and 4) resolution with anticipatory planning (evaluation). Crisis intervention modes of group process, family crisis counseling, telephone counseling, and home crisis visits were discussed. Basic legal aspects of crisis intervention were presented to inform the crisis worker of the potential for legal liabilities. Emergency admission to a psychiatric facility, by both voluntary admission and involuntary commitment, was explained.

LEARNING ACTIVITIES

I. Clinical activities
   A. Identify the crisis event that contributed to the hospitalization of your patient.
   B. Discuss the circumstances of the crisis in an effort to evaluate the patient's understanding of the situation.

    C. Identify coping mechanisms used by your patient in his or her effort to establish equilibrium.

    D. Identify the support systems of your patient.

    E. List the therapeutic interventive measures used by health care personnel.

    F. Evaluate effectiveness of interventive measures.

II. Independent activities

    A. Read Aguilera D, Messick J: Crisis Intervention: Theory and Methodology. St. Louis, CV Mosby, 1982.

    B. Review Swanson A: Crisis intervention. In Lego S: The American Handbook of Psychiatric Nursing. Philadelphia, JB Lippincott, 1984. Complete the following:

        1. State the basic concepts of crisis intervention.

        2. Describe the characteristics of crisis intervention.

        3. Compare developmental and situational crises.

        4. State general and specific guidelines during crisis intervention as described by Swanson.

SELF-TEST

1. Extraordinary stressful events that could affect a person regardless of sociocultural or socioeconomic status are called:

2. State the characteristics of a crisis.

3. Define the impact phase of a crisis.

4. Describe what happens during the defensive retreat phase of a crisis.

5. State the different levels of functioning that may occur in postcrisis.

6. Give examples of situational supports in your life.

7. List coping mechanisms that you think you would use if you were told you failed a final examination in psychiatric nursing.

8. State the purpose of crisis intervention.

9. Give the usual factors of developmental and situational crisis.

10. List examples of nursing diagnoses that may be formulated during the assessment process of crisis intervention.

11. Cite several therapeutic techniques the nurse can use during crisis intervention.

12. Explain the rationale for the following crisis intervention modes:
    Family crisis counseling
    Telephone hot-lines or counseling centers
    Home crisis visits

13. Differentiate between voluntary and involuntary admissions to a psychiatric facility.

REFERENCES

Aguilera D, Messick J: Crisis Intervention: Theory and Methodology, 4th ed. St. Louis, CV Mosby, 1982

Barry PD: Psychosocial Nursing Assessment and Intervention. Philadelphia, JB Lippincott, 1984

Carpenito L: Nursing Diagnosis: Application to Clinical Practice. Philadelphia, JB Lippincott, 1983

Dixon SL: Working with People in Crisis: Theory and Practice. St. Louis, CV Mosby, 1982

Garland L, Bush C: Coping Behaviors and Nursing. Reston, VA, Reston Publishing, 1982

Haber J et al: Comprehensive Psychiatric Nursing, 2nd ed. New York, McGraw–Hill, 1982

Hoff LA: People in Crisis: Understanding and Helping. Menlo Park, Addison–Wesley, 1978

Kreigh H, Perko J: Psychiatric and Mental Health Nursing: A Commitment to Care and Concern, 2nd ed. Reston, VA, Reston Publishing, 1983

Lancaster J: Adult Psychiatric Nursing. Garden City, NJ, Medical Examination Publishing, 1980

Lego S: The American Handbook of Psychiatric Nursing. Philadelphia, JB Lippincott, 1984

Lieb J et al: The Crisis Team. New York, Harper & Row, 1973

Mitchell J, Resnik HLP: Emergency Response to Crisis. Bowie, MD, Robert J Brady, 1981

Murray R, Zentner J: Nursing Assessment and Health Promotion Through the Life Span, 2nd ed. Englewood Cliffs, NJ, Prentice–Hall, 1979

Murray R, Zentner J: Nursing Concepts for Health Promotion, 2nd ed. Englewood Cliffs, NJ, Prentice–Hall, 1979

Murray R, Huelskoetter MM: Psychiatric Mental Health Nursing: Giving Emotional Care. Englewood Cliffs, NJ, Prentice–Hall, 1983

Nursing Skillbook Series King J (ed): Using Crisis Intervention Wisely. Horsham, PA, Intermed Communication, 1979

Parad HJ, Resnick HLP: A crisis intervention framework. In Resnick HLP, Rubed HL (eds): Emergency Psychiatric Care. Bowie, Charles Press, 1975

Stuart G, Sundeen S: Principles and Practice of Psychiatric Nursing, 2nd ed. St. Louis, CV Mosby, 1983

Wicks RJ: Crisis Intervention: A Practical Clinical Guide. Thorofare NJ, Charles B Slack, 1978

Wilson H, Kneisl C: Psychiatric Nursing, 2nd ed. Menlo Park, Addison–Wesley, 1983

Wright L, Leahey M: Nurses and Families: A Guide to Family Assessment and Intervention. Philadelphia, FA Davis, 1984

7

PSYCHOTROPIC DRUGS

Although as a nation we are concerned about the use of drugs, it is drug abuse, not therapeutic drug use, that distresses. Controlled drug therapy in psychiatry, accompanied by other therapies, has helped to change mental hospitals from "snake pits" to therapeutic communities.

Nathan S. Kline and John M. Davis (1973, p. 54)

Nurses often hold minimized roles regarding psychotropic drugs because the nurses usually do not prescribe the medication. However, since psychotropic medication frequently is an important part of the treatment, the professional nurse must maintain responsibility for the medication regimen whether she administers the medication herself or delegates this function.

Elaine Boettcher and Sylvia Anderson (1982, p. 12)

LEARNING OBJECTIVES

1. Define the term psychotropic drugs.
2. State the rationale for the administration of the following types of psychotropic medication:
   Antipsychotic drugs or neuroleptics
   Antianxiety agents and sedative–hypnotics
   Antidepressants or mood elevators
   Lithium salts
   Antiparkinsonism agents
3. Define the following terminology:
   Extrapyramidal side-effects
   Parkinsonism
   Akathisia
   Acute dystonic reactions
   Akinesia
   Tardive dyskinesia
4. List nursing actions for patients receiving the following psychotropic drug therapy:
   Phenothiazine agents: chlorpromazine hydrochloride (Thorazine) or thioridizine hydrochloride (Mellaril)
   Nonbarbiturate benzodiazepines or antianxiety agents: diazepam (Valium) and chlordiazepoxide hydrochloride (Librium)
   Sedative–hypnotics: sodium pentobarbital (Nembutal) and sodium butabarbital (Butisol)
   Tricyclic antidepressants: amitriptylline hydrochloride (Elavil) or doxepin hydrochloral (Sinequan)
   Monoamine oxidase (MAO) inhibitors: phenylzine sulfate (Nardil) or tranylcypromine sulfate (Parnate)
   Lithium salts: lithium carbonate (Eskalith or Lithane)
   Antiparkinsonism agents: benztropine mesylate (Cogentin), or biperidin hydrochloride (Akineton)

PSYCHOTROPIC or *psychoactive* drugs are chemicals that affect the brain and nervous system; alter feelings, emotions, and consciousness in various ways; and frequently are used therapeutically in the practice of psychiatry to treat a broad range of mental and emotional illnesses. "In the mid-1950s . . . 500,000 patients were hospitalized in the United States for mental illness. By 1973, the number of hospitalized mental patients had fallen to 250,000, largely due to the use of psychoactive drugs" (Walker, 1983, p. 209).

Categories of psychotropic drugs include 1) antipsychotic drugs, neuroleptics, or major tranquilizers; 2) antianxiety agents; minor tranquilizers and sedative–hypnotics; 3) antidepressants or mood elevators; and 4) lithium salts. Anticholinergic antiparkinsonism agents also are used in the chiatric setting. Each category will be discussed, focusing on principles or rationale for therapy; contraindications, precautions, and side-effects; and implications for nursing actions.

ANTIPSYCHOTIC AGENTS

The major clinical use of antipsychotic agents is in the treatment of psychoses such as schizophrenia, mania, paranoid disorders, organic dementia, and acute brain syndrome. Symptoms include impaired communication or the inability to relate to others, delusions, hallucinations, lack of responsiveness to the external environment, and the inability to identify reality. Antipsychotic agents provide symptomatic control of the patient by blocking the activity of dopamine, a chemical normally occurring in the brain and having the potential to produce psychotic thinking. Too much dopamine allows nerve impulses in the brain stem to be transmitted faster than normal, resulting in strange thoughts, hallucinations, and bizarre behavior. Blocking this activity of dopamine lessens or prohibits the development of such thoughts and behavior. In addition to this property, antipsychotic agents have antiemetic properties, have been used to treat intractable hiccoughs, and have been used in combination with other drugs for pain control. "Antipsychotic medication does not cure social withdrawal, apathy, and interpersonal difficulties that are found in schizophrenics and other psychotic individuals. Psychotherapy is needed to help with these problems" (Walker, 1980, p. 213).

Commonly used antipsychotic agents include: phenothiazines (*e.g.,* Thorazine, Mellaril, Prolixin, Trilafon, Serentil, Compazine, and Vesprin) and nonphenothiazines (*e.g.,* Taractan, Navane, Haldol, Loxitane, and Moban).

Contraindications and Side-Effects

Contraindications of the use of neuroleptics include a history of drug hypersensitivity, severe depression, bone marrow depression or blood dyscrasias, and brain damage.

Patients with a history of impaired liver function, cardiovascular disease, hypertension, glaucoma, diabetes, Parkinson's disease, peptic ulcer disease, epilepsy, or pregnancy should be observed closely when they are taking neuroleptics.

Side-effects of antipsychotic drugs include:

1. Drowsiness, lethargy and inactivity. Persons taking these drugs should avoid driving or operating hazardous machinery.

2. Dry mouth, nasal congestion, and blurred vision

3. Skin reactions such as urticaria and dermatitis

4. Pigmentation of the skin and eyes and photosensitivity or phototoxicity

5. Constipation or urinary retention

6. General orthostatic hypotension during the first 2 weeks of treatment.

7. Alteration in sexual functioning owing to a diminished sex drive

8. Seizures due to a lowering of the seizure threshold

9. Agranulocytosis (generally within first 8 weeks of treatment)

10. Hyperglycemia

11. Mild ECG changes

12. Gastrointestinal distress such as nausea or heartburn

13. Weight gain

14. Edema

Although the list of side-effects is lengthy, they are generally mild. They can be annoying, however, and should be treated as soon as they are recognized.

Extrapyramidal Side-Effects

Extrapyramidal side-effects or adverse neurologic effects may occur during the early phase of drug therapy. They are classified as parkinsonism, akathisia, and acute dystonic reactions. Tardive dyskinesia may occur following short-term use of moderate doses although it generally occurs after long-term use and high-dose therapy. A summary of these neurologic effects is presented here.

Parkinsonism	Akathisia (Motor Restlessness)	Acute Dystonic Reactions	Tardive Dyskinesia (Abnormal Movements)
Motor retardation or akinesia	Constant state of movement characterized by restlessness, difficulty sitting still, or strong urge to move about	Irregular, involuntary spastic muscle movement, wryneck or torticollis, facial grimacing, abnormal eye movements, backward rolling of eyes in the sockets (oculogyric crisis)	Most frequent serious side-effect occurring during abrupt termination of the drug, reduction in dosage or after long-term high-dose therapy
Masklike facies			
Rigidity			Characterized by involuntary rhythmic, stereotyped movements, protrusion of tongue, puffing of cheeks, chewing movements, involuntary movements of extremities and trunk.
Tremors			
"Pill rolling"	Referred to as the "walkies and talkies" by Harris (DeGennaro, 1981, p. 1326)		
Salivation			
Generally occurs after 1st week of treatment or before the 2nd month		May occur anytime after first dose of antipsychotic drug from a few minutes to several hours	
	Generally occurs 2 weeks after treatment begins		

Parkinsonism	Akathisia (Motor Restlessness)	Acute Dystonic Reactions	Tardive Dyskinesia (Abnormal Movements)
			Occurs in approximately 3% of the patients who take antipsychotic medication. If not detected early, symptoms may persist for years or the syndrome may be irreversible.

Implications for Nursing Actions

Patients receiving antipsychotic drug therapy should have an evaluation of blood pressure, complete blood count, liver function tests, and vision tests before therapy and at periodic intervals thereafter.

Nurses who administer antipsychotic drugs should be aware of the following precautions (Abrams, 1983):

1. If a single daily dose is ordered, give oral neuroleptics within 1 or 2 hours of bedtime whenever possible to aid sleep. Minor side-effects are less bothersome at this time.

2. Avoid contact with concentrated solutions while preparing them as they are irritating to the skin and may cause contact dermatitis.

3. Liquid concentrates should be mixed with at least 60 ml of fruit juice or water just before administration to mask the taste of the concentrate.

4. Do not give antipsychotic drugs subcutaneously (SC) unless specifically ordered since they may cause tissue irritation. They should be given as deep intramuscular (IM) injections.

Persons receiving neuroleptic medication should be observed for the following:

1. Therapeutic effects of the drugs, such as decreased agitation, decreased hallucinations, and increased socialization

2. A decrease in nausea and vomiting if the drug is given as an antiemetic

3. Drug-induced extrapyramidal side-effects and early signs of tardive dyskinesia

4. Anticholinergic effects, respiratory depression, and hypersensitivity

5. Drug interactions. Anticholinergics, tricyclic antidepressants, antihistamines, central nervous system (CNS) depressants, propranalol (Inderal), and thiazide diuretics (Hydrodiuril) increase the effects of neuroleptics.

6. Signs of agranulocytosis (*e.g.,* sore throat, fever, and discomfort)

7. Drug-induced, endocrine-related changes: Menstrual irregularities, breast enlargement, lactation, and changes in libido

8. Signs of jaundice, high fever, upper abdominal pain, nausea, diarrhea, and skin rash

Patient Education

Patients need to be informed about the planned drug therapy, length of time it takes to achieve therapeutic results, and possible side-effects of drug therapy. They should be instructed to report any physical illnesses or unusual side-effects and to avoid taking over-the-counter (OTC) drugs or any medications prescribed by another physician. The following is a list of instructions for patients receiving antipsychotic drug therapy:

1. Alcohol and sleeping pills cause drowsiness and decrease one's awareness of environmental hazards. Sleeping pills, alcohol, and other medication should be avoided during drug therapy. Driving or operating hazardous machinery also should be avoided while taking antipsychotic drugs.

2. Patients should avoid being in direct sunlight for an extended time to prevent sunburn or pigmentation of the skin.

3. Individuals should be instructed not to increase, decrease, or cease taking drugs without discussing this with the physician. The drug should be withdrawn slowly to avoid nausea or seizures.

4. The patient should be told that antacids may decrease the absorption of antipsychotic drugs from the intestinal tract, thus altering the effects.

5. To avoid falls or other injuries, the patient should be made aware of the possibility of dizziness and faintness from postural hypotension for about an hour after receiving medication or following an injection.

6. Good oral hygiene should be practiced to avoid mouth infections, dental caries, and ill-fitting dentures. An annual dental examination should be performed.

7. Tablets or capsules should be kept in a safe place if children are in the home to avoid their mistaking the medicine for candy.

Daily Dosage of Commonly Used Antipsychotic Agents

Generic Name	Trade Name	Dosage Range	
Chlorpromazine	Thorazine	30 mg–1000 mg	
Fluphenazine	Prolixin	0.5 mg–20 mg	
Haloperidol	Haldol	1 mg–15 mg	*(continued)*

Generic Name	Trade Name	Dosage Range
Mesoridazine	Serentil	30 mg–400 mg
Molendone	Moban	0.5 mg–225 mg
Perphenazine	Trilafon	12 mg–64 mg
Thioridazine	Mellaril	150 mg–800 mg
Trifluoperazine	Stelazine	2 mg–40 mg

ANTIANXIETY AGENTS AND SEDATIVE–HYPNOTICS

Antianxiety agents are used to relieve moderate to severe anxiety and tension associated with emotional disorders, physical disorders, excessive environmental stress, neuroses, and mild depressive states, without causing excessive sedation or drowsiness. They may also be used to manage persons experiencing withdrawal symptoms associated with chronic alcoholism, control convulsions, and produce skeletal muscle relaxation. These agents also are used for preoperative sedation, sedation before diagnostic tests, and insomnia.

Commonly used antianxiety agents include chlordiazepoxide (Librium), diazepam (Valium), oxazepam (Serax), chlorazepate (Tranxene), lorazepam (Ativan), prazepam (Centrax), and alprazolam (Xanax). They should be used for a short time, 1 or 2 weeks, because of their potential for abuse, toxicity, and lethal overdose. These nonbarbiturate benzodiazepines work selectively on the limbic system of the brain, which is responsible for emotions such as rage and anxiety. They produce tranquilizing effects without much sedation and may numb emotions, taking away one's enthusiasm and zest for life. Individuals who take 40mg or more of diazepam daily for several months may experience seizures and die if they stop taking it abruptly. When used in combination with alcohol, diazepam (Valium) can be lethal. Benzodiazepines interfere with normal coping mechanisms; increase irritability, aggressiveness, and hostility when taken over an extended time; and increase chances of depression.

Nonbenzodiazepines with sedative qualities include meprobamate (Equanil), hydroxyzine hydrochloride (Atarax), hydroxyzine pamoate (Vistaril), ethchlorvynol (Placidyl).These drugs present a high risk of abuse and physical dependence.

Sedatives alone ideally do not cause drowsiness, lethargy, decreased alertness or impaired mental or physical performance. Sedative–hypnotics are used to induce a state of natural sleep; reduce periods of involuntary awakenings during the night; and increase total sleep time. Examples of sedative–hypnotic barbiturates include secobarbital (Seconal), amobarbital (Amytal), pentobarbital (Nembutal), butabarbital (Butisol), phenobarbital (Lumenal).Tolerance can occur within 7 to 14 days resulting in physical dependence after a month or more of use.

Contraindications and Side-Effects

Persons diagnosed as having porphyria should not be placed on sedative–hypnotic therapy as those agents aggravate the symptoms of acute intermittent porphyria. Caution should be used when prescribing antianxiety agents for patients with impairment of respiratory, liver, or kidney function, as well as for depressed persons with possible suicidal tendencies.

Physical dependence may occur if these drugs are taken in large quantities for prolonged periods, and on abrupt withdrawal, an abstinence syndrome can occur. Symptoms include nausea, vomiting, hypotension, fatigue, sleep disturbance, fever, delirium, and potentially fatal grand mal seizures within 12 hours to 2 weeks.

Injections of barbiturates in children and elderly persons may result in excitement and confusion.

Implications for Nursing Actions

Before administering sedative–hypnotics, the nurse should assess the person's mental and physical status to avoid the risk of untoward side-effects. Pregnant women or those breast-feeding should not be placed on antianxiety agents to avoid untoward side-effects. If a patient complains of a sleep disturbance, the causative factor should be identified if possible. Appropriate nursing measures, for example, a warm drink or a backrub, should be tried to promote relaxation before the administration of sedative–hypnotics.

When administering antianxiety or sedative–hypnotic drugs, the nurse should

1. Give the daily dose at bedtime to promote sleep, minimize adverse reactions, and allow more normal daytime activities to occur.

2. Administer IM dosages deeply and slowly into large muscle masses because they are irritating to tissues and can cause pain at the site of injection.

3. Observe for therapeutic effects.

4. Observe for adverse side-effects such as oversedation, hypotension, pain at the injection site, skin rashes, and paradoxic excitement. Symptoms of paradoxic excitement include hostility, rage, confusion, depersonalization, or hyperactivity. Rare side-effects include gastrointestinal (GI) discomfort, nausea, vomiting, menstrual irregularities, blood dyscrasias, photosensitivity, and nonthrombocytopenic purpura.

5. Observe for symptoms of drug interactions, especially with elderly patients who often are taking a variety of medications.

Patient Education

Patients should be told the name of the drug, dose, and schedule of treatment, as well as the expected course of treatment. As with psychoactive drugs. patients on sedative–hypnotic therapy should not alter the dose of medication nor should they drive or operate hazardous equipment.

Other instructions include

1. Avoid mixing alcoholic beverages, antihistamines, or antipsychotic drugs with antianxiety agents because they can increase the depressant effects of those agents, possibly causing death.

2. Avoid ingesting large amounts of beverages containing caffeine, a stimulant, because it can decrease the effects of sedative–hypnotic agents.

3. Report symptoms of fever, malaise, sore throat, petechiae, easy brusing or bleeding, and skin rash.

4. Sudden cessation of these agents can cause rapid eye movement (REM) or rebound with insomnia, dreams, or nightmares, in addition to hyperexcitability, agitation, or convulsions.

5. Avoid excessive use of these drugs to prevent the onset of substance abuse or addiction.

6. Sedative–hypnotics are ineffective as analgesics.

Daily Dosage of Commonly Used Antianxiety Agents

Generic Name	Trade Name	Dosage Range
Alprazolam	Xanax	0.25 mg–4 mg
Chlordiazepoxide	Librium	15 mg–100 mg
Chlorazepate dipotassium	Tranxene	15 mg–60 mg
Diazepam	Valium	2.5 mg–40 mg
Lorazepam	Ativan	0.5 mg–10 mg
Oxazepam	Serax	30 mg–120 mg

Daily Dosage of Commonly Used Sedative–Hypnotics

Generic Name	Trade Name	Dosage Range
Amobarbital	Amytal	60 mg–150 mg
Butabarbital	Butisol	45 mg–120 mg
Pentobarbital	Nembutal	60 mg–120 mg
Secobarbital	Seconal	30 mg–200 mg

Antidepressants or Mood Elevators

Antidepressant agents are used to treat depressive disorders caused by emotional or environmental stressors, frustrations, losses, drugs, disease states such as Parkinson's disease or cancer, or depression that cannot be related to an identifiable cause. These drugs are classified as tricyclic antidepressants and monoamine oxidase inhibitors. Tricyclic antidepressants increase the level of the neurotransmitters, serotonin or norepinephrine, in the space between nerve endings, carrying messages from one nerve cell to another. A deficiency in these neurotransmitters is thought to cause depression. Choice of medication depends on which chemical is thought to be deficient in the nerve endings. Monoamine oxidase (MAO) inhibitors prevent the metabolism of neurotransmitters but are used less frequently than the tricyclics because they are less effective, must be given for longer periods of time before they are beneficial are more toxic, have a longer duration of action, and may cause adverse reactions if taken with tyramine-rich foods.

TRICYCLIC ANTIDEPRESSANTS

Tricyclic antidepressants generally are used to treat symptoms of depression, for example, insomnia, decreased appetite, decreased libido, excessive fatigue, indecisiveness, difficulty thinking and concentrating, somatic symptoms, irritability, and feelings of worthlessness. These agents are considered effective in 85% of those people who exhibit symptoms of depression. Those receiving tricyclic agents generally show an increased mental alertness and physical activity with mood elevation within a few days after initial therapy is begun. People on antidepressant drug therapy continue on the medication for several months to allow neurotransmitters to return to normal levels and to achieve a reversal of the depressive episode.

Contraindications and Side-Effects

Persons who are recovering from a myocardial infarction, are pregnant, are breast feeding, or have a severe liver or kidney disease should not be given tricyclic antidepressants. Caution should be used when administering these drugs to persons with asthma, urinary retention, hyperthyroidism, glaucoma, cardiovascular disorders, benign prostatic hypertrophy, alcoholism, epilepsy, and schizophrenia.

Common side-effects of tricyclic drugs include dry mouth, blurred vision, tachycardia, urinary retention, and constipation. Less frequently encountered side-effects include loss of appetite, insomnia, hypotension, anxiety, and increased intraocular pressure. Eisenhauer (1984) lists the following potentially dangerous side-effects of tricyclic drug therapy: agranulocytosis, jaundice, increased seizure susceptibility in epileptic patients, and prolongation of atrioventricular conduction time. Acute toxicity due to overdose may occur.

Implications for Nursing Actions

The nurse should 1) assess the patient's level or severity of depression, including the presence of suicidal ideation, 2) identify usual coping mechanisms, 3) observe for side-effects, 4) observe for drug interactions, and 5) observe for therapeutic effects of tricyclic antidepressants. Several drugs increase the effects of these agents. They include antihistamines, atropine, alcohol, narcotic analgesics, benzodiazepines, and urinary alkalizers, such as sodium bicarbonate. Barbiturates, nicotine, and chloral hydrate decrease the effects of tricyclic antidepressants (Abrams, 1983).

Within 2 to 3 weeks after the initial dose, tricyclic drugs should reach a serum plasma level at which optimal response occurs (therapeutic window); therefore, if no therapeutic response is observed within 4 to 8 weeks, another drug generally is prescribed.

Because these agents may cause urinary retention and constipation, the patient should be observed for abdominal distention. Patients on high doses should be observed for signs of seizure activity.

Patient Education

Patients undergoing antidepressant drug therapy should be instructed to

1. Take drugs as prescribed. No attempt should be made to alter the dosage. Therapeutic effects may not occur for 2 to 3 weeks after initial therapy.
2. Avoid taking OTC cold remedies or other drugs without the physician's knowledge.
3. Inform other professionals that may treat the patient, such as a dentist or surgeon, of the drug therapy.
4. Report any side-effects, such as fever, malaise, sore throat, sore mouth, urinary retention, fainting, irregular heartbeat, restlessness, mental confusion, or seizures.
5. Avoid excessive exercise and high temperatures because anticholinergic effects of these agents block perspiration.

Tricyclics are not addictive but some patients may have a chronic deficiency in neurotransmitters, requiring them to take these agents over an extended period.

Daily Dosage of Commonly Used Tricyclic Antidepressants

Generic Name	Trade Name	Dosage Range
Amitriptyline	Amitril, Elavil, Endep	75 mg–300 mg
Amoxapine	Asendin	100 mg–400 mg
Desipramine	Norpramin, Pertofrane	75 mg–300 mg
Doxepin	Sinequan, Adapin	75 mg–300 mg
Imipramine	Tofranil, Imavate, Presamine, Janimine	75 mg–300 mg
Moprotiline (tetrocyclic)	Ludiomil	75 mg–300 mg
Nortriptyline	Aventyl, Pamelor	40 mg–100 mg
Protriptyline	Vivactil	15 mg–60 mg
Trazodone	Desyrel	150 mg–600 mg
Trimipramine maleate	Surmontil	75 mg–300 mg

MONOAMINE OXIDASE (MAO) INHIBITORS

As stated earlier, MAO inhibitors are antidepressants that prevent the metabolism of neurotransmitters. They are generally effective when treating depression associated wtih acute anxiety attacks, phobic attacks, or many physical complaints; patients who fail to respond to tricyclic agents; and patients who are in the depressive phase of manic–depressive illnesses.

Contraindications and Side-Effects

The list of conditions that prohibit the use of MAO inhibitors is lengthy but is presented at this time to emphasize the caution that should be used when prescribing or administering these drugs:

1. Asthma
2. Cerebral vascular disease
3. Congestive heart failure
4. Hypertension
5. Hypernatremia
6. Impaired kidney function
7. Cardiac arrhythmias
8. Pheochromocytoma
9. Hyperthyroidism
10. Liver disease

11. Abnormal liver function tests

12. Severe headaches

13. Alcoholism

14. Glaucoma

15. Atonic colitis

16. Paranoid schizophrenia

17. Debilitated patients

18. Patients over age 60

19. Pregnancy

20. Children under age 16

Caution should be exercised when treating patients with a history of angina pectoris, pyloric stenosis, epilepsy, and diabetes mellitus.

Frequently seen side-effects include orthostatic hypertension, drowsiness or insomnia, abnormal heart rate, headache, dizziness, blurred vision, vertigo, constipation, weakness, dry mouth, nausea, vomiting, and loss of appetite.

Hypertensive crisis may result if MAO inhibitors are taken with tyramine-rich foods (*e.g.,* aged cheese, avocados, guacomole dip, bananas, chicken livers, fava bean pods, canned figs, meat tenderizers, pickled herring, raisins, sour cream, soy sauce, and yogurt). Patients also should avoid drinking beer, Chianti and other red wines, and any caffeine-containing beverages. Meat tenderizers and yeast supplements should be restricted. Drugs that should be avoided include amphetamines, antiallergy and antihistiminic preparations, antihypertensive agents, levodopa, and meperidine. Toxic symptoms may not occur until 12 hours or later after drug ingestion.

Implications for Nursing Actions

MAO inhibitors are nonaddictive and are considered safe and effective if taken as directed. As with tricyclic antidepressants, observe the patient for signs of adverse effects, drug or food interactions, and therapeutic effects.

Drugs that increase the effects of MAO inhibitors have been identified as anticholinergics, adrenergic agents, alcohol, levodopa, reserpine, meperidine, and guanethidine (Abrams, 1983).

To reach a maximum therapeutic effect, MAO inhibitors may require 2 to 6 weeks of therapy. Beneficial response should be evident within 3 to 4 weeks.

Medication for overdose includes phentolamine (Regitine) for excessive pressor response and diazepam (Valium) for excessive agitation.

Patient Education

The receiving MAO inhibitor therapy should be instructed to

1. Take the drug as prescribed. Avoid altering the dosage or discontinuing the use of the drug.

2. Avoid the ingestion of tyramine-containing foods, and caffeine-containing or certain alcoholic beverages.

3. Report any symptoms indicative of a hypertensive crisis, such as headache or heart palpitations.

4. Avoid overactivity because these agents may suppress anginal pain, a warning of myocardial ischemia.

5. Have vision checked periodically because optic toxicity may occur if therapy is given over an extended period.

Daily Dosage of Commonly Used MAO Inhibitors

Generic Name	Trade Name	Dosage Range
Isocarboxazid	Marplan	10 mg–30 mg
Phenelzine	Nardil	15 mg–90 mg
Tranylcypromine	Parnate	20 mg–30 mg

LITHIUM SALTS

Administration of lithium is considered the treatment of choice for the manic phase of the bipolar disorder formerly termed manic–depressive illness and for the long-term prophylaxis of this bipolar disorder. It has also been tried in the treatment of depressive and schizoaffective disorders.

The exact method of how lithium produces therapeutic effects is unknown. It is not metabolized by the body; approximately 80% of a lithium dose is reabsorbed in the proximal renal tubules and excreted by the kidneys. It is believed to level out the activity of neurotransmitters in the area of the brain that controls emotions, thus preventing a decreased activity of nerve impulses, resulting in depression, or an increased activity of nerve impulses, resulting in mania. Lithium also is thought to maintain a constant sodium concentration in the brain, regulating impulses along the nerve cells as well as mood swings.

Contraindications and Side-Effects

Lithium should not be prescribed during pregnancy or in the presence of severely impaired kidney function. Caution should be used when prescribing lithium for patients who have heart disease; perspire profusely; are on a sodium-restricted diet; are hypotensive; have epilepsy, parkinsonism, or other CNS disorders; or are dehydrated. Serum lithium concentrations may increase in the presence of extreme vomiting, diarrhea, or perspiration, resulting in lithium toxicity.

Common side-effects include nausea, metallic taste, abdominal discomfort, polydipsia, polyuria, muscle weakness, fine hand tremors, fatigue, and mild diarrhea, as well as edema of the feet, hands, abdominal wall, or face. These effects may occur as early as 2 hours after the first dose is taken.

Lithium toxicity occurs when serum lithium levels exceed 1.5 to 2.0 mEq/liter and include symptoms such as drowsiness; slurred speech; muscle spasms; blurred vision; diarrhea; dizziness; stupor; convulsions; coma; or death.

Implications for Nursing Actions

Patients undergoing lithium therapy should be given the drug during or after meals to decrease gastric irritation. Serum lithium levels should be taken at least twice a week during the initiation of therapy before stabilization of the manic episode. Following stabilization, they should be taken at monthly intervals. Serum samples should be drawn 12 hours after a dose is administered; desired levels should reach 1.0 to 1.5 mEq/liter.

Patients should be observed for decreases in manic behavior and mood swings, adverse side-effects, and drug interactions. Drugs that increase the effects of lithium include diuretics (*e.g.,* Lasix and anti-inflammatory agents such as Indocin). The effects of lithium are decreased by acetazolamide (Diamox), sodium bicarbonate, excessive amounts of sodium chloride, drugs with a high sodium content, and theophylline compounds.

Patient Education

Instructions should focus on the following information about lithium therapy during patient education:

1. Take the drug as directed. Do not alter the dosage or cease taking the prescribed drug.

2. Do not decrease dietary salt intake unless instructed to do so by the physician because it increases the risk of adverse effects from lithium.

3. Maintain a high intake of fluids (3 liters daily) unless contraindicated because of a physical disorder.

4. Avoid crash or fad diets.

5. Avoid excessive exercise in warm weather.

6. Regular blood lithium levels are necessary for safe, effective therapy. Blood samples should be taken 12 hours after the previous dose of lithium; therefore, do not take the morning dose until the serum sample has been taken.

7. Avoid taking other medications without the physician's knowledge because these may increase or decrease the effects of lithium.

8. Report any unusual symptoms, illness, or loss of appetite immediately to the physician.

9. Continue to take the drug despite an occasional relapse. Some patients respond slowly to lithium therapy.

10. Notify the doctor whenever a change in diet occurs because this may affect the lithium level.

11. Women should not breast-feed while taking lithium.

12. Schedule an annual physical examination.

Daily Dosage of Lithium Salts

Generic Name	Trade Name	Dosage Range
Lithium carbonate	Eskalith Lithane Lithobid Lithonate Lithotabs	900–1800 mg/day in divided doses until serum levels reach 1.0–1.5 mEq/liter 300 mg t.i.d. or q.i.d. as a maintenance dose with serum levels at 0.6–1.2 mEq/liter

ANTIPARKINSONISM AGENTS

Anticholinergic antiparkinsonism agents are the drugs of choice to treat extrapyramidal effects, including akathisia, acute dystonia, and parkinsonism. Benadryl, an antihistamine, and Symmetrel may be used, but these are classified as secondary agents.

Contraindications and Side-Effects

Anticholinergic drugs are contraindicated in the following conditions: hypersensitivity reactions; prostatic hypertrophy; glaucoma; and obstruction of the GI biliary, or urinary tracts. Caution must be exercised when prescribing these agents for patients with cardiac disease, chronic respiratory disease, and myasthenia gravis, as well as for elderly patients with atherosclerosis or mental impairment, nursing mothers, and children under age 6 (Eisenhauer, 1984).

Side-effects include dry mouth, blurred vision, dizziness, drowsiness, constipation, tachycardia, and urinary retention. When anticholinergic drugs are administered with antihistamines, more pronounced sedation occurs.

Implications for Nursing Actions

Nursing actions for anticholinergic drug therapy include

1. Monitor intake, urinary output, and bowel elimination to prevent urinary retention and constipation. Provide an adequate intake of fluids and bulk in the patient's diet.

2. Monitor blood pressure and pulse every 4 hours when the patient first is started on anticholinergic agents, when the dosage is changed, or when other medications are added.

3. Observe for other adverse side-effects, such as tachycardia and palpitations; excessive CNS stimulation; sedation and drowsiness; dilated pupils; blurred vision; and photophobia.

4. Observe for drug interactions. Antihistamines, disopyramide phosphate (Norpace), phenothiazines, thioxanthene agents, and tricyclic antidepressants all increase the effects of anticholinergic agents.

Patient Education

As is true of other types of drug therapy, the patient receiving medication to lessen or reverse extrapyramidal side-effects of psychotropic drugs should be instructed to follow the physician's instructions regarding dosage. Other instructions to the patient include

1. Maintain an adequate amount of fluid intake unless contraindicated to prevent excessive dryness of the mouth. Taking the medication just before meals, chewing gum, or sucking on hard candies may alleviate this side-effect.

2. Avoid operating potentially hazardous machinery or driving an automobile if symptoms of blurred vision or drowsiness occur.

3. Report any side-effects of unusual symptoms to the family physician.

4. Use caution when rising from a sitting or reclining position because of the possibility of postural hypotension and drowsiness.

5. Limit strenuous activities in hot weather as anticholinergic drugs may cause anhidrosis (the inability to sweat).

6. Have routine vision examinations to eliminate the possibility of the presence of glaucoma.

Daily Dosage of Commonly Used Antiparkinsonism Agents

Generic Name	Trade Name	Dosage Range
Benztropine	Cogentin	1 mg–6 mg
Biperiden	Akineton	2 mg–8 mg
Trihexyphenidyl	Artane	2 mg–15 mg
Diphenhydramine	Benadryl	25 mg–200 mg
Amantadine	Symmetrel	100 mg–300 mg

SUMMARY

Psychotropic drugs are chemicals used therapeutically in the practice of psychiatry to treat a wide range of mental and emotional illness and are categorized as antipsychotic drugs, antianxiety agents, sedative–hypnotics, antidepressants, and lithium salts. Antiparkinsonism agents also are used in the psychiatric setting. Each category was presented, focusing on the principle or rationale for therapy; contraindications, precautions, and side-effects; and implications for nursing actions. Patient education was discussed, and examples of commonly used drugs and the daily dosage were given.

LEARNING ACTIVITIES

I. Clinical activities
    A. Identify several psychotropic drugs prescribed in the clinical setting.
    B. State the rationale for the administration of each identified drug.
    C. Identify any side-effects.
    D. List nursing implications for each drug identified.
II. Independent activities
    A. Read the series of articles on Psychotropic Drug Therapy in the *American Journal of Nursing,* July, 1981.
    B. Complete the following self-test on psychotropic drugs.

SELF-TEST

1. List five types of psychotropic drugs.

2. Explain the action of tricyclic antidepressants.

3. List the trade names of various tricyclic antidepressants.

4. Explain the action of MAO inhibitor antidepressants.

5. List the trade names of various MAO medications.

6. Explain the term *therapeutic window*.

7. List common side-effects of antidepressant medications.

8. List conditions, other than depression, that appear to respond to antidepressant medications.

9. Explain why lithium is the drug of choice in the treatment of manic disorders.

10. State two reasons why lithium is considered a potentially dangerous drug.

11. List the disorders that appear to respond to lithium.

12. List side-effects and toxicity levels of lithium.

13. List drug classifications that interact dangerously with lithium.

14. What are the absolute and relative contraindications in the use of lithium?

15. Compare the terms *neuroleptics, major tranquilizers,* and *antipsychotic medications.*

16. List causes of those psychotic conditions that respond to the antipsychotic medications.

17. State symptoms that *do* and *do not* respond to antipsychotic medication.

18. List other disorders that respond to the use of an antipsychotic medication.

19. Explain the action of an antipsychotic medication.

20. Note drug interactions of various agents with antipsychotic medications.

21. List the trade names of various antipsychotic medications.

22. List the side-effects of antipsychotic medications.

23. Define the term *extrapyramidal*.

24. Cite examples of extrapyramidal side-effects.

25. State two classifications of antiparkinsonism agents.

26. List common antiparkinsonism medications.

27. Compare the terms *anxiolytic, minor tranquilizer,* and *sedative–hypnotic.*

28. Explain the difference between the terms *sedative* and *hypnotic.*

29. Discuss the terms tolerance and physical–emotional dependence in relationship to the sedative–hypnotic agents.

30. State the two classifications of the sedative–hypnotic medications.

31. List the trade names of various sedative–hypnotic medications.

32. List common side effects of sedative–hypnotic medications.

33. State conditions that contraindicate the use of sedative–hypnotic medications.

REFERENCES

Abrams AC: Clinical Drug Therapy: Rationales for Nursing Practice. Philadelphia, JB Lippincott, 1983

Boettcher E, Alderson S: Psychotropic medications and the nursing process. J Psych Nurs: Nov, 1982

Clark J et al: Pharmacological Basis of Nursing Practice. St. Louis, CV Mosby, 1982

Cohen M, Amdur M: Medication groups for psychiatric patients. Am J Nurs: Feb, 1981

DeGennaro MD, et al: Psychotropic drug therapy. Am J Nurs: July, 1981

Eisenhauer L, Gerald M: The Nurses' 1984–1985 Guide to Drug Therapy. Englewood Cliffs, NJ, Prentice–Hall, 1984

Hahn AB et al: Pharmacology in Nursing, 15th ed. St. Louis, CV Mosby, 1982

Kline N, Davis J: Psychotropic Drugs. Am J Nurs: Jan, 1973

Liska K: Drugs and the Human Body with Implications for Society. New York, Macmillan, 1981

Newton M et al: How you can improve the effectiveness of psychotropic drug therapy. Nurs 78: July 1978

Scherer JC: Lippincott's Nurse's Drug Manual. Philadelphia, JB Lippincott, 1985

Swonger AK: Nursing Pharmacology: A Systems Approach to Drug Therapy and Nursing Practice. Boston, Little, Brown & Co, 1978

Tardive Dyskinesia and EPS: Recent Findings. East Hanover, Sandoz Pharmaceuticals, Feb 28, 1978

Vernon AW: Classification of psychotherapeutic drugs, J Psychosoc Nurs: Nov, 1981

Walker J: Everybody's Guide to Emotional Well-Being. San Francisco, Harbor Publishing, 1982

THE PATIENT

AS A

PERSON

8

THEORIES OF PERSONALITY

DEVELOPMENT

There are two lasting gifts
we can give our children—
One is roots,
the other is wings.

Anonymous

LEARNING OBJECTIVES

1. Define personality.
2. Summarize the following developmental theories:
   Freud's psychoanalytic theory
   Erikson's psychosocial theory
   Piaget's cognitive developmental theory
   Duvall's theory of the family life cycle
3. State the common feelings, behavioral patterns, and social considerations to be assessed when one is working with minority groups.
4. Differentiate between a functional and nonfunctional American Indian.
5. List distinctive characteristics of black families.
6. Describe briefly the traditional role and power structure of a Chicano family.
7. Explain why the understanding of a person's cultural background (e.g., Asian Americans) is crucial for appropriate nursing interventions.
8. Discuss the importance of a working knowledge of personality growth and development in the mental health setting.

PERSONALITY is the total of a person's internal and external patterns of adjustment to life, determined in part by genetically transmitted organic endowment and life experiences. Thus, the dynamics of personality development become increasingly complex throughout the life span as one continually interacts with the environment and experiences various stages of physical and psychological maturation. Factors influencing psychological maturation have been identified as genetic stressors, such as Down's syndrome; environmental stressors, including parental relationships, peer relationships, and cultural and social experiences; individual accomplishments that are a result of learning and adaptation; and one's mental health status at each developmental stage. Thus a newborn infant reacts differently to a given environmental stimulus than does an adolescent, young adult, or elderly person.

Various theories of personality maturation are presented in developmental psychology classes as part of the curriculum in nursing programs. Generally, they are categorized as psychoanalytical, cognitive, behavioristic, and humanistic. It is not the intent of this book to provide an in-depth chapter on these theories; but, rather, to present a summary of the more common theorists such as Freud, Erikson, and Piaget. Duvall's theory describing family developmental tasks also will be presented because it provides ways of anticipating the overall pattern of a family's activities and the influence of these activities on a person's psychological maturation.

FREUD'S PSYCHOANALYTIC THEORY

Freud's theory of personality development describes three major categories: the organization or structure of personality, the dynamics of personality, and the development of personality.

The organization or structure of the personality consists of the *id,* which is an unconscious reservoir of primitive drives and instincts dominated by thinking and the pleasure principle; *ego,* which meets and interacts with the outside world as an integrator or mediator and is the executive function of the personality that functions at all three levels of consciousness; and *superego,* which acts as the censoring force or conscience of the personality and is composed of morals, mores, values, and ethics largely derived from one's parents. The superego operates at all three levels of consciousness also.

According to Freud's explanation of the dynamics of the personality, each person has a certain amount of psychic energy to cope with the problems of everyday living. The id's energy is used to reduce tension and may be exhibited, for example, by frequency of urination, daydreaming, or eating. The ego's energy controls the impulsive actions of the id and the moralistic or idealistic actions of the superego. One whose energy is controlled primarily by the superego generally behaves in an overly moralistic manner because the system monopolizing the psychic energy governs the person's behavior.

Freud explains the development of the personality by describing three levels of consciousness: the unconscious, preconscious (subconscious), and conscious. The unconscious level consists of drives, feelings, ideas, and urges outside of the person's awareness. This is the most significant level of consciousness because of the effect it has on one's behavior. A considerable amount of psychic energy is utilized to keep unpleasant memories stored in the unconscious level of the mind. The preconscious or subconscious level, midway between the conscious and unconscious levels, consists of feelings, ideals, drives, and ideas that are out of one's ongoing awareness but can be recalled readily. The conscious level of the personality is aware of the present and controls purposeful behavior.

Freud also describes five phases of psychobiologic process (psychosexual theory) that have a great impact upon personality development: oral; anal; phallic; latency; and genital. These stages are discussed more fully in Chapter 18. The oral phase (0–18 mo) is a period in which pleasure is derived mainly through the mouth by the actions of sucking or biting. During the anal phase (18 mo–3 yrs), attention focuses on excretory function, and the foundation is laid for the development of the superego. The phallic phase (3–7 yrs) is a stage of growth and development in which the child identifies with the parent of the same sex. During the latency phase (7 yrs to adolescence) the person learns to recognize and handle reality.

The final stage of psychosexual development is the genital phase (puberty or adolescence into adult life), in which the individual develops the capacity for object love and mature heterosexuality.

ERIKSON'S PSYCHOSOCIAL THEORY

Erikson emphasizes the concepts of identity or an inner sense of sameness that perseveres despite external changes, identity crisis, and identity confusion in the dynamics of personality development. He has identified eight psychosocial stages during one's life span: 1) sensory–oral (birth to 18 months), characterized by the central task of trust versus mistrust; 2) muscular–anal (18 mon–3 yrs), characterized by autonomy versus shame and doubt; 3) locomotor–genital (3–5 yrs), characterized by initiative versus guilt; 4) latency (6–11 yrs), characterized by industry versus inferiority; 5) puberty and adolescence (12–18 yrs), involving identity versus role confusion; 6) young adulthood (19–40 yrs), characterized by intimacy versus isolation; adulthood (41–64 yrs), characterized by generativity versus stagnation or self-absorption; and 8) late adulthood or maturity (65 years to death), characterized by ego integrity versus despair. These developmental stages are a series of normative conflicts that every person must handle. The two opposing energies (developmental crisis) must be synthesized in a constructive manner to produce positive expectations for new experiences. If the crisis is unresolved, the person does not develop attitudes that will be helpful in meeting future developmental tasks. The following is a summary of Erikson's psychosocial theory, focusing on the developmental stage, area of conflict and resolution; basic virtues, or qualities acquired; and positive behavior. Failure to resolve a challenge or conflict will result in negative behavior, but an opportunity to resolve it recurs later in one's life span.

Developmental Stage	Area of Conflict and Resolution	Basic Virtues or Qualities	Positive Behavior or Resolution of Conflict
Sensory–oral or early infancy (0–1½ yrs)	Trust vs mistrust	Drive and hope	Displays affection, gratification, recognition, and the ability to trust others
Muscular-oral or later infancy (1½–3 years)	Autonomy vs shame and doubt	Self-control and willpower	Cooperative, expresses oneself, displays self-control, views self apart from parents
Locomotor-genital or early childhood (3–5 years)	Initiative vs guilt	Direction and purpose	Tests reality. Shows imagination, displays some ability to evaluate

(continued)

Developmental Stage	Area of Conflict and Resolution	Basic Virtues or Qualities	Positive Behavior or Resolution of Conflict
			own behavior, exerts positive controls over self
Latency or middle childhood (6–11 yrs)	Industry vs inferiority	Method and competence	Develops a sense of duty, scholastic and social competencies. Displays perseverance and interacts with peers in a less infantile manner
Puberty and adolescence (12–18 yrs)	Identity vs role confusion	Devotion and fidelity	Displays self-certainty, experiments with role, expresses ideologic commitments, chooses a career or vocation, and develops interpersonal relationships
Young adulthood (29–40 yrs)	Intimacy vs isolation	Affiliation and love	Establishes mature relationship with a member of the opposite sex, chooses a suitable marital partner, performs work and social roles in a socially acceptable manner
Middle adulthood (41–64 yrs)	Generativity vs stagnation	Productivity and ability to care for others	Spends time wisely by engaging in helpful activities such as teaching, counseling, community activities, and volunteer work. Displays creativity
Late adulthood or maturity (65 years to death)	Ego integrity vs despair	Renunciation, or "letting go," and wisdom	Reviews life realistically, accepts past failures and limitations, helps members of younger generations view life positively and realistically, accepts death with dignity

PIAGET'S COGNITIVE DEVELOPMENTAL THEORY

Piaget's theory views intellectual development as a result of constant interaction between environmental influences and genetically determined attributes. Piaget's research focused on four stages of intellectual growth during childhood, with emphasis on how a child learns and adapts what is learned to the adult world. The four stages are sensorimotor, preoperational, concrete operational, and formal operational.

During the sensorimotor stage, ages 0 to 2 years, the infant uses the senses as he learns about self and the environment by exploration of objects and events, and by imitation. He also develops schemata, or methods for assimilating and accommodating incoming information; these include looking schema, hearing schema, and sucking schema.

The preoperational thought stage, ages 2 to 7 or 8, is subdivided into the preconceptual and intuitive phases. Learning to think in mental images and the development of expressive languages and symbolic play occurs between the ages of 2 and 4. During the ages of 4 to 7 the child exhibits egocentrism while seeing things from his own point of view. He is unable to comprehend the ideas of others if they differ from his own. As he matures, he realizes that other people see things differently.

The concrete operational stage begins at about age 8 and lasts until age 12. The child is able to think more logically as he develops the concepts of moral judgment, numbers, and spatial relationships.

The formal operational stage occurs during age 12 and lasts to adulthood. The person develops adult logic and is able to reason, form conclusions, plan for the future, think abstractly, and build ideals.

DUVALL'S THEORY OF THE FAMILY LIFE CYCLE

The family is a developing system that must progress in the right way for the child's development to be healthy. According to Duvall's theory, there are predictable successive stages of growth and development within the life cycle of every family. Family developmental tasks refer to growth responsibilities achieved by a family unit as well as individual developmental requisites. The interfacing of individual developmental needs and family tasks is not always possible and may lead to conflict, resulting in poor interpersonal relationships, the development of individual emotional problems, or a family crisis. An understanding of these eight stages of the family life cycle provides the nurse with guidelines to analyze family growth and health promotion needs as well as the ability to provide therapeutic intervention when conflict arises. The following is a summary of each of the eight stages as described by Duvall, including the age and school placement of the oldest child, which impacts on the responsibilities of family members.

STAGE	DESCRIPTION OF FAMILY TASKS
I. Beginning families (no children; commitment to each other)	Establishing a mutually satisfying marriage by learning to live together and provide for each other's personality needs Relating harmoniously to three families; each respective family and the one being created by marriage

(continued)

STAGE	DESCRIPTION OF FAMILY TASKS
	Family planning: whether to have children and when
	Developing a satisfactory sexual and marital role adjustment
II. Early childbearing (begins with birth of first child and continues until infant is 30 months)	Developing a stable family unit with new parent roles
	Reconciling conflicting developmental tasks of various family members
	Jointly facilitating developmental needs of family members to strengthen each other and the family unit
	Accepting the new child's personality
III. Families with preschool children (firstborn child 2½ years old, continues until age 5	Exploration of environment by children
	Establishment of privacy, housing, and adequate space
	Husband–father becomes more involved in household responsibilities
	Preschooler develops a more mature role and assumes responsibility for self-care
	Socialization of children such as attending school, church, sports
	Integration of new family members (second or third child)
	Separation from children as they enter school
IV. Families with school-aged children (firstborn child ages 6–13)	Promoting school achievement of children
	Maintaining a satisfying marital relationship as this is a period when it diminishes
	Promoting open communication within the family
	Accepting adolescence
V. The family with teenagers	Maintaining a satisfying marital relationship while handling parental responsibilities
	Maintaining open communication between generation gaps
	Maintaining family ethical and moral standards by the parents while the teenagers search for their own beliefs and values
	Allowing children to experiment with independence
VI. Launching center families (covers the first child through last child leaving home)	Expanding the family circle to include new members by marriage
	Accepting the new couple's own life style and values
	Devoting time to other activities and relationships by the parents
	Reestablishing the wife and husband roles as the children achieve independent roles
	Assisting aging and ill parents of the husband and wife

STAGE	DESCRIPTION OF FAMILY TASKS
VII. Families of middle years ("empty nest" period through retirement)	Maintaining a sense of well-being psychologically and physiologically by living in a healthy environment Attaining and enjoying a career or other creative accomplishments by cultivating leisure-time activities and interests Sustaining satisfying and meaningful relationships with aging parents and children Strengthening the marital relationship
VIII. Family in retirement and old age (begins with retirement of one or both spouses, continues through the loss of one spouse, and terminates with the death of the other spouse)	Maintaining satisfying living arrangements Maintaining marital relationships Adjusting to a reduced income Adjusting to the loss of a spouse

CULTURAL CONSIDERATIONS IN PERSONALITY DEVELOPMENT

Culture is an important variable in the assessment of individuals in addition to the structural and functional aspects of the family. To understand an ethnic group and to be able to work with individuals or family members, the nurse must be aware of a culture's unique, distinctive qualities and the variety of life styles, values, and structures within a given group that influence the development of one's personality. Cultural differences are often the cause of poor communication, interpersonal tensions, avoidance in working effectively with others, and the poor assessment of health problems; therefore, the racial identity and unique cultural experiences of members of minority cultures cannot be ignored in mental health nursing.

Kozier (1983) lists common feelings, behavioral patterns and social considerations to be assessed when working with minority groups:

1. Feelings of inferiority and inadequacy
2. Anger and hostility
3. Selective inattention
4. Incompetent behavior
5. Withholding feelings and experiences
6. Denial of the existence of a situation
7. Attempt to perform in a superior way to succeed in society
8. Language barrier
9. Food habits
10. Perception of illness
11. Illness practices
12. Here-and-now time orientation

13. Concept of family

14. Male/female norms or roles

Cultural practices of American Indians, blacks, Chicanos, and Asian Americans will be discussed to assist the reader in developing an understanding of personality development in these minority families.

American Indians

Cultural identity of Native Americans is no longer determined by physical appearance but rather by the classification of functional or nonfunctional. The functional Indian has an intimate understanding of heritage obtained through socialization from childhood and considers himself to be Indian. His behavior is dictated by accepted patterns of other Indians. The nonfunctional Indian may appear to be full blooded but may have little or no knowledge of the traditions of culture of Indian people. He follows the cultural practices of the white race and considers himself a non-Indian.

Beliefs and practices that influence the personality of a member of this minority are summarized by Kozier (1979):

1. Believe that illness is the result of an imbalance between a person and natural or supernatural forces rather than an altered physiologic state. Illness may result from abusing another person, thinking bad thoughts, or entertaining thoughts of jealousy or anger.

2. Are less concerned about the future than are whites

3. Do not maintain direct eye contact because this is a disrespectful practice and an invasion of one's privacy

4. Maintain a large kinship structure. Family, relatives, and friends play an important part in their support system.

5. Are casual about time because their lives are less rigidly controlled by the clock

6. Have a suicide rate twice as high as other races

7. Have a homicide rate three times greater than that of any other races

8. Have a mortality rate related to alcohol that is six times greater than that of any other race

9. Experience an increase in the rate of emotional problems of childhood

10. Practice healing ceremonies referred to as "sings" or prayers to restore homeostasis.

Blacks

During the era of slavery, the black family was allowed to exist only by the consent of the slave owner and was not autonomous or self-sufficient. Today blacks have been able to maintain two-parent nuclear families while they adapt to a larger society and become members of the middle class. Distinctive characteristics of black families include: 1) households have a larger number of extended family members living with them owing to strong kinship bonds; 2) black children often are expected to assume responsible duties such as helping with housework, running errands, and caring for younger siblings since both parents work; 3) young children often hold odd jobs to supplement family incomes; 4) poor families have survival needs that often supercede the resolution of health problems; and 5) poor black families often experience feelings of discomfort and alienation toward white health care providers (Friedman, 1981). Health practices and beliefs that still exist to some extent include voodoo and witchcraft.

Chicanos

Chicano (Mexican–Americans or those of Hispanic background) families exhibit a significant characteristic referred to as familism. The family is the single most important social unit, wherein individual needs are subordinated to familial needs. The father, who is the head of the family, will work long hours to provide for a large family to be economically self-sufficient. The wife frequently is ambivalent about her marital role owing to sexual inhibitions and beliefs; thus, the marital relationship becomes formal and distant because the husband is free culturally to have extramarital affairs to prove his machismo (manliness). In response to this relationship, the wife often turns to her children and female relatives to meet her needs for affection and companionship.

Children often are expected to assist with household chores and jobs outside the home. They are taught to place family needs before individual ambitions. The world of the adolescent girl generally consists of the family and home; whereas adolescent sons are encouraged to gain worldly experience.

Family power is exhibited by men over women and the older order over the younger family members; therefore, the younger females have the least power in the family.

Chicano beliefs about health practices are significant: 1) specific foods can cause good or poor health; 2) being in tune with God fosters good health; 3) health is described as being free of pain; 4) certain illnesses are considered to be hot or cold and are treated by eating particular herbs; 5) the hospital is a place to die; and 6) illness is a family affair, during which time many relatives gather around.

Asian Americans: Chinese

Due to the recent influx of immigrants from Asia, nurses must be aware of the personality traits and cultural practices of the Chinese. In the past traditional family structure was that of a patriarchal system, in which the Chinese displayed respect for an obedience toward their ancestors. As the Chinese began immigrating to the United States, family ties continued to be strong but traditional family practices and superstitions became less obvious.

Chinese folk medicine proposes that health is regulated by two opposing forces, yin and yang. They must be in perfect balance for physical, mental, and social well-being to occur. Yang, the positive force, represents the male, as well as light, warmth, and fullness, whereas, yin is a negative, female force characterized by darkness, cold, and emptiness. Excessive yin predisposes one to nervousness and digestive disorders, and excessive yang contributes to dehydration, fever, and irritability.

The Chinese use hot foods to treat yin illnesses and cold foods for yang disorders. They may contact an herb pharmacist or herbalist to treat yin and yang disorders or an acupuncturist to treat musculoskeletal disorders. Family customs may promote the use of herbs, pills, and food to treat mental or physical disorders. The nurse should be aware that Chinese patients may follow both Western and Asian medical advice simultaneously, resulting in double doses of medication (Kozier, 1979, and Wilson and Kneisl, 1983).

IMPLICATIONS FOR NURSING INTERVENTIONS

A working knowledge of personality growth and development is important when the nurse cares for patients in the mental health setting. She participates in the individual's treatment plan in several ways: 1) identifying developmental needs through close observation and assessment of developmental tasks that have or have not been resolved; 2) assisting the person in understanding problem areas; 3) planning interventions that will decrease the continuance of maladaptive behavior; 4) anticipating future developmental stressors; and 5) evaluating the patient's progress during the course of treatment.

In pediatric settings, the psychiatric nurse works with parents and significant others to assess the cognitive and behavioral development of children. The nursing role generally focuses on assessing and evaluating opportunities for the child's growth and development; assessing and evaluating the outcome of a child's development related to life experiences; and making recommendations or providing teaching pertaining to ways positive, cognitive, and behavioral development can be fostered and enhanced.

Without knowledge of differences in cultural norms and patterns, the mental health nurse may be unable to recognize the meaning of a person's behavior or actions. Normal patterns of behavior are often labeled as deviant, immoral, illegal, or crazy, depending on the type of behavior violated. Communication styles, the establishment of rapport, goal expectations, and the acceptance of ideas often are impaired because of cultural dissimilarity. Personal feelings, beliefs, and attitudes must be identified, discussed, and accepted before one can work effectively with people seeking assistance.

SUMMARY

The dynamics of personality development were discussed, as well as factors influencing psychological maturation. Various theories of personality development presented were 1) Freud's psychoanalytic theory, 2) Erikson's psychosocial theory, 3) Piaget's cognitive developmental theory, and 4) Duvall's theory of the family life cycle. Cultural considerations pertaining to the personality development of American Indians, blacks, Chicanos, and Asian Americans were stated. Implications for nursing interventions focusing on personality growth and development were given.

LEARNING ACTIVITIES

I. Clinical activities
   A. Assess the developmental level of at least two assigned patients by applying one of the following theories of personality development:
      1. Freud's psychoanalytic theory
      2. Erikson's psychosocial theory
      3. Piaget's cognitive developmental theory
      4. Duvall's theory of the family life cycle
   B. Discuss the developmental tasks appropriate for each patient's chronological age.
   C. List any tasks that may be stress producing for each patient.
   D. State nursing interventions appropriate to assist the patient in resolving any identified conflicts.
   E. Assess each of the patient's cultural background:
      1. Do they belong to minority groups?
      2. Identify feelings, behavioral patterns, or social considerations (as discussed in this chapter) that may impair nursing interventions.
II. Independent activities
   A. Read one of the following to increase your knowledge base of personality development:
      1. Erikson's *Childhood and Society*
      2. Murray's *Nursing Assessment and Health Promotion Through the Life Span* (2nd ed).

    3. Murray's *The Nursing Process in Later Maturity*.
    4. Barry's *Psychosocial Nursing Assessment and Intervention*.
  B. Using Duvall's Theory of Family Life Cycle, compare your family's growth and development to the eight states described by Duvall.

SELF-TEST

Match the following:

1. Id
2. Freud's psychoanalytic theory
3. Piaget's cognitive developmental theory
4. Duvall's theory of family life cycle
5. Ego
6. Erikson's psychosocial theory

a. Censoring force of the personality
b. Eight stages of one's life span characterized by a central task
c. Discusses organization, dynamics, and development of one's personality
d. Integrator or mediator of the personality
e. Discusses eight stages of growth and development and the impact of children on the predictable stages
f. Describes intellectual growth and development
g. Unconscious reservoir of primitive drives and instincts

7. Cite examples of failure to resolve the following conflicts.

a. Trust versus mistrust

b. Autonomy versus shame and doubt

c. Initiative versus guilt

d. Industry versus inferiority

e. Ego identity versus role confusion

f. Intimacy versus isolation

g. Generativity versus stagnation

h. Ego integrity versus despair

8. Discuss cultural practices of American Indians, blacks, Chicanos, and Asian Americans and the relationship of these practices to the assessment process.

REFERENCES

Altrocchi J: Abnormal Behavior. New York, Harcourt Brace Jovanovich, 1980
Barker P: Basic Child Psychiatry, 4th ed. Baltimore, University Park Press, 1983
Barry PD: Psychosocial Nursing Assessment and Intervention. Philadelphia, JB
    Lippincott, 1984

Deaux: Social Psychology in the 80s, 3rd ed. Monterey, CA, Brooks/Cole Publishing, 1981

Donlon PT, Rockwell DA: Psychiatric Disorders: Diagnosis and Treatment. Bowie, MD, Robert J. Brady, 1982

Erikson EH: Childhood and Society, 2nd ed. New York: WW Norton & Co., 1963

Friedman MM: Family Nursing: Theory and Assessment. Norwalk, Appleton Century Crofts, 1981

Haber J et al: Comprehensive Psychiatric Nursing, 2nd ed. New York, McGraw-Hill, 1982

Kolb LC: Modern Clinical Psychiatry. Philadelphia, WB Saunders, 1977

Kozier B, Erb G: Fundamentals of Nursing: Concepts and Procedures. Menlo Park, Addison-Wesley, 1983

Lancaster J: Adult Psychiatric Nursing. Garden City, NJ, Medical Examination Publishing, 1980

Murray R et al.: The Nursing Process in Later Maturity. Englewood Cliffs, NJ, Prentice-Hall, 1980

Murray R, Heulskoetter M: Psychiatric/Mental Health Nursing: Giving Emotional Care. Englewood Cliffs, NJ, Prentice-Hall, 1983

Murray R, Zentner J: Nursing Assessment and Health Promotion Through the Life Span, 2nd ed. Englewood Cliffs, NJ, Prentice-Hall, 1979

Rowe CJ: An Outline of Psychiatry. Dubuque, William C. Brown, 1980

Stuart GW, Sundeen SJ: Principles and Practice of Psychiatric Nursing, 2nd ed. St. Louis, CV Mosby, 1983

Wilson HS, Kneisl CR: Psychiatric Nursing, 2nd ed. Menlo Park, Addison-Wesley, 1983

9

EMOTIONAL REACTIONS TO

ILLNESS AND

HOSPITALIZATION

LEARNING OBJECTIVES

1. Discuss why a person assumes the "sick role".
2. State the psychological or emotional needs of most people.
3. List nursing interventions for the needs identified in objective No. 2.
4. Explain the following emotional reactions to illness:
   Anxiety
   Fear
   Loneliness
   Powerlessness
   Helplessness
   Hopelessness
5. State nursing interventions for each of the emotional reactions listed in objective No. 4.
6. Discuss the concept of humor as it relates to illness.
7. Describe the impact of hospitalization on an adolescent.

CHANGE, such as illness and hospitalization, is a threatening experience that elicits various emotional reactions from patients as well as from family members or significant others. A questionnaire developed by the author was distributed to approximately 200 hospitals and patients in an attempt to obtain first-hand information about their reactions to illness, hospitalization and nursing care. The results revealed some important factors regarding the psychological or emotional needs of hospitalized patients, their emotional reactions to illness, and their impressions of members of the health care team. A summary of the questionnaire follows.

Type of facility in which hospitalization occurred:

General community hospital: 90%

Private hospital: 10%

Length of hospitalization:

A week or less: 60%

Two weeks or less: 30%

Other: 10%

Reason for hospitalization:

Illness: 52%

Surgery: 35%

Accident: 8%

Other: 5%

Area of hospital admitted to:

Medical unit: 40%

Surgical unit: 52%

Intensive care: 6%

Psychiatric unit: 0%

Other: 2%

Eighty-one percent of those surveyed felt they were treated as a person rather than as a patient with an illness, whereas nineteen percent felt they were not. Ninety-one percent of the respondees stated they were permitted to maintain independence and participate in their own care, whereas nine percent felt they were placed in a dependent position.

Of the persons asked, 84% stated that they were given a satisfactory explanation of treatment, equipment, and nursing care; 66% felt they were given the opportunity to make decisions regarding their treatment. Of the hospitalized patients responding, 44% felt that the nurses were aware of their spiritual needs; however, 56% did not. Fifty percent of the patients felt their need for privacy was respected. Forty-two percent felt the nursing personnel were aware of their fears during hospitalization.

Respondents also commented about the quality of nursing care they received. Several of the hospitalized persons:

Stated the nurses took time to talk with them: 60%

Felt their complaints were ignored: 65%

Were given an explanation of their illness or surgery: 37%

Felt their family was informed of their progress: 37%

Felt the nurses were friendly: 68%

Felt the nurses were professional: 64%

Felt the nurses were competent: 64%

Reactions to hospitalization were listed as:

Loneliness: 17%

Helplessness: 17%

Hopelessness: 2%

Fear: 25%

Anxiety: 52%

Depression: 15%

Anger: 8%

Powerlessness: 17%

Need for spiritual care: 27%

Specific comments included the following:

> "We were not informed that so many doctors would be caring for my mother. The doctors were not always available to let us know how she was doing."

> "Most of my contact was with LPNs. The RNs were busy giving medication."

> "The nurses were rude to me and my family. Two of them attempted to physically prevent me from leaving the floor, claiming my *bill* had to be paid first!"

> "I learned to do anything to avoid being in that position (hospitalization) again!"

> "Felt like I was in a business with no power over any solutions. Get in, get it done, don't ask questions, but make sure you pay."

> "When he died there, all of us were satisfied that everything that could be done for him had been done and he died in peace."

> " . . . completely satisfied with this hospital, personnel, treatment and everything pertaining to the patient—nurse relationship!"

> "My minister provided me *much* spiritual support. The chaplains in the hospital stopped by daily."

This chapter will discuss psychological or emotional needs, behavioral or emotional reactions, and nursing interventions as they pertain to the person who becomes a patient.

HOSPITALIZATION AND THE SICK ROLE

Various aspects of care occur within the hospital setting, such as diagnostic tests, medical treatment, surgical intervention, nursing interventions, rehabilitative care and research. Holistic health care has emerged recently, focusing on the physical, psychological, social, cultural and spiritual needs of patients and involves several disciplines.

When a person is hospitalized, he is influenced by several factors: 1) the extent or seriousness of the illness; 2) the manner in which he is admitted to the hospital; 3) his feelings, thoughts and attitudes about the hospital and personnel; and 4) information given by friends, acquaintances, and the attending physician. Experiences during childhood also influence a person's reaction to hospitalization. If the parents have been matter of fact about visits to the doctor's office, the child is likely to accept the nurse, doctor, and other health care-givers as caring persons. He learns to trust their judgment and cooperate with them while receiving care. If parents have used health care as a threat to reprimand a child, for example, "The nurse will give you a shot if you don't behave!", the child will expect the nurse or doctor to be punitive or sadistic in treatment approaches. These beliefs are carried into one's adult life, influencing reactions to illness and hospitalization.

The sick role is assumed by people for many reasons. They may perceive themselves as helpless, requiring the assistance of others to meet their needs or modify their condition. Such persons often turn their lives over to the care of the nurse or doctor, expecting them to "fix" their problems and send them home when they are improved. One man acted unconcerned about his illness and treatment. He never questioned the attending physician about his condition or various medications and treatments that were ordered, nor did he mention going home. When the student nurse asked the patient if he was eager to get home, the patient stated that he would stay as long as the doctor thought he should. "He'll tell me when I'm ready to go home. That's his job." The student was amazed at the lack of concern displayed by the patient during hospitalization.

Illness relieves one of social responsibilities and often produces secondary gains, such as personal attention or disability benefits. The sick role may become a way of life. A 35-year-old man had complained of an industrial back injury at age 24 and was able to collect industrial compensation and disability benefits. For 11 years he was unable to work but did manage to travel to attend sporting events, and to lead a relatively active life. When questioned by the student nurse whether he ever thought of trying another vocation, he informed her that he was "an industrial injury and the company is paying my way. I don't want to lose my benefits by becoming gainfully employed!"

The sick role may be a manipulative ploy when a person attempts to cope with various emotional conflicts. For example, a 54-year-old woman whose children had left home was hospitalized several times in one year for vague symptons, including dizziness, heartburn, headaches, and chest pain. She was unable to work and was placed on sick leave. Her children and neighbors were quick to to respond to her needs each time she was hospitalized. The attending physician explored the patient's vague complaints with her and identified underlying feelings of loneliness and depression. Her complaints were producing a secondary gain of attention and concern displayed by her children and neighbors. She was, to a degree, manipulating their lives since they planned their social and recreational activities around her needs while she assumed the sick role.

PSYCHOLOGICAL OR EMOTIONAL NEEDS

Most people experience the following common emotional needs at some point in their lives: to be loved and to love others, to feel secure, to feel important or good about themselves, to be self-sufficient and to be productive or develop one's full potential. Consider the impact of illness or hospitalization on these needs.

A person with terminal cancer who is hospitalized over an extensive period experiences separation from loved ones at a critical time in life. It is difficult for family members or significant others to spend all of their time at the bedside of a seriously ill person. They may be absent at times when their presence would provide a feeling of security to the patient: during bone marrow aspirations, chemotherapy treatments, and other serious procedures.

Cancer affects a person's self-concept, or the ability to feel good about oneself, especially if one's physical appearance is altered by weight loss or disfigurement. It can also cause a self-sufficient person to become dependent on others, experiencing feelings of helplessness and powerlessness as his physical condition deteriorates. Terminal cancer, generally accompanied by pain and weakness, interferes with one's ability to be productive or develop one's full potential.

The impact of cancer on a 26-year-old woman's emotional needs is given as an example. MJ, mother of 3 children, developed uterine cancer that was treated surgically but not before it had metastasized to the lungs and brain. She had undergone chemotherapy and cobalt treatments in hopes of prolonging her life. Her husband refused to visit her at the hospital; instead, he stayed home with the children waiting for "mommy to come home." As a result of her husband's decision, MJ was denied the presence of her loved ones during her last hospitalization. On one occasion MJ told the student she felt like "an apple being peeled away one layer at a time." She was referring to the surgery, chemotherapy, and side-effects of alopecia, nausea, vomiting, and weight loss. MJ also expressed a concern that she would not be able to see her children go to school, become teenagers, and attend college. She felt that she was being denied the right to be a wife and mother. As her strength failed, MJ became dependent on the student nurse to bathe, feed and turn her. She stated that she "hated to be dependent on others and wished she could at least wash her face and feed herself." MJ had become a lonely, insecure, dependent person with a negative self-concept. She was unable to develop her full potential as a wife, mother, and a woman.

The role of a nurse is very important because she plans interventions to meet these emotional or psychological needs of hospitalized people. A list of the needs and appropriate nursing interventions follows:

NEED	NURSING INTERVENTIONS
To be loved	Display a sincere interest in the patient by setting aside time each day to be with that person. Encourage the patient to verbalize feelings about loved ones. Identify significant others, such as family members, friends and pastor.

(continued)

NEED	NURSING INTERVENTIONS
To feel secure	Assist the patient, family , or friends in planning scheduled visits whenever possible. Encourage verbalization of feelings about hospitalization. Explore feelings about security. Promote feelings of security by orienting the patient to the unit, explaining hospital policies, routines, and procedures. Answer questions honestly. Direct them to the attending physician whenever necessary.
To feel important or *good* about oneself	Convey to the patient that you care about him. Encourage verbalization of feelings about the self. Provide feedback by focusing attention on positive traits identified during hospitalization; (i.e., nice voice, pretty hair, nice smile, interesting job).
To be self-sufficient and to have control	Promote independence by encouraging the patient to participate in self-care as much as possible. Encourage decision making regarding menu selection, treatment plan, which pain medication (if a choice is available), and so forth. Give positive recognition for any independency exhibited.
To be productive	Encourage patient to discuss feelings about role as an individual, spouse, parent, patient. Explore ways to be productive while hospitalized: oil painting, writing poetry, needlepoint, crewel work, plan household chores for family members, write or dictate letters, read, plan grocery list.

If the nurse is aware that each person experiences the needs just described and implements nursing interventions to meet these needs, negative comments, such as those listed with the questionnaire described earlier, will become less common. Meeting such needs also will influence a person's emotional reactions to illness and hospitalization.

EMOTIONAL REACTIONS TO ILLNESS

Numerous books and articles have been written about emotional reactions to illness. (see References)

The following is a list of identified emotional reactions to illness as described by various authors:

Lambert (1979)	Robinson (1984)	Carlson (1978)	Barry (1984)
Behavioral reactions to physical illness:	*Psychological aspects of hospitalized patients:*	*Responses to change in health status:*	*Personality styles of general hospital patients:*
Anxiety		Alienation	
Denial	Anxiety	Hostility	Dependent,
Ambivalence	Crying	Restlessness	demanding
Suspicion	Frightened	Boredom	Controlled,
Hostility	Disoriented	Trust	orderly
Regression	Depressed	Hope	Dramatizing,
Loneliness	Demanding	Humor	emotionally
Rejection	Regression	Denial	involved,
Depression	Dependency	Privacy	captivating
Withdrawal	Helplessness	Relaxation	Suspicious,
	Hopelessness		complaining
	Denial		Long-suffering,
			self-sacrificing
			Superiority
			Uninvolved, aloof
			Antisocial
			Inadequate

Anxiety

Over 30 descriptive words have been used to describe emotional reactions manifested during illness, the most common being anxiety. Anxiety has been described as a fear of the unknown or unrecognized. The person experiences feelings of apprehension, tension, or uneasiness. Persons who assume the sick role cannot always identify the source of anxiety in their lives. They may experience anxiety as they 1) are told hospitalization is necessary, 2) arrive in a hospital setting, 3) undergo diagnostic tests, 4) face impending surgery, 5) undergo various treatment approaches, or 6) prepare to return home after hospitalization. One patient, a 44-year-old man was playing basketball in the community center's gymnasium when he experienced severe chest pains. The emergency squad was called when his condition did not improve. He was rushed to the local community hospital to be admitted for treatment of a possible myocardial infarction. This was the first time that the man had experienced chest pains; as a result, feelings of anxiety occurred. He was uncertain what was contributing to his severe chest pains because he appeared to be in good physical health. Admission to the intensive care unit increased his anxiety because he was in unfamiliar surroundings, including tubes, oxygen equipment, monitors, and personnel. As the student nurse cared for him, the patient told her that he had never been hospitalized before. She recognized his feelings of insecurity and, once the patient was stabilized, she took time to explain why he was admitted to the unit. She also gave him a verbal orientation to the unit, described his treatment regimen, and asked if he had any questions. The patient thanked her for taking the time to discuss his illness, treatment, and nursing care.

Fear

Fear is another common reaction identified in hospitalized patients. "I'm afraid I might have cancer," "Ted's afraid of shots", "My husband's afraid to be put to sleep by the anesthesiologist" are some of the comments made by patients or their relatives in the hospital setting. They are referring to *recognized* sources of danger. Such fear can have an immobilizing or irrational influence on people during illness. Nurses can help patients to explore the reasons for their fears and plan appropriate interventions to alleviate them. An 18-year-old female patient was in labor for 10 hours when her labor failed to progress. X-ray pelvimetry revealed cephalopelvic disproportion and an emergency caesarean section was scheduled. She was quite upset and admitted that she was "scared." The nurse and the anesthesiologist explained general anesthesia to the patient before her caesarean section, how it is performed and the nursing care that she would receive. After surgery the student cared for the patient as she recovered from the general anesthetic. After she recovered, the patient thanked the student for taking time to "explain everything to me. I'm not so afraid now." The patient was discharged approximately a week after caesarean section and voiced excitement about taking her newborn infant home. No evidence of fear was noted.

Loneliness

Everyone experiences loneliness at some point in life in this fast-paced, mobile, and changing society. Feelings of loneliness appear to increase during hospitalization. People feel lonely because of a need for contact with a person, place or object. When hospitalized, the person is removed from his normal environment, containing familiar persons, places, and objects. He experiences a desire for contact but is unable to make it. Feelings of unexplained dread, desperation or extreme restlessness may be noted in the patient as a result of inability to make contact. Loneliness, like fear, can immobilize a person.

During clinical rotation through a nursing home for geriatric nursing experience, student nurses were asked to assess assigned patients regarding loneliness. They observed the patients' rooms for familiar items brought from home, such as pictures, radios, televisions, pieces of furniture, or quilts and pillows. They also observed who visited the patients and how frequently. The results of their assessment revealed that a majority of the patients had brought personal items with them, but few patients had regular visitors such as family members, neighbors, or friends. Feelings of loneliness were voiced by many of the elder patients as they spent much of their time sitting or sleeping, showing little interest in their environment, unless stimulated by others. Another group of students in the medical–surgical setting were instructed to observe patients' rooms for flowers, get-well cards, gifts, personal items brought from home, and visitors. It was interesting to note the students' reactions to the patients' rooms. One student stated "Her room is so cold and barren looking. She looks so lonely", "It looks like everyone's deserted him since his surgery for cancer. Why doesn't his family visit?", and "Her room is so warm and friendly looking. She has flowers and cards all over the place," are other comments by students. A discussion followed pertaining to the influence of familiar items and visitors on the mood of hospitalized persons.

Powerlessness

"The ability to affect, to influence, and to change others" is one definition of power (Roberts, 1978, p. 125). Powerlessness occurs in the clinical setting owing to loss of control over oneself, one's behavior, and one's environment. It also can result when one has lack of sufficient knowledge regarding illness and how it affects one's being, family, and future (Roberts, 1978, p. 127). Hospitalization encourages a person to be passive or dependent on the health care team both for nursing care and for obtaining knowledge about one's illness. Roberts (1978) states that the patient: 1) is powerless to influence information obtained and recorded during the history-taking process when admitted; 2) has little power over what is placed in the chart and who reads it; 3) relinquishes the ability to make decisions; 4) may become aggressive to compensate for the loss of power; and 5) may become violent because of feelings of aggression and anger that are not expressed verbally.

Feelings of powerlessness, then, may result in withdrawn, demanding, or manipulative behavior as the person struggles to maintain control while hospitalized. A nurse was assigned to care for a patient who had undergone diagnostic tests for symptoms of dizziness, blurred vision, weight loss, weakness, chest pain, and insomnia. He had expected to be in and out of the hospital within 3 days. Inconclusive tests necessitated a longer stay in the hospital. The patient asked his attending physician if the tests could be continued on an outpatient basis. After the physician informed him that he would need to stay at least two more days, the nursing staff noticed a change in this compliant patient's behavior. He became quite demanding and tried to manipulate the staff to persuade the doctor to discharge him early. The nurse spent time with the patient in an attempt to explore the meaning behind his change in behavior. He told her that he was the sole owner of a small business and felt that he was losing business while he was hospitalized. He was afraid that his business would fail if he wasn't at the office daily to oversee his office help.

Helplessness and Hopelessness

When a person reaches the point in his reasoning process that he believes everything that can be done has been done, he is experiencing helplessness. Persons who are ill generally realize that they need help; whether they seek it depends upon the presence of hope or the knowledge and feeling that there is treatment for or a solution to their illness. Helplessness also can occur when a person is forced into the position of temporary or permanent dependency on others. Nurses working in rehabilitative units often see people express helplessness owing to dependency and the knowledge that nothing more can be done at present for their physical condition. Some persons refuse to give in to helplessness or hopelessness, exhibited by two members of the 1984 Olympic team. A woman paraplegic qualified for the archery competition, and a young man diagnosed with Hodgkin's disease qualified for and won a gold medal in wrestling. Both did not succumb to feelings of helplessness; they maintained hope, used their inner strength or energy, and overcame their disabilities.

Helplessness or hopelessness may contribute to regressive behavior, ambivalence, and feelings of rejection, as well as to dependent behavior.

Family members or significant others also may experience feelings of helplessness when they hear about the patient's prognosis. Comments such as "I feel so helpless," "Please tell me what I can do to help," and "I've done everything I can think of. What more can I do?" all transmit the message of helplessness.

Nurses who maintain hope and inspire it in patients are a motivational force creating energy and the desire to achieve health. Lange (Carlson, 1978, pp. 182–184) discusses the importance of hope in maternal–child nursing, medical–surgical nursing, and psychiatric–mental health nursing. She discusses the impact of hope on birth defects, chronic disabling illness, severe illness or injury, and psychiatric disorders that are emotional in origin. Seven coping skills and their impact on the degree of hope are presented by Lange:

1. Denying or minimizing the seriousness of an illness or disorder. People arrive at this skill to avoid facing the worst situation.
   Example: A diabetic refers to his illness as "just a little inconvenience."

2. Asking relevant questions about one's condition to relieve anxiety.
   Example: A woman experiencing tachycardia asks the nurse if "nerves" could be the cause of it.

3. Seeking reassurance and emotional support by reaching out to others. Family, friends, clergy, and health team members may be available to listen, thus lessening worry and uncertainty and reinforcing hope.
   Example: A woman asks her pastor to stop by to discuss her son's sudden change in behavior.

4. Learning an effective action to do necessary procedures or provide

self-care. Such coping instills a sense of pride in one's ac-complishments.
Example: A patient with chronic kidney failure is taught the portable dialysis technique.

5. Setting specific goals. The patient is encouraged to be as independent as possible, meeting one goal at a time.
   Example: The orthopedic patient is taught to "logroll" himself following surgery until he is able to increase his activity level.

6. Rehearsing alternative outcomes with staff and family. Hope is restored or maintained by considering previous successes or failures when faced with difficulties.
   Example: A patient scheduled to undergo surgery has a 50% change of surviving. He shares his feelings with his family about his future *if* the surgery is successful.

7. Finding meaning in experiences such as a crisis, illness, or prognosis of an illness.
   Example: A woman undergoing frequent bone marrow aspirations during hospitalization for leukemia stated that she hoped the research findings would help other patients as well as herself.

CLINICAL EXAMPLES OF EMOTIONAL REACTIONS TO ILLNESS

Clinical examples denoting regression, dependency, a struggle to maintain independence, withdrawal due to fear, and hope, follow.

Regression: Clinical Example

A 32-year-old woman was admitted for an emergency cholecystectomy. During her postoperative period, the patient became whining, demanding, and manipulative. When interviewed, the patient revealed ambivalent feelings toward her mother. She stated that she loved her but did not get along with her. (Her mother had been staying with her during the recovery period.) She also stated that she was afraid she would continue to have pain when she returned home. She had regressed to a developmental level of a 10- or 11-year-old child in which she assumed the sick role, relieving her of any social responsibilities that she might have. It also produced a secondary gain of her mother's attention and concern about her pain.

Dependency: Clinical Example

A 59-year-old woman, a newly diagnosed diabetic patient, was identified as being "overly"dependent on the staff. She was quite obese and did not participate in her care. During an interview she confided in the student that her husband washed and set her hair, did the housework, and prepared the meals. She stated that she had been sick and unable to work for a long time and enjoyed being taken care of by her family. She had assumed the sick role to relieve herself of social responsibilities and to allow her husband and family to meet her needs.

Independency or Maintaining Power: Clinical Example

A 71-year-old woman with the diagnosis of angina refused to have student nurses assigned to her. She was active in her community, very independent, had never been hospitalized, and was "capable of caring for herself." When procedures were scheduled, the patient became upset if they were not done "on time" and insisted on knowing why they were delayed. She would complain that the hospital was not run efficiently. When staff personnel entered her room she would dismiss them verbally and state that she would let them know "if and when she needed anything." On the second day of hospitalization the patient was observed to have tears in her eyes. She related that she was scared, saying she had never had "anything like this happen to me before" and she didn't like being sick. She further stated that she had "tons of work waiting for me at home." This patient demonstrated a valiant attempt to reject the sick role rather than to assume it. The passive manipulation and demanding behavior exhibited by this patient were her attempts to maintain control and independence during her hospitalization.

Withdrawal Due to Fear: Clinical Example

A 62-year-old man admitted to the hospital with gastritis, spent much of the time in his room, although he was permitted and encouraged to walk in the halls. He responded briefly when spoken to and never initiated conversation with the staff. On the second day he disclosed to a student nurse that his wife had Parkinson's disease and he was having difficulty watching her symptoms progress. He had kept his emotions to himself, in an attempt to reassure his wife that she would be okay. During the interview his fear of the unknown (his wife's prognosis) was identified and the patient appeared relieved that he was able to discuss his wife's illness with someone.

Hope: Clinical Example

A 16-year-old pregnant girl was in an auto accident during her third month of pregnancy. She was comatose as the result of injuries sustained in the accident and delivered a 5 lb 6 oz, premature infant by caesarean section in her eighth month of pregnancy. Immediately after the accident, her husband, who was in the service, was transferred to the city where she was hospitalized. He kept a daily vigil throughout his wife's hospitalization. After the birth of his daughter, the young serviceman stated that he would be waiting for "the second miracle to happen, my wife's return to good health." He stated, "All I have left is hope and a lot of prayers."

HUMOR

"To be able to joke may spell the difference between sinking and swimming, psychologically. The capacity to laugh about things, including ourselves at times, means that we are still masters of our fate" (Harrower 1971).

Norman Cousins used the concept of humor to overcome a chronic debilitating illness. When his condition did not respond to traditional treatment measures, he decided to view movies by comedians such as Laurel and Hardy, read humorous articles and books, and tell jokes. Journal articles, a book, and a movie describe Cousins' controversial method of treating his illness and his recovery.

Humor has been called a coping mechanism or outlet for feelings of tension, anger, aggression and embarrassment. It serves as a tool for communication, illustrated in the following example. A student nurse was caring for a patient who had just returned from physical therapy. She wanted to straighten the linens before he returned to bed. Innocently, she stated to the patient "Let me tighten your draw strings before you get into bed." The patient and his roommate responded with laughter while the student nurse's face turned several shades of red. Later the patient apologized for his response and told the student he hadn't been able to laugh since he was admitted to the hospital. Although the student had not planned to be funny, the situation provided the patient with an opportunity ro relate his feelings. He discussed a problem that was bothering him at work during his hospitalization. Other nurses have related humorous situations that "broke the ice", in their nurse–patient relationships.

Robinson (Carlson, 1978) states that humor is a "natural phenomenon within the humanistic approach to patient care" and lists the following nursing situations in which humor may be used by patients and/or staff (Carlson, 1978, p. 175): 1) to establish interpersonal relationships; 2) to relieve or release feelings of tension, anxiety, anger, hostility and aggression; 3) to cope with feelings that are too painful or stressful to handle at that moment; and 4) to promote the learning process.

The following headline appeared in a local newspaper: "Laughter Cures Patients' Blues, Therapist Finds." An occupational therapist in Seattle, Washington uses various humorous techniques to "heal emotional wounds." Patients who have difficulty expressing their feelings are encouraged to draw cartoons and wear Halloween masks that depict their mood for the day. Persons who have difficulty with interpersonal relationships watch a daytime soap opera that "borders on humor" and discuss how the characters interact with each other. The patients are able to identify with various humorous or stressful situations and coping behaviors used by the actors and actresses.

Humor occurs in the general hospital setting in various ways. The patient may receive amusing get-well cards, joke with people about hospitalization, or receive cheery gifts, such as balloon flower bouquets, smiling chrysanthemums, or singing telegrams. Rooms have been decorated by family members in an attempt to "cheer up" patients. One patient displayed a cartoon and joke scrap book given to her by a friend. It was the topic of many conversations among the hospital staff and patients. Students have walked into rooms on several occasions while patients were watching cartoons or situation comedies. Such television shows serve as a coping mechanism for the hospitalized patient, who is lonely, depressed, or needs to be distracted from everyday conflicts.

Staff members also use humor. Paraphrased poems and cartoons have been put on bulletin boards or placed in locker rooms. Students have stated several times that surgical staff exchange jokes or "joke around a lot" as they prepare for surgery. One student nurse, who was quite nervous as she cared for her first postoperative patient, bumped into the IV pole and dropped the nurse's call button. When she uncontrollably passed flatus, she quickly stated, "Oops, I just tore my panty hose!" The instructor, who was present during the entire scenario, had to stifle a smile until she left the room. The embarrassed student stated she was "mortified by her actions" but, as other students heard about her embarrassment, the situation turned into a laughing matter and the student saw the humor in her behavior. She stated, "I guess it doesn't pay to get uptight when taking care of a patient."

Robinson (Carlson, 1978) discusses the use of humor in the nursing care plan for an elderly widow, who became depressed following major surgery. She attributes the success of humor to the patient's life-style and the tone of the ward. The patient was referred to as a person "with a good sense of humor who was the cut-up of the senior citizen's club" (p. 203). The health care team was able to use humor therapeutically by creating a warm climate and promoting positive interpersonal relationships.

Humor is to be used cautiously because not all people are able to respond to this approach. They may not possess a sense of humor or the timing may be inappropriate. Approaching problems from "the bright side" does not always work, at least not immediately.

HOSPITALIZED ADOLESCENTS: SPECIAL NEEDS

Adolescent behavior during hospitalization can be frustrating as well as challenging to the care-giver. Common health problems contributing to the hospitalization of the adolescent include: 1) auto accidents, sports related accidents, or accidents that result from unsuccessful suicide attempts; 2) obesity; 3) teenage pregnancy; 4) alcoholism; 5) drug abuse; 6) depression; 7) venereal diseases; and 8) acne vulgaris. Anorexia nervosa and bulimia, indirect self-destructive behaviors, are rapidly growing adolescent health problems that often are treated on an out-patient basis, unless a life-threatening situation occurs.

During adolescence, the teenager faces two major conflicts: identity versus role confusion and independence versus dependence as he attempts to establish a stable self-concept, make a career or vocational choice, and adjust to a comfortable sexual role.

Psychological needs that must be met during hospitalization include peer interactions, privacy, autonomy, and the opportunity to verbalize concern about body image, sexual identity, and self-worth. Such concerns often result in the following emotional reactions: anger or hostility, resentment, fear, guilt, dependency, regression, and embarrassment. The hospitalized adolescent may reject hospital rules and regulations and even physical care because he fears loss of control. Illness often interrupts school and social life, resulting in behavior such as resentment, hostility, anger, manipulation, or aggressiveness. Fear and guilt may occur as the adolescent is overwhelmed by the disease process or illness. A 15-year-old girl diagnosed with diabetes thought she was being punished for promiscuous behavior. She felt guilty and "confessed" her behavior to the student nurse. The same patient also expressed a fear of diabetes and how it would affect her life. Another teenage patient displayed fear and embarrassment because she was scheduled for an inguinal herniorrhaphy. He was concerned about his self-image and sexual role identity. A nurse explained the surgery to the young man and allayed his fears.

Homesickness also may occur if the teenager has never been separated from parents or family. Such feelings may result in undue dependency needs or regressive behavior.

If an adolescent is admitted to an adult unit, the nurse should be aware of the following effects of hospitalization:

1. Emotional trauma may occur owing to erroneous advice or information given by adult patients.

2. The adolescent's imagination may result in fear since he exaggerates sights and sounds.

3. The adolescent's need for peer interactions may not be met if placed in a room with an adult patient.

4. Strict visiting regulations may not allow visitors under age 16 on an adult unit.

5. Defense mechanisms commonly seen include: denial, projection, displacement, regression, and isolation.

Nursing interventions for emotional reactions and common behaviors of adolescents during hospitalization follow:

REACTIONS	NURSING INTERVENTIONS
Fear	Accept defenses or behavior used to retain control. Discuss with the patient when able. Give detailed explanations regarding treatment, nursing care, and progress. Encourage participation in care. Encourage questions and discuss concerns. Interpret medical terminology to decrease fears.

(continued)

REACTIONS	NURSING INTERVENTIONS
	Maintain consistency in care to discourage manipulative behavior.
Resentment	Explore feelings of resentment to identify underlying cause.
	Encourage visits with peers.
	Allow young siblings to visit.
	Permit flexible visiting hours when appropriate.
	Make arrangements for school work to continue.
	Do not "side" with parents if the adolescent displays hostility.
Embarrassment	Explain and maintain confidentiality.
	Provide an opportunity to discuss concerns without family present if necessary.
	Be alert to feelings regarding body image and need for privacy.
	Encourage as much self-care as able.
	Provide for personal space and minimal body exposure during care.
	Explain treatments, procedures, or surgery and impact on the body.
	Give positive reinforcement when possible.
Homesickness	Provide for home conveniences such as TV, telephone and snacks as able.
	Arrange for dietary preferences when appropriate.
	Allow family members to bring in favorite foods if they are part of the diet prescribed by the attending physician.
	See that the patient is kept informed of news at home.
Guilt	Give detailed explanations regarding illness and causative factors if appropriate.
	Be positive in approaches and comments to reinforce interest in the patient.
	Explain that hospitals are to help people, not punish them.
Manipulative behavior	Be consistent in expectations regarding rules and regulations for all patients.
	State the limits and behavior expected from the patient.
	Explore the patient's perceptions and feelings.
	Avoid arguing, debating or bargaining with the patient.
	Confront the patient, if necessary, regarding any manipulative ploys.
	Avoid a personal relationship.

REACTIONS	NURSING INTERVENTIONS
Hostile, aggressive behavior	Be firm and consistent in treatment approaches.
	Accept the patient but tell him that certain behaviors are unacceptable.
	Try to determine what precipitated these feelings.
	Assist the patient to explore alternative ways in handling feelings.
	Inform the patient that he is to take responsibility for his actions.
	Be supportive and provide positive feedback when the patient controls hostile or aggressive behavior.

IMPACT OF PHYSICAL ILLNESS

Lambert (1979) uses a unique approach to emotional or behavioral reactions to illness. Alterations in body structure and life-sustaining functions are discussed with specific attention to emotional, somatic, sexual, occupational, and social impact on the person. A patient undergoing a mastectomy may cry frequently owing to depression (emotional impact of a mastectomy); express concern about her body image because of the need to wear a prosthesis (somatic impact); avoid sexual contact with her husband owing to a poor self-concept (sexual impact); express feelings of incompetency as a housewife and mother (occupational impact); and refuse to socialize owing to feelings of embarrassment or shame (social impact). Nursing care plans focus on the various impacts due to physical illness.

Barry (1984) devotes three chapters to the areas of personality styles of hospitalized patients, psychosocial aspects of illness, and coping challenges in chronic illness. She discusses the development of trust; the impact of illness on the patient's self-esteem; alteration in body image during various developmental stages and illness; the ability to be in control of one's environment, especially during illness; plus the issues of loss, guilt, and intimacy as underlying dynamics in the patient's attempts to adapt to illness. Nursing approaches are given for specific physical conditions, such as menopause, amputation, mastectomy, severe burns, isolation due to immunosuppressive conditions, and congenital anomaly.

NURSING INTERVENTIONS FOR EMOTIONAL REACTIONS

Nursing interventions for the following emotional reactions to illness are presented here, including anxiety, fear, loneliness, powerlessness, helplessness, and hopelessness. (The emotional reactions of denial, anger or hostility, and depression as well as spiritual needs of hospitalized patients are discussed in the chapter on loss and grief.)

EMOTIONAL REACTIONS	NURSING INTERVENTIONS
Anxiety and fear (anxiety disorders are discussed in a separate chapter)	Accept the patient. Display a nonjudgmental attitude. Assess the patient's level of anxiety to behavioral and physiological responses. (See Chapter 15 for classification of levels of anxiety as well as symptons of anxiety). Recognize the patient's feelings by encouraging verbalization of feelings readily. Assess and support the patient's strengths. Be readily available to assist the patient in meeting his needs. Explain procedures, treatments and nursing care to decrease anxiety. Give only necessary details because too many may make the procedure appear complicated and may frighten the patient. Increasing awareness and control of a situation generally reduces anxiety and fear. Utilize relaxation techniques to decrease anxiety.
Loneliness	Encourage verbalization of feelings about hospitalization. Recognize the need for contact with others. Be readily available by making routine periodic visits. Use touch as a therapeutic intervention when appropriate. Identify significant others and encourage visitation. Extend visiting hours or provide for special visitation if the situation warrants the presence of a family member or significant other. Minimize physiologic pain as loneliness generally increases when pain is present.
Powerlessness and helplessness	Promote independence as the patient's physiologic or psychological problems subside by encouraging: 1) verbalization of feelings such as frustration, anger, hostility and fear; 2) participation in self-care; 3) decision making; and 4) allowing the patient to organize and control his environment when appropriate; that is placement of call light, bedside table, bringing personal items from home. Educate the patient about his illness and treatment; promote self-care; and encourage a return demonstration when appropriate.
Hopelessness	Assess the patient's behavior for signs of suicidal ideation owing to feelings of doom, fail-

EMOTIONAL REACTIONS	NURSING INTERVENTIONS
	ure, poor self-concept, and then intervene accordingly.
	Express a sincere interest in wanting to help the patient.
	Encourage the patient to relate to other patients such as roommates, or people with similar conditions, the Reach for Recovery program and ostomy clubs. Recovered mastectomy patients visit hospitalized patients shortly after surgery. Ostomy patients are encouraged to participate in self-care by members of ostomy clubs.

SUMMARY

Illness and hospitalization can be a life-threatening situation when a person undergoes diagnostic tests, medical treatment, surgical intervention, nursing interventions, rehabilitative care, and participates in research. Several factors influence the patient's behavior as he is hospitalized, including the extent or seriousness of the illness, the manner in which hospitalization occurs, personal feelings, thoughts, and attitudes, and information given by others. Childhood experiences also influence one's response to hospitalization and members of the health care team. People assume the sick role for various reasons, among them helplessness, relief of social responsibilities, and manipulation of one's environment. Most people experience common emotional needs that are influenced by illness and hospitalization. They include the need to love and be loved, to feel secure, to feel good about oneself, to be self-sufficient, and to be productive. Examples of nursing interventions to meet these needs were discussed. An explanation of the more common emotional reactions to illness, as well as appropriate nursing interventions, are given. These include anxiety, fear, loneliness, powerlessness, helplessness and hopelessness. Clinical examples of regression, dependency, a struggle to maintain independence, withdrawal due to fear and hope also are given. The concept of humor as it relates to illness was discussed. Special attention was given to the psychological needs, emotional reactions, and coping behaviors of hospitalized adolescents, as well as nursing interventions for fear, resentment, embarrassment, homesickness, guilt, manipulative behavior, and hostile, aggressive behavior.

LEARNING ACTIVITIES

I. Clinical activities
  A. Identify the following pertaining to one of your assigned patients:
    1. Psychological needs during hospitalization

2. Emotional reactions to illness. Consider the somatic, sexual, occupational, and social impact of the patient's physical illness.
   B. Plan nursing interventions for each need and emotional reaction identified.
   C. Observe your patient for any expressions of humor. If such responses do occur, what purpose do you think they serve?
II. Independent activity
   A. Read one or more of the following articles listed in the references:
      1. Gluck M: Learning a therapeutic verbal response to anger. J Psych Nurs: Mar, 1981
      2. Greenwood B: Check your patient's presurgery tears. Nursing 82: July, 1982
      3. Hein E: Providing emotional support to patients. Nursing 82: June, 1982
      4. McHugh M: When everything is fine. Nursing 80: July, 1980
      5. McMorrow ME: The manipulative patient. Am J Nurs: June, 1981
      6. Murray R: What to do with crying, clinging, demanding, seductive, abusive and withdrawn patients. Nursing Life: Sept/Oct, 1982
   B. List nursing interventions for a demanding, manipulative adolescent.
   C. State nursing interventions to reduce fear in the surgical patient.
   D. Plan nursing interventions for a 55-year-old woman who has never been hospitalized and politely tells you that she can take care of herself. (Diagnosis: Possible myocardial infarction). Focus on possible emotional reactions and psychological needs.

SELF-TEST

1. Explain why a person assumes the sick role.
2. List the common emotional needs experienced by most individuals.
3. State nursing interventions for each of the needs listed in question No. 2.
4. Discuss how illness and hospitalization can create anxiety.
5. List nursing interventions to alleviate fear in a 12-year-old boy hospitalized for an emergency appendectomy.
6. List nursing interventions to decrease loneliness in a nursing home resident with emphysema.
7. Discuss how feelings of powerlessness can occur during hospitalization.
8. Differentiate between helplessness and hopelessness.
9. Explain how humor can be therapeutic in the hospital setting.
10. List the five impacts of physical illness as described by Lambert.

REFERENCES

American Cancer Society: The Psychological Impact of Cancer. Professional Education Publication, May, 1977

Barry PD: Psychosocial Nursing Assessment and Intervention. Philadelphia, JB Lippincott, 1984

Billings CV: Providing better emergency care when behaviors bar the way. Nursing 82: May, 1982

Brallier L: Successfully Managing Stress. Los Altos, National Nursing Review, 1982

Carlson C, Blackwell B (eds): Behavioral Concepts and Nursing Intervention. Philadelphia, JB Lippincott, 1978

Ciuca et al: When a disaster happens, how do you meet emotional needs? Am J Nurs: Mar, 1977

Dericks V: The psychological hurdles of new ostomates: Helping them up . . . and over. Nursing 76: Nov, 1976

Elliot E: My Name is Mrs. Simon. Ladies' Home Journal: Aug, 1984

Elliott S: Denial as an effective mechanism to allay anxiety following a stressful event. J Psych Nurs: Oct, 1980

"Feelings . . . How to Make a Rational Response to Emotional Behavior." Nursing 79: Oct, 1979

Frances GM, Munjas B: Promoting Psychological Comfort. Dubuque, William C Brown, 1975

Garland L, Bush C: Coping Behaviors and Nursing. Reston, VA, Prentice–Hall, 1982

Gluck M: Learning a therapeutic verbal response to anger. J Psych Nurs: Mar, 1981

Greenwood B: Check your patients presurgery fears. Nursing 82: July, 1982

Harrower M: Mental Health and M.S. (pamphlet). New York, National Multiple Scleroses Society, 1971

Hein E, Leavitt M: Providing emotional support to patients. Nursing 82: June 1982

Kimball CP: Reactions to illness: The acute phases: The interplay of environmental factors in intensive care units. The Psychiatric Clinics of North Am: Aug, 1979

Knowles RD: Dealing with feelings: Preventing anger. Am J Nurs: Jan, 1982

Kozier B, Erb G: Fundamentals of Nursing: Concepts and Procedures. Menlo Park, Addison–Wesley Publishing, 1983

Lambert V, Lambert C: The Impact of Physical Illness and Related Mental Health Concepts. Englewood Cliffs, Prentice–Hall, 1979

Luckman J, Sorensen K: Medical–Surgical Nursing: A Psychophysiologic Approach. Philadelphia: WB Saunders, 1980

Maynard C, Chitty K: Dealing with anger: Guidelines for nursing intervention. J Psych Nurs: June, 1979

McHugh M: When everything is fine. Nursing 80: June, 1980

McMorrow ME: The manipulative patient. Am J Nurs: June, 1981

Murray R: What to do with crying, clinging, demanding, seductive, abusive, and withdrawn patients. Nursing Life: Sept/Oct, 1982

Osterlund H: Humor: A serious approach to patient care. Nursing 83: Dec, 1983

Ranken N: Name that feeling: An innovative teaching tool. J Psychosoc Nurs: Dec, 1981

Richardson JI, Berline-Naumah D: In the face of anger. Nursing 84: Feb, 1984

Roberts L, Keniston E: Lottie tried to do everything for her husband—including our job. Nursing 82: July, 1982

Roberts S: Behavioral Concepts and Nursing Throughout the Life Span. Englewood Cliffs, Prentice–Hall, 1978.

Robinson L: Psychological Aspects of the Care of Hospitalized Patients. Philadelphia, FA Davis, 1984.

Schultz J, Dark S: Manual of Psychiatric Nursing Care Plans. Boston, Little, Brown, & Co, 1982

Sloboda S: Understanding patient behavior. Nursing 77: Sept, 1977

Weidner C: From model patient to little tyrant. Nursing 78: Apr, 1978

Williams J, Zugler J: Why did Annie hate us so? Nursing 78: May, 1978

LOSS AND GRIEF

To everything there is a season,
    And a time to every person under the heaven;
A time to be born,
    And a time to die.

Ecclesiastes 3:1

I walked a mile with Pleasure,
    She chattered all the way;
But left me none the wiser
    For all she had to say.

I walked a mile with Sorrow
    And ne'er a word said she;
But oh, the things I learned from her
    When sorrow walked with me.

Robert Browning

LEARNING OBJECTIVES

1. Discuss the concept of loss.
2. State the types of losses an individual can experience.
3. Explain the stages of grief identified by Westberg.
4. Differentiate between normal and pathologic or dysfunctional grief.
5. Describe Kübler–Ross' five stages of dying.
6. List the needs of dying persons and their survivors.
7. State the rationale for "The Dying Person's Bill of Rights."
8. Discuss the role of a chaplain or clergyman in the hospital setting.
9. Compare the perceptions of death by children during various growth stages.
10. Plan nursing interventions for emotional and spiritual needs of a terminally ill patient.

EVERYONE has experienced some type of major loss at one time or another, for example, the loss of a spouse, relative, friend, job, pet, home or personal item. The following definitions have been selected to familiarize the reader with the concept of loss:

"Change in status of a significant object" (Barry, 1984, p. 69)

"Any change in an individual's situation that reduces the probability of achieving implicit or explicit goals" (Carlson, 1978, p. 73)

"An actual or potential situation in which a valued object, person, etc. is inaccessible or changed so that it is no longer perceived as valuable" (Kozier, 1983, p. 913)

"A condition whereby an individual experiences deprivation of, or complete lack of, something that was previously present" (Lambert, 1979, p. 33)

A loss may occur suddenly or gradually, be predictable or unexpected, and be viewed as traumatic or temperate. For example, a 35-year-old cancer victim has been told he has approximately 2 years to live. He is experiencing a gradual loss of self that has been predicted by his physician. Whether the loss is traumatic or temperate to the patient and significant others "depends upon past experiences with loss, the value placed on the lost object, and the cultural, psychosocial, economic, and family supports available" (Lambert, 1979, p. 34).

Loss also has been referred to as actual, perceived, anticipatory, temporary or permanent. Kozier (1983) described actual loss as loss that "can be defined by others"; whereas perceived loss "cannot be verified by others" (p. 914). The death of a spouse is obvious to others and therefore is considered an *actual* loss. A recent college graduate who is unable to find employment and returns home may be experiencing a loss of freedom or independence. Unless he shares his feelings with others, such loss of free-dom or independence cannot be identified or verified by others and, there-fore, is considered a *perceived* loss. Anticipatory loss is experienced before the time a loss occurs. Family members of a chronically or termi-nally ill person may anticipate the loss of a loved one before his or her death due to the prognosis or severity of the person's illness. The wife of a cancer patient stated that she was "relieved that he doesn't have to suf-fer anymore. I knew it was just a matter of a week or two so I told my children not to be surprised if I called and told them he had died.'" She had anticipated the permanent loss of her husband. Temporary loss can occur in numerous ways, such as misplacing one's wedding rings or watch while working in obstetrics or the nursery, a child wandering off to a neighbor's house without letting the mother know where he has gone, being laid off from work for a specific period because of a decrease in sales, and hospitalization for emergency surgery. Such losses could be a condi-tion in which the person is deprived temporarily of something that was previously present.

Student nurses were instructed to assess their assigned patients for any losses before or during hospitalization. They identified these examples:

1. Loss of body image and social role because of a below-the-knee ampu-tation. The patient was a 19-year-old girl who was involved in a motorcycle accident. She had shared her feelings with the student nurse about her body image and dating after hospitalization.

2. Loss of a loved one owing to fetal demise or intrauterine death. The student nurse had been assigned to a young woman, who was in her 28th week of pregnancy. The following day, the patient expressed a sincere thanks to the student nurse for supporting her during such a difficult time in her life.

3. Loss of a job, as well as of body image and social role. The patient had lost his right arm in a farming accident and would be unable to return to his job as a telephone lineman. He has been recently married and was concerned about the impact of his accident on their relationship. The student nurse encouraged the patient to verbalize his feelings about his accident and to discuss his concerns with his wife. A few days later the wife told the student nurse that she was glad that her husband was able to talk to her about his feelings and that the acci-dent had drawn them "closer together."

4. Loss of physiologic function, social role, and independence because of kidney failure. One student cared for a 49-year-old woman who was undergoing renal dialysis every other day. She was admitted to the hospital for improper functioning of a shunt in her left forearm. The woman was depressed and asked that no visitors be permitted in her private room. She shared feelings of loneliness, helplessness, and

hopelessness with the student nurse as she described the impact of kidney failure and frequent dialysis treatment on her life-style. Once an outgoing, independent person, she was housebound due to her physical condition and "resented what her kidneys were doing to her."

GRIEF

Various emotional or psychologic responses occur when one experiences a loss. These emotional experiences are referred to as grief and may result in maladaptive behavior or pathological grief if the person is unable to work through the grieving process.

Many articles and books have been written about the subject of grief. *Good Grief* (Westberg, 1979) discusses what happens to people when they lose someone or something important (e.g. health, security, money, material comforts, a home, job, or a spouse). Westberg, who is a Lutheran minister, states that there are healthy and unhealthy ways to grieve and that people should be familiar with the good aspects of grief. He contends that people who handle daily "little griefs" in a positive manner prepare themselves for healthy reactions to larger griefs when they occur. The following is a summary of the ten stages of grief as described by Westberg.

Stage One: State of Shock

During the first stage the grieving person experiences a state of temporary anesthesia that may last anywhere from a few minutes to a few days. If the state of shock lasts over a week or two, it is a sign of unhealthy grief and professional help should be obtained before maladaptive behavior occurs. For example, a woman whose husband was killed unexpectedly in an automobile accident appears "cool, calm, and collected" at the funeral home while greeting people who have come to offer their sympathy. If within a week or two, she does not openly express feelings such as disbelief, anger, or loneliness, she may need support and encouragement to verbalize her emotions. Care-givers should be near and available during this stage of grief but are advised not to take over tasks that the person can perform. Self-care is therapeutic and enables the person to proceed to the next stage.

Stage Two: Expressing Emotion

People are encouraged to express pent-up emotions after a significant loss occurs. Westberg (1979) states, "We have been given tear glands, and we are supposed to use them when we have good reason to use them" (p. 26). Men have difficulty expressing emotion because they have been conditioned not to cry; it is looked on as a sign of weakness. Members of the health care team should encourage the expression of emotions and should not be ashamed to cry with the patients.

Stage Three: Depression and Loneliness

During the third stage, the person experiences feelings of utter depression and isolation. The care-giver is advised to "stand by" in quiet confidence and reassure the grieving person that loneliness and depression are normal reactions and eventually do pass.

Stage Four: Physical Symptoms of Distress

Physical symptoms such as insomnia, chest pain, abdominal pain, and shortness of breath may occur when someone stops at one of the stages of the grief process. If no one helps the person to explore the reason for emotional and physical complaints associated with unresolved grief, an illness can develop. The classic example is the death of a widow or widower within a year of the spouse's death. Such persons are said to have died of "broken hearts," or they just gave up because they were unable to live without their mate. The physical consequences of distress resulted in death.

Stage Five: Panic

During the fifth stage the person is unable to think of anything except the loss. Concentration and productivity are impaired because of obsessive thoughts, causing the person to think he is "losing his mind". The helping person should encourage the grieving person in this stage to develop new and different interests and interpersonal relationships rather than to stay at home and prolong grief work.

Stage Six: Guilt Feelings

Normal guilt is guilt that we feel when we have done something or neglected to do something for which we ought, by the standards of society, to feel guilty. On more than one occasion, survivors of deceased persons have made comments such as "If only I had insisted he see a doctor" or "I should have realized he was sicker than he looked." Such statements express guilt feelings. The person who says that he will "never forgive himself" and continually berates his actions out of proportion to the real situation is exhibiting symptoms of guilt. Such people should be encouraged to talk about guilt feelings so that they begin to handle them effectively and resume living.

Stage Seven: Anger and Resentment

Once the grieving person overcomes guilt feelings and is able to express emotions, stronger feelings, such as anger and resentment, may emerge. (Repressed or buried feelings of anger and resentment are unhealthy and can be very harmful to a person's personality). During this stage the person may blame anyone or everyone for the loss. Most nurses have heard family members on at least one occasion question whether the attending physician did everything possible for the patient. "If only he had operated sooner. He waited too long," or "He should have called in a consultant when my husband didn't respond to treatment"; these are examples of comments made by angry family members who resented the loss of a loved one. Such feelings are a normal part of grief work and can be overcome in time.

Stage Eight: Resistance

During this stage, grieving persons resist returning to normal daily living. They are intent on keeping the memory of a loved one or thing alive. Returning to normal activities may be too painful for some people because they experience an emptiness in the world about them. Too many times grieving persons are forced to carry all the grief within themselves since they find it difficult to grieve in the presence of others. Society says "Okay, you had time to grieve. Now get back to work!" and expects the person to return to a normal state very shortly after a loss has occurred. Friends and relatives are encouraged to help keep the memory of the loss alive because this facilitates progress toward the stage of hope.

Stage Nine: Hope

After a few weeks or many months of grief work, hope generally emerges. Life does go on; opportunities do exist for change or improvement in one's life in spite of the recently experienced loss. New friends can gradually help one find meaning again in life.

Stage Ten: Affirming Reality

Grieving persons generally realize that life will never be the same again, but they begin to sense that there is much in life that can be appreciated and enjoyed. To affirm something is to say that it is good and worth living for.

People who have a mature faith or belief in God often demonstrate an inner strength that helps them to face a serious loss without feeling that they have lost everything. Nurses must be aware of the religious beliefs and spiritual needs of their patients so that nursing interventions can address these areas. As stated in Chapter 9, 27% of those patients surveyed felt they had a need for spiritual care as well as physical care. Fifty-six percent did not feel nurses were aware of their spiritual needs during hospitalization.

PATHOLOGIC OR DYSFUNCTIONAL GRIEF

The cause of pathologic or dysfunctional grief is usually an actual or perceived loss of someone or something of great value to a person. Clinical features or characterestics include expressions of distress or denial of the loss; changes in eating and sleeping habits; mood disturbances, such as anger, hostility, or crying; and alterations in activity levels, including libido. The person experiencing dysfunctional grief idealizes the lost person or object, relives past experiences, loses the ability to concentrate, and is unable to work purposefully because developmental regression occurs. The grieving person may exhibit neurotic or psychotic symptoms in an attempt to cope with stress and anxiety owing to the actual or perceived loss. Examples of such behavior include development of physical symptoms similar to those experienced by the deceased person before death; progressive social isolation and interrupted interpersonal relationships with friends and relatives; extreme anger or hostility, directed at people associated with the lost person or object; agitated depression; or activities that are detrimental to one's social or economic existence.

DEATH AND DYING

Kübler–Ross (1969) has identified five stages of the grieving process. The following basic premise has evolved as a result of her work with dying persons: Patients know when they are dying (with the exception of the patient who is seriously ill and dies within a very short time or is the victim of a fatal accident). She feels that the helping persons experience two reactions as they care for dying patients: 1) gut reactions and 2) mental reactions. Gut reactions are spontaneous thoughts and ideas that occur such as "I hope he doesn't die on me," or "Please let him live until my shift is over," or "What will I do if she dies on me?" The mental reactions that nurses experience depend on whether the care-giver is able to comprehend the patient's feelings about death and dying and the care-giver has resolved any feelings about her own mortality or death. Many times the care-giver attempts to satisfy her own needs when talking with the patient. To work effectively with the dying patient, the nurse must be aware of her own feelings regarding death and the patient's condition. Kübler–Ross has stated that the higher the education, the less capable we are of dealing with dying since too many educational responses have been learned; individual responses are not used. In addition, a nurse cannot help a dying patient to work through the grieving process if she pushes the patient to communicate when the patient isn't ready to talk; pushes herself on the patient although the patient does not want the support; or genuinely does not like the patient. A summary of Kübler–Ross' well-known stages of dying follows.

First Stage: Denial

During this first stage the person displays a disbelief in his prognosis of inevitable death. This stage serves as a temporary escape from reality. Fewer than 1% of all dying patients remain in this stage. Typical responses are "No, it can't be true," "It isn't possible," and "not me." Denial generally subsides when the person realizes that someone will help him to express his feelings while facing reality.

Second Stage: Anger

"Why me?", "Why now?", and "It's not fair!" are a few of the comments commonly expressed during this stage. The nurse must remember that she represents a picture of health whenever she enters the patient's room and should be prepared for hostile responses or complaints. The patient appears to be difficult, demanding, and ungrateful during this stage. Holst (1984) states the dying need to "pour out their anger and frustration at the unjustice of it all, while maintaining an image of bravery and serenity for all to remember" (p. 12).

Stage Three: Bargaining

"Just one more chance, please!", "If I get better, I'll never miss church again", or "If I promise to take my medicine, will I get better?" are all examples of attempts at bargaining to prolong one's life. The dying person acknowledges his fate but is not quite ready to die at this time. He is ready to take care of unfinished business, such as writing a will, deeding a house over to a wife or child, or making funeral arrangements.

Stage Four: Depression

"The dying patient is about to lose not just one loved person but everyone he has ever loved and everything that has been meaningful to him" (Ross, 1971, p. 58). This stage is a very difficult period for the family and physician also because they feel so helpless watching the depressed patient mourn present and future losses. Treatment should not be forced on the depressed person. He should be supported and encouraged to voice his feelings *if* he feels comfortable doing so.

Stage Five: Acceptance

At this stage the dying person has achieved an inner and outer peace owing to a personal victory over fear: "I'm ready to die. I have said all the goodbyes and have finished unfinished business." During the acceptance stage, the patient may want only one or two significant people to sit quietly by his side, touching and comforting him. Kübler–Ross states that during this stage, little physical pain and discomfort is felt. Tender loving care and compassion by one person generally meets the physical needs of the dying.

The following are paraphrased comments about death and dying made by Kübler–Ross during a seminar the author attended at Providence Hospital, Sandusky, Ohio in 1974:

1. Patients conceive death as a killer; a catastrophic, destructive bearing force over which they have no control.

2. During the acceptance stage, death is like an old acquaintance returning for a final visit.

3. We as a society deprive children of the knowledge of death and dying by not allowing them to view it as a normal part of life.

4. The less one knows about a dying patient's condition, initially, the better equipped one is to listen. One displays a "gut reaction" rather than a conditioned response.

5. The care-giver learns to sense when he is needed and accepts when he is not wanted. This behavior should not be taken as a personal rejection of one's ability to establish rapport with the dying person.

6. The "needy time," when psychological defenses are down, is generally 2:00 to 3:00 AM. Nurses and clergy should be readily available during these hours should the patient need to talk.

7. The most neglected persons are the patient's family. Many times caregivers are involved in meeting the needs of the dying person and overlook the needs of the survivors.

8. We are a death-denying society.

9. People who reach a stage of acceptance lead a very different type of life, focusing on quality of life, rather than quantity.

10. Children have a right to know that a loved one is dying and should be allowed to act out emotions. Psychological problems often result when children are not permitted to express their emotions.

11. Professional groups need a "screaming room" to ventilate pent-up emotions when handling death and dying persons.

NEEDS OF THE DYING AND SURVIVORS

Holst (1984) describes a list of needs experienced by dying persons as well as their survivors while they face conflicts and dilemmas during this critical time in their lives. Holst, who is chairman of the division of pastoral care at a major hospital states that families and patients may "die to many things before the disease finally takes life" (p. 11). Optimism, spontaneity, holidays, long-range planning, dreams, retirement, and grandparenthood are just a few of the many things that die as a person and his family live with a terminal illness. The following are the needs stated by Holst (1984, pp. 12 and 13):

DYING PERSON'S NEEDS	SURVIVOR'S NEEDS
1. To vent anger and frustration	1. To provide a quality of life for the dying person while preparing for a life without that loved person
2. To share the knowledge that the end is near	2. To be available to offer comfort and care even though the survivor feels like running away to escape the pain of death
3. To assure the well-being of loved ones who will be left behind because they resent the fact that life will go on without them	3. To hope that the loved one will somehow live in spite of obvious deterioration and inability to function. At this time, the survivor may pray for the peace of death.
4. To vent feelings or irritation at omissions or neglect although they feel guilty over the pain this causes others	4. To vent feelings of irritation and guilt over the dying person's demands and increased dependency needs
5. To remain as independent as possible fearing they will become unlovable	5. To live and appreciate each day as one plans for a future without the loved one
6. To be normal and natural at a time when nothing appears to be normal or natural. The dying patient generally experiences the fear of pain, loss of control, and of dying alone. He has a need to maintain security, self-confidence, and dignity.	6. To reassure the dying person that they will "continue in his footsteps" by holding the family together, raising the children or managing the business, while knowing such talk about the future is painful to the dying person

From Holst L: To love is to grieve. The Lutheran Standard, Apr 6, 1984

Holst also shares the following six "lessons learned" while dealing with dying: 1) respect one another's needs for distance or spatial territory; 2) trust your feelings when expressing your emotions since there are few rights and wrongs; 3) respect the feelings each moment brings without deflating, defending, or defusing them; 4) respect each person's limits by not demanding more than a person can give; 5) respect and accept the life you shared with others; and 6) accept the fact that as a human, who is capable of love, you are also vulnerable. Love must end at some time in one's life.

THE DYING PERSON'S BILL OF RIGHTS*

I have the right to be treated as a living human being until I die.

I have the right to maintain a sense of hopefulness however changing its focus may be.

I have the right to be cared for by those who can maintain a sense of hopefulness, however changing this might be.

.I have the right to express my feelings and emotions about my approaching death in my own way.

I have the right to participate in decisions concerning my care.

I have the right to expect continuing medical and nursing attention even though "cure" goals must be changed to "comfort goals."

I have the right not to die alone.

I have the right to be free from pain.

I have the right to have my questions answered honestly.

I have the right not to be deceived.

I have the right to have help from and for my family in accepting my death.

I have the right to die in peace and dignity.

I have the right to retain my individuality and not be judged for my decisions, which may be contrary to beliefs of others.

I have the right to discuss and enlarge my religious and/or spiritual experiences, whatever these may mean to others.

I have the right to expect that the sanctity of the human body will be respected after death.

I have the right to be cared for by caring, sensitive, knowledgeable people who will attempt to understand my needs and will be able to gain some satisfaction in helping me face my death.

(Taken from the *American Journal of Nursing*, January, 1975, p. 99).

This document was included at this time to familiarize the care-giver with the needs and rights of dying persons. Every nursing unit should have this Bill of Rights posted in a readily accessible area to remind members of the health care team of their responsibilities in providing holistic health care. If the nurse feels uncomfortable in planning care to meet

*The Dying Person's Bill of Rights' was created at a workshop on "The Terminally Ill Patient and the Helping Person" in Lansing, Michigan, sponsored by the Southwestern Michigan Inservice Education Council and conducted by Amelia J. Barbus, associate professor of nursing at Wayne State University in Detroit, Michigan.

these rights or needs, a team conference should be held to enlist suggestions or help from other members of the team.

SPIRITUAL NEEDS OF THE PERSON SUFFERING A LOSS

As stated earlier, people suffer many types of loss including health. It is at this time in one's life that the person reaches out for support from significant others, such as friends, family, or clergymen. Recognizing this need, the author enlisted the support of Rev. Peter Brown, Faith Lutheran Church, Orlando, Florida, to survey clergymen in a specific area to obtain information regarding the role of the minister in the health care setting. The results of the survey showed that 97.14% of the respondents considered themselves to be primary members of the health care team in the clinical setting; 88.57% felt they were members of the health care team on the medical–surgical unit; 94.28% in the psychiatric setting. According to the survey, 82.57% of the clergy were informed of the patient's physical condition or diagnosis during hospitalization by family members, whereas 57.14% were informed by the patient; 22.85% by the chaplain's office or by directly contacting the hospital; 17.14% by friends of the patient; 5.7% by the patient's physician. Regarding the presence of a minister when a patient is informed of the prognosis of his illness, 94.28% of the clergy surveyed felt they should be present at that time to provide support to the patient and family members. All the respondents replied that they would like to be informed of a physician's decision not to tell the patient he has a terminal illness. Comments such as "but this is rarely done" and "Although we should be told, no one informs us" were written in the survey. In support of Kübler–Ross' basic premise that patients know when they are dying, as nurses, we need to respond to any spiritual needs by securing the help of the patient's minister or the hospital chaplain when the patient is informed.

The American Cancer Society (1975) has published a booklet, *The Clergy and the Cancer Patient,* that addresses the topic of the pastor's role during a terminal illness. The tasks are defined as being an active listener, facilitating good communication between the patient and family or significant others, and providing spiritual support, including last rites, communion, annointing and blessing the sick, and baptism.

Pumphrey (1977) discusses how patients search for an understanding listener and spiritual support by "sending out feelers," or remarks such as "I haven't gone to church much lately" or "My pastor is so busy, I hate to bother him while I'm in the hospital." Pumphrey states "Ideally, you (the nurse) should be able to respond to each patient's spiritual needs as naturally as you respond to his physical needs" (p.64). Nurses need to familiarize themselves with the attitudes and requirements of various religious groups as described by Pumphrey (1977). If uncomfortable with addressing various spiritual concerns, the nurse can suggest that the patient talk to the hospital chaplain, his own minister, members of his congregation, or other patients with similar religious beliefs. If none of these options seems appropriate, the nurse can provide quiet time for private meditation or prayer.

CHILDREN AND DEATH

Although children grow at varied paces, both physically and emotionally, books that discuss children and the impact of dying outline general growth stages, citing the needs and understanding of children in each phase of development. Preschool children between ages 3 and 5 have a fear of separation from their parents and are unable to think of death as a final separation. They perceive death as a temporary trip to heaven or some other place in which the person still functions actively by eating, sleeping, and so forth. If a child displays guilt feelings because he "wished something awful would happen when he was angry at mommy," he needs to be told that wishes do not kill. Conversely, the "well-adjusted" child who appears to be "a brave little boy" and displays little emotion while appearing to accept a parent's death should be seen by a professional counselor to be certain that no psychological problem is developing. Fear of death may occur due to parental expression of anger, stress, the use of physical restraints during an illness, or punishment for wrongdoing (Murray, 1979).

Children between ages 5 and 9 begin to accept death as a final state. It is conceptualized as a destructive force, a frightening figure, a bogeyman, or an angel who comes during the night "to get bad people." Children of this age believe they will not die if they avoid the death figure. One dying child drew a picture of death as a tank with its gun barrel aiming directly at him, a destructive force he could no longer avoid.

By age 10 children begin to realize death is an inevitable state that all human beings experience due to an internal process. They also believe that the body of a dead person is slowly rotting or turning to bones as insects infest the coffin and prey on the body. Words such as afterlife, cremation, rebirth, and reunion may be verbalized by the child at this age.

Murray (1979) states that not all children think about death as described in basic textbooks. She describes the following additional conceptions about death voiced by young children:

1. Parental death is a deliberate abandonment that the child caused, and he will die next.

2. Death occurs while one sleeps; therefore, do not go to sleep or take naps.

3. The surviving parent caused the other parent to die.

4. Death is catching; don't associate with anyone who just lost a parent or relative or you will be the next person to die.

Adolescents are able to intellectualize their awareness to death although they generally repress any feelings about their own death. As one adolescent commented, "My life is just beginning. I have a lot of years ahead of me before I need to think about dying." Death at this age is considered to be a lack of fulfillment; the adolescent "has too much to lose" if he dies. Adolescents often hide the fact that they are mourning; they may listen to records, withdraw, or bury themselves in activities. They are inexperienced in coping with such a crisis and may not shed tears or voice emotions such as " I miss mom already", "I loved dad so much", "It hurts so much to lose someone you love", "I'm scared what will happen now that dad is dead. Who will take care of us?" or "It's not fair. He was too young to die." Frank (Haber, 1982) states that children "are capable of feeling the great loss of a loved one one moment and yet becoming fully absorbed in something funny the next" (p. 116). Adults need to be aware of this capability so that they do not misinterpret such behavior as disrespect or lack of love for the deceased person.

ASSESSMENT AND NURSING CARE OF THE DYING PATIENT

Perhaps we need to remind ourselves from time to time that patients who are dying are not just dying. They are also living. Whether or not they have the opportunity to live this final human experience to the fullest—each in his own way—is influenced in a great measure by those who take care of them (Browning and Lewis 1972).

The philosophy of an institution about the dying process can be one of the most important factors in the quality of a patient's death. (Barry, 1984)

Care-givers need to reflect on both of these views as they work with terminally ill persons. Nurses are conditioned to do all they can to help a patient recover to a state of wellness and have very little experience on how to cope with something beyond their control. They need to examine their own reactions to loss, grief, death, and dying before they can deal with the psychological needs of dying patients and survivors. Once the nurse has explored any personal feelings and accepted her own mortality, she is better prepared to provide an atmosphere of acceptance, love, and concern.

Dying persons provide a unique challenge to nurses. Consider the following questions raised by family, friends, and health care providers:

1. Should the patient be informed that he is dying? When? What if his family does not want him to know?

2. How much information should be given about his condition? Should this take the form of minimal information or a description of how death will occur?

3. What can I say to comfort a dying patient?

4. What environment would be the best suited to a dying patient (*i.e.,* home, hospice, or hospital)?

5. How frequently should the patient be given pain medication? What if it depresses respirations or causes other untoward effects?

6. Should pastoral care be offered even if the patient indicates little or no interest in religion?

The nurse needs to assess the dying patient's knowledge about his illness and prognosis. Does he know what is wrong with him? How much longer does he think he will be hospitalized? What has his physician told him about his illness? How does his family feel about his hospitalization? As the patient responds to such questions, the nurse should observe for signs of the grieving process so that she can plan appropriate interventions.

Nonverbal communication may provide a clue to the patient's emotions. The nurse also should observe the patient's interactions with family, friends, as well as the doctor and minister. These people may constitute the "task force" to meet the patient's needs. The age of the patient needs to be considered because views toward death vary at different developmental stages. An adolescent may feel robbed of life, whereas an elderly cancer patient may welcome death as a release from pain. Mood swings may occur frequently as the patient wrestles with emotional responses such as denial, anger, fear, or depression. The patient's role in the family, marital status, and religious beliefs play an important part in providing support systems as the patient attempts to cope. The type of illness, symptoms that the patient exhibits, and predicted type of death all influence the patient's reactions to dying. For instance, the patient who knows he will be medicated frequently to minimize pain and that he will slip into a "deep sleep" before death will probably face death more readily than will the patient who has excruciating pain and loss of body functions.

Several fears have been voiced by dying persons. The nurse needs to be cognizant of these fears so that nursing interventions will be planned to alleviate them. They are fear of the unknown, abandonment, loss of self-control or independence, pain, loss of identity, worthlessness or meaninglessness in one's life, and dying alone. Dolan (1983) discusses the importance of one's environment during death. Although the suggestions are for the patient who chooses to die at home, they are appropriate for a variety of settings and are worth mentioning at this time. Many of the potential fears could be alleviated by altering the environment as follows:

1. Select a room with plenty of fresh air and sunshine.

2. Provide a readily accessible bathroom.

3. Decorate the room with familiar personal objects so that the patient can see them from the bed.

4. Provide access to music if the patient enjoys it.

5. Keep the room tidy and provide colorful bed linen as well as occassional fresh-cut flowers.

6. Keep medical supplies, bedside commode and other sickroom out of sight unless necessity dictates their presence.

7. Allow children to visit if the patient desires their company.

8. Allow pets to be enjoyed by the patient, if possible.

If the patient desires special snacks or food from home, the nurse should make every effort to grant this wish when possible.

There are privileges or rewards for nurses who care for terminally ill persons. Dying people often display dignity, courage, and an appreciation for life that one is unaccustomed to seeing. A simple telephone call, surprise anniversary or birthday party, or ride outdoors in a wheelchair constitute a new quality of life for the dying person and survivors. The nurse matures while observing valiant efforts to sustain life in spite of pain, anxiety, or fear. Family interactions can teach helping persons a lot about support systems, family dynamics, and the will to live. Each family has its own unique way of relating and reacting to change or loss. Listening to the patient share emotions, being sensitive to and showing respect for the patient's needs, and providing privacy all constitute an atmosphere of love and concern that promote successful grieving.

Examples of nursing diagnoses and nursing interventions for patients experiencing loss and grief follow:

NURSING DIAGNOSES	NURSING INTERVENTIONS
Grieving related to actual loss	Assess for causative or contributing factors that may hinder or delay any grief work (*i.e.*, denial, anger, depression, or inability to grieve).
	Establish rapport by promoting a trust relationship.
	Convey to the patient that although feelings may be uncomfortable, they are a normal and necessary part of the grief process.
	Explain grief reactions.

(continued)

NURSING DIAGNOSES	NURSING INTERVENTIONS
	Promote grief work by encouraging ventilation of feelings and exploration of reasons for behavior such as fear or denial. Maintain a safe, secure environment.
Ineffective individual coping related to depression	Assess for causative or contributing factors such as loss, negative self-concept, or lack of support systems. Assess present coping status to determine risk of inflicting self-harm and intervene appropriately (see Chapter 24). Offer support by reassuring the patient and teaching problem-solving techniques. Help to establish a support system of people who understand the patient's situation. Maintain a sense of humor as depression subsides.
Social isolation related to depression and loss	Identify causative and contributing factors. Encourage verbalization of feelings. Promote social interaction by mobilizing the person's support systems. Identify activities that the patient likes to help to keep him busy during periods of loneliness (*i.e.,* reading, sewing, shopping, pets, or church activities).

SUMMARY

Loss is experienced by all of us at one time or another when we are deprived of something valuable that was previously present in our lives. Loss of one's health, spouse, home, job, or pet may occur suddenly or gradually, may be predictable or unexpected, and may be viewed as traumatic or temperate. The descriptive terms actual, perceived, anticipatory, temporary, and permanent loss were explained. Examples of loss of physiologic function or part of self, environment or objects external to self, and loved or valued person were given. The ten states of grief as described by Westberg (1971) were discussed, as well as Kübler–Ross' five stages of the grieving process. Needs of the dying and their survivors as identified by Holst (1984) were stated. A copy of "The Dying Person's Bill of Rights" was included to familiarize the reader with this document. Spiritual needs of the person suffering a loss were addressed, as well as the role or tasks of the clergyman on the health care team. The understanding or perception of death by children at various growth stages was explained. Suggestions for nursing care of dying persons were listed with an emphasis on the nurse's need to examine personal reactions to loss, grief, death, and dying. The privileges and rewards for nursing personnel who care for terminally ill patients were noted. Examples of nursing interventions for grieving related to actual loss, ineffective individual coping related to depression, and social isolation related to depression and loss were presented.

LEARNING ACTIVITIES

I. Clinical activities
   A. Assess your assigned patient for any losses.
   1. Is the loss considered to be an actual, perceived, anticipatory, temporary, or permanent loss?
   2. Explain the type of loss. Is it physiologic, environmental, or the loss of a person?
   3. Identify which state of the grieving process the patient is experiencing. Compare to the stages described by Westberg or Kübler–Ross.
   4. List any needs that your patient presents.
   5. Are the patient's rights being honored? (Review "The Dying Person's Bill of Rights.")
   B. Plan nursing interventions appropriate for the stage of grief identified, focusing on emotional and spiritual needs of the patient.
II. Independent activity
   A. Read one or more of the following books about children and death listed in the references:
   1. Gordon A, Keass D: They Need to Know: How to Teach Children About Death. Englewood Cliffs, Prentice–Hall, 1979
   2. Jackson E: Telling a Child About Death. New York, Dutton, 1965
   3. Stein SB: About Dying: An Open Book for Parents and Children Together. New York, Walker & Co, 1974
   B. Read Engel's "Grief and Grieving" article to familiarize yourself with his three stages of grieving.
   C. Plan therapeutic interventions for a 9-year-old child whose mother just died.
   D. Read Klagsbrun S: Communications in the Treatment of Cancer. Am J Nurs: May, 1971.

SELF-TEST

1. Differentiate between loss and grief.
2. List the emotional or behavioral reactions to loss as described by Kübler–Ross.
3. State the needs of a dying person.

4. List nursing interventions for each need identified in question No. 3.
5. State the survivor's needs.
6. Explain the purpose of "The Dying Person's Bill of Rights."
7. Describe the tasks of the clergyman as he relates to people experiencing a loss.
8. Discuss how the following age groups perceive death:
   Ages 3 to 5
   Ages 5 to 10
   Ages 10 to adolescence
9. You are assigned to a 21-year-old woman who has approximately 2 weeks to live and feel uncomfortable with this assignment. What would you do?
10. List ways to alter the environment of a dying patient to promote a homelike atmosphere.
11. State the rewards of caring for terminally ill persons.

REFERENCES

American Cancer Society: A Cancer Source Book for Nurses. Professional Education Publications, 1975

American Cancer Society: The Clergy and the Cancer Patient. Professional Education Publications, 1975

Barckley V: Grief, a Part of Living. Ohio's Health: 20, 1968.

Barry P: Psychosocial Nursing Assessment and Intervention. Philadelphia, JB Lippincott, 1984

Browning M, Lewis E: The Dying Patient: A Nursing Perspective. New York, American Journal of Nursing, 1972

Bryer K: The Amish way of death: A study of Family Support Systems. Am Psychol: Mar, 1979

Chetwood L: A Lesson in Living. Nursing 84: Jan, 1984

Craft M et al: Coping. Am J Nurs: Mar, 1982

Crout T: Caring for the mother of a stillborn baby. Nursing 80: Apr, 1980

Death in the first person. Am J Nurs: Feb, 1970

Dolan M: If your patient wants to die at home. Nursing 83: Apr, 1983

Encounters With Grief Series: Am J Nurs: Mar, 1978

Engel G: Grief and grieving. Am J Nurs: Sept, 1964

Erikson BL: With all my heart. The Lutheran Standard, May 6, 1983

Florida Hospital Health Education Department: When dreams are shattered (pamphlet). Orlando, Florida, 1982

Forsyth D: The hardest job of all. Nursing 82: Apr, 1982

Goffnett C: Your patient's dying. Now what? Nursing 79: Nov, 1979

Gordon A, Keass D: They Need to Know: How to Teach Children About Death. Englewood Cliffs, Prentice–Hall, 1979

Groff B: Death and I. Am J Nurs: July, 1982

Gyulay J: Care of the dying child. Nurs Clin North Am: Mar, 1976

Haber J et al: Comprehensive Psychiatric Nursing, 2nd ed. New York, McGraw-Hill, 1982

Hoffman E: Don't give up on me! Am J Nurs: Jan, 1971

Holst L: To Love Is To Grieve. The Lutheran Standard: Apr 6, 1984

Jackson EW: Nursing Skillbook Series: Dealing with Death and Dying. Springhouse, Intermed Communications, 1983

Jackson E: Telling A Child About Death. New York, Dutton, 1965

Kavanaugh R: Dealing naturally with the dying. Nursing 76: Oct, 1976

Kavanaugh R: Helping patients who are facing death. Nursing 74: May, 1974

Klepser MJ: Grief: How long does grief go on? Am J Nurs: Mar,

Kozier B, Erb G: Fundamentals of Nursing, 2nd ed. Menlo Park, Addison–Wesley, 1983

Kübler–Ross E: Death, The Final Stage of Growth. Englewood Cliffs, Prentice–Hall, 1978

Kübler–Ross E: On Death and Dying. New York, MacMillan, 1969

Kübler–Ross E: To Live Until We Say Good-bye, Englewood Cliffs, Prentice–Hall, 1978

Kübler–Ross E: What is it like to be dying? Am J Nurs: Jan, 1971

Lambert V, Lambert C: The Impact of Physical Illness and Related Mental Health Concepts. Englewood Cliffs, Prentice–Hall, 1979

Left E: Dilemmas in practice: Keeping a promise. Am J Nurs: July, 1982

Manning D: Don't Take My Grief Away from Me. Springfield, IL, Creative marketing human services division, 1979

Martocchio B: Living While Dying. Bowie, Robert J Brady, 1982

Mills GC: Books to help children understand death. Am J Nurs: Feb, 1979

Murray R, Zentner J: Nursing Assessment and Health Promotion Through the Life Span. Englewood Cliffs, Prentice–Hall, 1979

Nelson J: Adolescence: Helping the teenage cope with cancer . . . Am J Nurs: Mar, 1982

Popoff D: What are your feelings about death and dying? Parts I, II, and III. Nursing 75: Aug, Sept, Oct, 1975

Poslusny E et al: Nursing and Thanatology. New York, Arno Press, 1978

Pumphrey J: Recognizing your patient's spiritual needs. Nursing 77: Dec, 1977

Raymond M, Laube JD: Time to say good-bye. Am J Nurs: June, 1982

Robinson L: Psychological Aspects of the Care of Hospitalized Patients. Philadelphia, FA Davis, 1984

Schmale AH: Reactions to illness: Convalescence and grieving. Psychiatr Clin North Am: Aug, 1979

Sharer P: Helping survivors cope with the shock of sudden death. Nursing 79: Jan, 1979

Smith M: When a child dies at home. Nursing 82: Aug, 1982

Sobol D: Death and dying. Am J Nurs: Jan, 1974

Stein SB: About Dying: An Open Book for Parents and Children Together. New York, Walker & Co, 1974

Stickney SK, Gardner E: Companions in suffering. Am J Nurs: Dec, 1984

Stuart MS: Dear Paula. Journal of Psychiatric Nursing and Mental Health Services: July, 1977

Westburg G: Good Grief. Philadelphia, Fortress Press, 1979

White R, Gotham L: The syndrome of ordinary grief. Am Fam Physician: Aug, 1975

Zopf D: The dying patient: Meeting his needs could be easier than you think. Nursing 79: Mar, 1979

NURSING INTERVENTIONS
FOR PERSONS WITH
PSYCHIATRIC DISORDERS

11

ASSESSMENT OF THE

PATIENT WITH

DYSFUNCTIONAL COPING

LEARNING OBJECTIVES

1. Define assessment.
2. List the components of a psychiatric interview.
3. List data obtained during the mental status examination.
4. Define the following terminology:
    Blocking
    Circumstantiality
    Flight of ideas
    Perseveration
    Verbigeration
    Neologism
    Mutism
    Inappropriate affect
5. Differentiate between *flat* and *blunt* affect.
6. Differentiate delusions of reference, grandeur, self-deprecation, alien control, nihilism, and somatic concerns.
7. Describe auditory, visual, olfactory, gustatory, and tactile hallucinations.
8. Differentiate between obsessions and compulsions.
9. State how information obtained during the assessment process is transmitted to members of the health care team.
10. List the criteria for charting psychiatric nurses' notes.

T HE psychiatric–mental health nurse initially interviews the patient to establish rapport and to gain knowledge of usual activities, including how he perceives himself and those in his environment. The interview provides factual information about the patient as the nurse observes appearance, speech, and nonverbal communication. This assessment process focuses on the patient's psychosocial history and includes a mental status examination.

The psychosocial history provides a profile of the patient as it includes identifying or demographic data such as age, sex, race, marital status, religion, education, and occupation; chief complaint or presenting problem stated in the patient's own words for which the person has sought professional help; history of the present problem; and relevant information pertaining to psychiatric, medical, surgical, sociocultural, and family history. This chapter will focus on the mental status assessment of patients with dysfunctional coping and includes a psychiatric nursing observation guide to be used in the general hospital setting while assessing a patient's basic human needs.

Mosby's *Medical and Nursing Dictionary* (1983) defines assessment as "an evaluation or appraisal of a condition . . . an examiner's evaluation of the disease or condition based on the patient's subjective report of the symptoms and course of the illness or condition, and the examiner's objective findings ... " (p 89). Psychiatric assessment or determination of a person's mental status is the psychologic counterpart of a physical examination. It serves as the basis for diagnoses and as an understanding of dynamic factors that contribute to the patient's maladjustment, dysfunctional coping, or illness as it exists at the time of examination. Data obtained during an interview should include (Small, 1980):

1. Appearance

2. Behavior

3. Attitude

4. Ability to communicate

5. Emotional state or affect

6. Content of thought

7. Orientation

8. Memory

9. Intellectual ability

10. Insight regarding illness or condition

Barry (1984 p. 10) lists eight psychosocial assessment factors that should be considered to "provide structure as you work with the patient in order for him to return to his presickness level of psychosocial, as well as physical, functioning":

1. Social history

2. Level of stress during the year before admission

3. Normal coping patterns

4. Neurovegetative changes

6. Patient's understanding of illness

6. Mental status

7. Personality style

8. Major issues of illness

These factors constitute a very comprehensive psychiatric assessment and will be discussed in detail.

APPEARANCE

General appearance includes physical characteristics, apparent age, peculiarity of dress, cleanliness, and use of cosmetics (Small, 1980). The examiner may consider questions similar to the following while assessing the person's appearance:

1. Is the patient neat, clean, and tidy, or does he appear dirty and unkempt?

2. Is his attire or manner of dress appropriate or bizarre?

3. Is the patient overly anxious or meticulous about his appearance to the extent that it interferes with his activities of daily living (ADL)?

4. Are the patient's eyes bright or dull; pupils round, equal, and regular; skin clear or unhealthy looking; hair neatly groomed or disheveled looking?

5. Are there any noticeable or outstanding physical characteristics such as extreme obesity or cachexia? Does the patient were a prosthesis?

6. Does the person appear to be older or younger than his chronological age?

A person's general appearance, including facial expressions, is a manner of nonverbal communication in which emotions, feelings, and moods are related. For example, depressed people often neglect their personal appearance, appear disheveled, and wear drab-looking clothes generally dark in color, reflecting a depressed mood. The facial expression may appear sad, worried, tense, frightened, or distraught. Manic patients may dress in bizarre, or overly colorful outfits, wear heavy layers of cosmetics, and don several pieces of jewelry.

BEHAVIOR, ATTITUDE, AND NORMAL COPING PATTERNS

The interviewer assesses the person's actions or behavior by considering the following factors:

1. Does he exhibit strange, threatening, or violent behavior? Is he making an effort to control his emotions?

2. Is there evidence of any unusual mannerisms or motor activity, such as grimacing, tremors, tics, impaired gait, psychomotor retardation, or agitation? Does he pace excessively?

3. Does the person appear friendly, embarrassed, evasive, fearful, resentful, angry, negativistic, or impulsive? His attitude toward the interviewer or helping persons can facilitate or impair the assessment process.

4. Is his behavior overactive or underactive? Is it purposeful, disorganized, or stereotyped? Are reactions fairly consistent?

The patient should be asked how he normally copes with a serious problem or with high levels of stress if he is in contact with reality and able to respond to such a question. Responses to this question enable the interviewer to assess the person's present ability to cope as well as his judgment. Has he lost this ability? Does he need to develop new coping measures? His behavior may be the result of inadequate coping patterns.

The paranoid or suspicious person may isolate himself, appear evasive during a conversation, and demonstrate a negativistic attitude toward the nursing staff. Such activity is an attempt to protect oneself by maintaining control of a stressful environment.

PERSONALITY STYLE AND COMMUNICATION ABILITY

"The manner in which the patient talks enables us to appreciate difficulties with his thought processes. It is desirable to obtain a verbatim sample of the stream of speech to illustrate psychopathologic disturbances" (Small, 1980, p. 8).

Factors to be considered while one is assessing the person's ability to communicate and interact socially include:

1. Does he speak coherently? Does the flow of speech seem natural or logical, or is it illogical, vague, and loosely organized? Does he enunciate clearly?

2. Is the rate of speech slow, retarded, or rapid? Does he fail to speak at all or respond only when questioned?

3. Does the patient whisper, speak softly, or does he speak loudly or shout?

4. Is there a delay in answers or responses or does the patient break off his conversation in the middle of a sentence and refuse to talk further?

5. Does he repeat certain words and phrases over and over?

6. Does he make up new words that have no meaning to others?

7. Is his language obscene?

8. Does his conversation jump from one topic to another?

9. Does he stutter, lisp, or regress in his speech?

10. Does he exhibit any unusual personality traits or characteristics that may interfere with his ability to socialize with others or adapt to hospitalization? For example, does he associate freely with others or does he consider himself a "loner"? Does he appear aggressive or domineering during the interview? Does he feel that people like him or reject him? How does he spend his personal time?

The following terminology generally is used to describe impaired communication observed during the assessment process: 1) blocking, 2) circumstantiality, 3) flight of ideas, 4) perseveration, 5) verbigeration, 6) neologisms, and 7) mutism. They are defined by the American Psychiatric Association (1980) as follows:

BLOCKING. This impairment is a sudden stoppage in the spontaneous flow or stream of thinking or speaking for no apparent external or environmental reason. Blocking may be due to preoccupation, delusional thoughts, or hallucinations; for example, while talking to the nurse, a patient stated, "My favorite restaurant is Chi-Chi's. I like it because the atmosphere is so nice and the food is . . . ."

CIRCUMSTANTIALITY. This is a pattern of speech in which the person gives much unnecessary detail that delays meeting a goal or stating a point. For example, when asked to state his occupation, a patient gave a very detailed description of the type of work he did.

FLIGHT OF IDEAS. This is an impairment characterized by overproductivity of talk and verbal skipping from one idea to another. The ideas are fragmentary, although talk is continuous. Connections between the parts of speech often are determined by chance of associations; for example: "I like the color blue. Do you ever feel blue? Feelings can change from day to day. The days are getting longer."

PERSEVERATION. "A tendency to emit the same verbal or motor response again and again to verbal stimuli" (American Psychiatric Association, 1980, p. 70). Smith (p. 9) states that perseveration is "repetition of speech (or movement) despite patient's efforts to produce a new answer." Verbigeration is a severe or extreme form of perseveration.

NEOLOGISM. A new word or combination of several words coined or self-invented by a person and not readily understood by others; for example: "His *phenologs* are in the dryer."

MUTISM. This is refusal to speak even though the person may give indications of being aware of the environment. Mutism may occur from conscious or unconscious reasons.

Other terminology such as loose association, echolalia, and clang association are described in the chapter discussing schizophrenic disorders.

EMOTIONAL STATE OR AFFECT

Affect is defined as "the outward manifestation of a person's feelings, tone, or mood. Affect and emotion are commonly used interchangeably" (American Psychiatric Association, 1980, p. 3). "The relationship between mood and the content of thought is of particular significance. There may be a wide divergence between what the patient says or does on the one hand and his emotional state as expressed objectively in his face or attitudes . . . " (Small, 1980, p. 10).

A lead question such as "What are you feeling?" may elicit responses as "nervous," "angry," "frustrated," "depressed," or "confused." The person should be asked to describe the nervousness, frustration, or confusion. Is the person's emotional response constant or does it fluctuate during the assessment? The interviewer should record a verbatim reply to questions concerning the patient's mood and note whether an intense emotional response accompanies the discussion of specific topics. Affective responses may be appropriate, inappropriate, flat, or blunt. An emotional response out of proportion to a situation is considered inappropriate. For example, a 45-year-old man's mailbox and newly planted rose bushes are run over by a car driven by a teenager while under the influence of alcohol. The man becomes extremely angry, to the point of hysteria, and yells obscenities at the teenager. If the same man registered no emotional response although extensive damage was done to the yard, he would be demonstrating a flat affect. A subdued or suppressed response to the situation would be considered an example of blunt affect.

Under ordinary circumstances, a person's affect varies according to the situation or subject under discussion. The person with emotional conflict may have a persistent emotional reaction based on this conflict. It is imperative that the examiner or observer identify the abnormal emotional reaction and explore its depth, intensity, and persistence. Such an inquiry could prevent a depressed person from attempting suicide.

CONTENT OF THOUGHT OR THINKING PROCESS

The American Psychiatric Association (1980, p. 131) defines thought disorder as "a disturbance of speech, communication, or content of thought, such as delusions, ideas of reference . . . A thought disorder can be caused by a functional emotional disorder or an organic condition." Small (1980) discusses those thought contents more readily exhibitied during a psychiatric examination: 1) delusions, 2) hallucinations, 3) depersonalization, 4) obsessions, and 5) compulsions.

Delusions

A *delusion* is a false belief not true to fact and is not ordinarily accepted by other members of the person's culture. The delusion cannot be corrected by an appeal to the reason of the person experiencing it. Following is a brief description of various types of delusions:

TYPE	DESCRIPTION
Delusions of reference or persecution	One believes that he is the object of environmental attention or that he is singled out for harassment. "The police are watching my every move. They're out to get me."

TYPE	DESCRIPTION
Delusions of alien control	The person believes his feelings, thoughts, impulses, or actions are controlled by an external source. "A space man sends me messages by TV and tells me what to to."
Nihilistic delusions	The person denies reality or existence of self, part of self, or some external object. "I have no head."
Delusions of self-deprecation	The individual feels unworthy, ugly, or sinful. "I don't deserve to live. I'm so unworthy of your love."
Delusions of grandeur	A person experiences exaggerated ideas of his importance or identity. "I am Napoleon!"
Somatic delusions	False belief pertaining to body image or body function. The person actually believes that he has cancer, leprosy, or some other terminal illness.

Hallucinations

Hallucinations are sensory perceptions that occur in the absence of an actual external stimulus. They may be auditory, visual, olfactory, gustatory, or tactile in nature. Examples of each follow:

TYPE	EXAMPLE
Auditory hallucination	AS tells you that he hears voices frequently while he sits quietly in his lounge chair. He states, "The voices tell me when to eat, dress, and go to bed each night!"
Visual hallucination	Ninety-year-old EK describes seeing spiders and snakes on the ceiling of his room late one evening as you make rounds.
Olfactory hallucination	AJ, a 65-year-old psychotic patient, states that she smells "rotten garbage" in her bedroom, although there is no evidence of any foul-smelling material.
Gustatory (taste) hallucination	MY, a young patient with organic brain syndrome, complains of a constant metallic taste in her mouth.
Tactile hallucination	NX, a middle-aged woman undergoing symptoms of alcohol withdrawal and delirium tremens, complains of feeling "worms crawling all over [her] body."

Depersonalization

Depersonalization is described as a feeling of unreality or strangeness concerning self, the environment, or both; for example, patients have described out-of-body sensations in which they view themselves from a few feet overhead. These people may feel they are "going crazy." Causes of depersonalization include prolonged stress and psychological fatigue, as well as substance abuse.

Obsessions

"Obsessions are insistent thoughts, recognized as arising from the self, usually regarded by the patient as absurd and relatively meaningless, yet they persist despite his endeavors to rid himself of them" (Small, 1980, p. 13). Persons who experience obsessions generally describe their thoughts as "thoughts I can't get rid of" or "I can't stop thinking of things . . . they keep going on in my mind over and over again."

Compulsions

"An insistent, repetitive, intrusive and unwanted urge to perform an act contrary to one's ordinary wishes or standards" (American Psychiatric Association, 1980, p. 21). If the person does not engage in the repetitive act due to an inner need or drive, he generally experiences feelings of tension and anxiety.

ORIENTATION

During the assessment, the person is asked questions regarding his ability to grasp the significance of his environment, an existing situation, or the clearness of conscious processes. In other words, is he oriented to person, place, and time? Does he know who he is, where he is, or what the date is? Levels of orientation and consciousness are subdivided as follows: confusion, clouding of consciousness, stupor, delirium, dream state, and coma. A brief description of each (Barry, 1984 and Kolb, 1977) follows:

TERMINOLOGY	DESCRIPTION
Confusion	Disorientation to person, place or time characterized by bewilderment and complexity.
Clouding of consciousness	Disturbance in perception or thought that is slight to moderate in degree, usually owing to physical or chemical factors producing functional impairment of the cerebrum.
Stupor	A state in which the person does not react to or is unaware of the surroundings. He may be motionless and mute but conscious.

TERMINOLOGY	DESCRIPTION
Delirium, or acute brain syndrome	Confusion accompanied by altered or fluctuating consciousness. Disturbance in emotion, thought, and perception is moderate to severe. Usually associated with infections, toxic states, head trauma, and so forth
Dream state	Disturbed, clouded, or confused consciousness in which the person may not be aware of his surroundings. Visual or auditory hallucinations may occur. May last several minutes to a few days
Coma	Loss of consciousness

MEMORY

Memory, or the ability to recall past experiences, is divided into categories: recent and long-term. Recent memory is the ability to recall events in the immediate past and up to 2 weeks previously. Long-term memory is the ability to recall remote past experiences such as the time and place of birth, names of schools attended, occupational history, and chronological data relating to the patient's previous illnesses. Small (1980) states that memory defects may be because of lack of attention, difficulty with retention, difficulty with recall, or any combination of these factors. Loss of recent memory may be seen in patients with chronic organic brain syndrome, acute organic brain syndrome, or depression. Long-term memory loss generally is due to a physiologic disorder resulting in brain dysfunction. Three disorders of memory are 1) hypermnesia or an abnormally pronounced memory, 2) amnesia or loss of memory, and 3) paramnesia or falsification of memory.

INTELLECTUAL ABILITY

The person's ability to use facts comprehensively is an indication of his intellectual ability. During the assessment he may be asked general information such as 1) to name the last three presidents, 2) to calculate simple arithmetical problems, and 3) "to correctly estimate and form opinions concerning objective matters" (Small, 1980, p. 16). He may be asked a question such as "What would you do if you found a wallet in front of your house?" The examiner is able to evaluate the person's reasoning ability and judgment by the response given. His abstract and concrete thinking abilities are evaluated by his responses to proverbs such as "an eye for an eye and a tooth for a tooth."

INSIGHT REGARDING ILLNESS OR CONDITION

Does the person consider himself ill or not? Does he understand what is happening? Is the illness threatening to the patient? Insight is defined as self-understanding, or the extent of a person's understanding of the origin, nature, and mechanisms of his attitudes and behavior. Patients' insights into their illness or condition range from poor to good, depending on the degree of psychopathology present.

NEUROVEGETATIVE CHANGES

Does the patient exhibit changes in psychophysiologic functions such as sleep patterns, eating patterns, energy levels, sexual functioning, or bowel functioning? Depressed persons usually complain of insomnia or hypersomnia, loss of appetite or increased appetite, loss of energy or anergia, decreased libido, and constipation, exhibiting neurovegetative changes. Persons who are diagnosed as psychotic may neglect their nutritional intake, appear fatigued, sleep excessively, and ignore elimination habits (sometimes to the point of developing a fecal impaction.)

MAJOR ISSUES OF ILLNESS

Barry refers to "disruptions in his ability to trust, maintain self-esteem, retain a sense of control, tolerate a major loss, avoid feelings of guilt, and maintain intimacy in his close relationships" (1980 p. 11) as major issues of illnesses. A patient who is alcoholic, a substance abuser, anorectic, bulimic, or depressed often presents with symptoms of a low self-concept, guilt, the inability to maintain control, or to develop positive interpersonal relationships. Similarly, trust is a major issue with a paranoid patient, who is often suspicious of everyone.

SOCIAL HISTORY

Information obtained during a social history focuses on the person's lifestyle, including hobbies, interests, ability to socialize, and availability of support persons during a difficult situation. Does he have many, few, or no friends? Does he participate in activities outside the home? How frequently? What are his interests or hobbies? Who does he seek as a support person when he is upset? Support persons may include spouse, significant other, pastor, or employer, and these people should be identified during treatment so that the person does not feel alone when faced with a difficult situation.

STRESS LEVEL BEFORE ADMISSION

Holmes and Rahe (1967) developed the social readjustment rating scale, which ranks 43 critical life events within a single year, according to their severity of stress on a person. By using this scale, the examiner can assess the severity of environmental stress, such as financial, marital, job insecurity, or acute illness that the person has been enduring before admission (see Chapter 14).

In summary, the assessment of a person's mental status focuses on appearance, behavior, communication skills, emotional state, thought processes, insight regarding illness, stress level, and social history. The information obtained should be objective, descriptive, and noninterpretive. Objective data state what the patient says and does, not what the examiner feels about his behavior. Descriptive data give a picture of the patient's behavior, appearance, and conversation in the situation in which it occurs. Noninterpretive data describes what the patient says and does without using terms that state the meaning of his behavior, whereas interpretive data is subjective in nature. Following is a comparison of interpretive or subjective data and of descriptive or noninterpretive data:

INTERPRETIVE OR SUBJECTIVE	DESCRIPTIVE OR NONINTERPRETIVE
Refuses to eat; is uncooperative at mealtime	MJ does not do what he is asked. "Why should I eat? I'm not hungry. This food is poisoned" was his response at mealtime.
Appears confused and disoriented	MJ was found walking in the hall attempting to use the elevator. He stated "Can you help me? I'm ready to go home but can't remember how I came here. What day is this, anyhow?"
Appears depressed	MJ was sitting in his room with the drapes closed and the lights off. "Leave me alone. I'm not worth all this attention. Go help those people who want help," was his response to the nurse as she entered his room.
Appears anxious	MJ was pacing the hallway, wringing his hands and perspiring. He stated "I feel so jittery inside. I can't sit still. Why do you think I feel this way?"
Dresses sloppily	MJ was dressed in a faded blue T-shirt with several cigarette burns on the lower front. His green slacks were torn at both knees and spotted with white paint. He was unshaven and his hair appeared to be uncombed, Nicotine stains were noted on his right forefinger and thumb.

(continued)

INTERPRETIVE OR SUBJECTIVE	DESCRIPTIVE OR NONINTERPRETIVE
Restless	MJ was unable to sit still during the 30-minute therapeutic community meeting. He would sit still for approximately 3 minutes and then stand up and ask if he could return to his room. After two attempts to sit still, MJ was permitted to leave the meeting. He paced the hall for approximately 15 minutes, asking the staff for cigarettes whenever they greeted him.

NURSING OBSERVATION GUIDE

The following nursing observation guide has been designed for the student nurse caring for the patient in the hospital setting and assesses the patient's basic human needs. Information obtained from the chart and by nursing assessment can be used to develop an individualized nursing care plan.

Patient's initials: _____

Diagnosis and presenting symptoms: _____

Date of birth: _____

Age: _____

Sex: _____

Occupation: _____

Information obtained from: _____

I. Safety and security
  A. General overall appearance
     1. Is the patient clean, neat, or tidy, and dressed appropriately?
        _____ Yes _____ No Comment _____
     2. Are the patient's eyes bright _____ dull _____ ?
     3. Describe the condition of the skin and hair.
     4. Does the patient's concern about personal appearance interfere with daily living? _____ Yes _____ No Comment _____
  B. Thought content
     1. Is the patient oriented to time, place, and person?
        _____ Yes _____ No Comment _____
     2. Evaluate the patient's memory regarding recent and long-term events.
     3. Does the patient demonstrate any of the following symptoms or behaviors? If so, give an example of each.
        a. Delusions (paranoid or grandiose)
        b. Ideas of reference
        c. Hallucinations
        d. Illusions
        e. Obsessions or compulsions
        f. Phobias
        g. Suicidal ideation

       h. Somatic concerns

       i. Other

    4. Does the patient display good insight about his current problem?_____ Yes _____ No   Comment _____

II. Activity and rest

  A. Activities and sociability

    1. Describe the patient's posture and gait. Include any unusual mannerisms present.

    2. Does he appear to be underactive or overactive?
    _____ Yes _____ No   Comment _____

    3. Does the atmosphere on the unit influence his activity?
    Comment _____

    4. Does the patient appear to participate freely in recreation and other scheduled activities?_____ Yes _____ No
    Does the patient appear to enjoy participating?_____ Yes _____ No

    5. Is the patient passive, assertive, or aggressive when participating in activities?

    6. Does he associate with other patients and the staff? Does he have any close friends? Do other clients like him? Do they reject him?

    7. How does he spend his time?

  B. Sleep

    1. Describe the patient's sleeping habits.

    2. Does he offer any complaints about dreaming (e.g., being afraid)?

    3. Does he object to getting out of bed in the morning?
    _____ Yes _____ No

III. Nutrition and elimination

  A. Does the patient eat willingly or must he be coaxed, spoon-fed, or fed by gavage or IV?

  B. Does the patient overeat?_____ Yes _____ No

  C. Describe the patient's eating habits including whether he

    1. conducts any ritualistic habits?

    2. eats certain foods first?

    3. displays elaborate motions?

    4. complains that food is poisoned?

    5. eats alone or in a group?

    6. eats fast or slow?

    7. is messy or neat?

  D. Describe the patient's bowel habits: Frequency_____
  Constipation _____
  Diarrhea _____

  E. Does the patient have any difficulty passing urine (water)? Last menstrual period _____

  F. Patient's weight? _____ Underweight _____ Overweight _____ Normal limits

  G. Is the patient on any specific diet?

IV. Oxygenation

  A. Vital signs: T _____   P _____   R _____   BP _____

  B. Any observations or information related to oxygenation? Comment _____

V. Sexual role satisfaction

  A. Marital status: M   W   S   D

  B. Describe the patient's role in the family unit.

(continued)

    C. Is there any support system provided by family or friends?

    D. Is the patient able to talk about or describe his body?

    E. Observations or information related to sexual role satisfaction?

VI. Mental health and behavioral adjustments

  A. Emotional reactions

    1. Does the patient make any effort to control his emotions?

        _____ Yes _____ No

        List any defense mechanisms he uses. Give examples.

        _____

    2. Are the patient's reactions fairly consistent?

        _____ Yes _____ No

    3. Does the patient display any sudden impulsive actions or outbursts of excitement?

    4. Do rules appear to upset the patient?

        _____ Yes _____ No

    5. Discuss the development tasks appropriate for this patient. How is the client handling these tasks?

  B. Speech

    1. Describe the patient's flow of speech:

      a. Natural

      b. Flighty, rapid, and disconnected

      c. Slow

      d. Breaks off conversation midsentence

      e. Other

    2. Is speech loud, noisy, soft, or quiet?

    3. Are the patient's answers appropriate according to questions asked?

    4. Does he speak voluntarily?

    5. Does he include any obscenity in his speech?

  C. Physical complaints

    1. Does the patient complain of such things as pains in the stomach, pains and weakness in the legs, suffocation, difficulty breathing, nausea, heart irregularity, headaches, or dizziness?

    2. Does the patient repeat one set of symptoms, or do they change from time to time?

    3. Does he feel that these symptoms are caused by some influence coming from outside his own body?

    4. Does he feel that he is unable to accomplish anything or to eat because of these symptoms?

    5. List any pertinent laboratory values, x-ray reports, or other diagnostic tests.

    6. List any medical problems that the patient may be experiencing.

  D. From available information, determine how many times this patient has been hospitalized for emotional problems or the inability to function outside the hospital setting. List the dates, where hospitalized, and diagnosis.

    Date _____ Hospital   or   Clinic _____

    Diagnosis

VII. Medication

  A. List all medications the patient has taken—prescribed or nonprescribed—before admission.

  B. List the medication prescribed during this hospitalization.

RECORDING OF ASSESSMENTS

In addition to evaluating one's mental status, assessment is done by nurses, doctors, dietitians, social workers, psychologists, and consultants to 1) identify the etiology of a disorder, 2) establish a medical or psychiatric diagnosis and prognosis, 3) obtain information pertaining to previous mental and physical illnesses, 4) establish a treatment program or plan intervention appropriate for specific problems, 5) monitor the patient's response to treatment, 6) evaluate the results of treatment, and 7) plan follow-up care or discharge planning after treatment is terminated.

Information obtained is relayed to the members of the health care team in the form of a summary of history and physical examination, a summary of social history, summary of psychological testing, progress notes, and nurses' notes. Examples of subjective or interpretive, and descriptive or noninterpretive, documentation of data were given earlier. Nurses can provide invaluable pertinent information if they follow the criteria of good recording. Such information is significant to the members of the interdisciplinary team who use these notes as an aid in planning treatment and disposition of patients. Thorough charting shows progress, lack of progress, or regression on the part of the patient. The details of the patient's conduct, appearance, and attitude are significant. Increased skill in observation and recording will result in concise charting. Charting is also important in research because it is an accurate record of the symptoms, behavior, treatment, and reactions of the patient. Charting is recognized by legal authorities, who frequently use the notes for testimony in court.

The basic criteria for charting psychiatric nurse's notes are listed here. The notes should be

1. *Objective:* The nurse records what the patient says and does by stating facts and quoting the patient's conversation.

2. *Descriptive:* The nurse describes the patient's appearance, behavior, and conversation as seen and heard.

3. *Nondiagnostic:* The nurse avoids the use of medical or psychiatric diagnoses. She can use acceptable nursing diagnoses such as "noncompliance," "potential for violence," "ineffective individual coping," and "sexual dysfunction."

4. *Complete:* A record of examinations, treatments, medications, therapies, nursing interventions, and the patient's reaction to each should be made on the patient's chart. Samples of the patient's writing or drawing should be preserved.

5. *Legible:* Psychiatric nursing notes should be written legibly, with the use of acceptable abbreviations only, and no erasures. Correct grammar and spelling are important and complete sentences should be used.

6. *Dated:* With a notation of the time entry was made. It is very important to note the time of entry. For example, MS has been quiet and withdrawn all day; however, later in the evening she becomes agitated. The nurse needs to state the time at which Mary's behavior has changed as well as describe any pertinent situations that might be identified as the cause of her behavioral change.

7. *Logical:* Presented in logical sequence

8. *Signed:* By the person making the entry

EXAMPLES OF CHARTING

Example 1

8 AM RK was eating breakfast when she began to perspire profusely and stated, "I don't know what's wrong with me, but I feel jittery inside. I feel like something terrible is going to happen." When asked to describe her feelings, RK replied, "I can't. I just have an awful feeling inside." Dr. Smith notified of RK's behavior.

J. Jones, RN

8:30 AM Valium 10 mg PO per order Dr. Smith.

J. Jones, RN

9:30 AM RK was seated calmly in a wicker chair near the nurses' station. When asked how she felt, she replied "A lot better. I don't know what came over me. I hope it doesn't happen again." No evidence of profuse diaphoresis noted.

J. Jones, RN

Example 2

9 PM JY was watching television when he yelled the following at EZ, "I'll get you for that comment. Don't you ever call me that name again!" JY picked up a potted plant and threw it at the floor. When asked what upset him, JY stated, "The television set told me EZ was out to get me. I tried to protect myself." JY went to his room cooperatively when asked to do so. Dr. Smith notified of JY's behavior.

J. Jones, RN

9:20 PM Librium 25 mg PO given per order Dr. Smith.

J. Jones, RN

10:20 PM JY is lying in bed snoring loudly.

J. Jones, RN

Example 3

10:00 AM NA arrived at art therapy wearing heavy makeup, several items of jewelry around her neck and on her left arm. She wore a purple blouse and red skirt with pink high heels. Her manner of speech was fast and loud. She talked continuously about her grandson, who plays football. NA was unable to sit still for more than 5 minutes at a time during art therapy and after approximately 15 minutes, stated, "I want to go back to my room."

J. Jones, RN

SUMMARY

Assessment of the patient with dysfunctional coping includes a mental status examination, the psychological counterpart of a physical examination. Data obtained during this assessment were discussed in depth, including: appearance; behavior, attitude, and normal coping patterns; ability to communicate and personality style; emotional state or affect; content of thought, or thinking process; orientation; memory; intellectual ability; insight regarding illness or condition; and social history. A comparison was made between interpretive or subjective data, and descriptive or noninterpretive data. A sample nursing observation guide focusing on the following basic human needs of the hospitalized psychiatric patient was discussed: safety and security, activity and rest, nutrition and elimination, oxygenation, sexual role satisfaction, and mental health and behavioral adjustments. Several purposes of assessment were stated. Criteria for charting psychiatric nursing notes were listed and examples given.

LEARNING ACTIVITIES

I. Clinical activities
   A. Assess the following areas on your assigned patient:
      1. Appearance
      2. Behavior
      3. Attitude
      4. Ability to communicate
      5. Emotional state or affect
      6. Content of thought
      7. Orientation
      8. Memory
      9. Intellectual ability
      10. Insight regarding illness
   B. Summarize the data obtained to give an informative report about the patient's mental health status.
   C. Chart pertinent information using descriptive, noninterpretive data.

II. Independent activity
   A. Use the following nonverbal behavior assessment guide while communicating with fellow students or friends:
      1. State any significant nonverbal behavior, such as finger tapping, tics, or poor eye contact.
      2. State the possible reason for or meaning of the behavior, such as fear, anxiety, boredom, or impatience.
      3. List nursing interventions pertaining to the reason for the identified behavior.
   B. Review the programmed instruction "Mental Status Assessment" in the August, 1981 issue of the *American Journal of Nursing*.
III. Case study behavioral assessment
   A. WJ, a 45-year-old patient admitted for emergency surgery for a bleeding ulcer, is referred to the psychiatric unit for a consultation because of symptoms of depression and anxiety. This married man has four children, two of whom are still living at home while attending college. He runs his own business, but often works 10 to 12 hours each day. He has had one previous hospitalization two years ago when he had surgery for cancer of the colon.

   WJ is alert and oriented in ICU but gets little sleep at night. While awake, he watches the nurses carefully and is very pleasant when he converses with them. When he calls for a nurse and one does not respond immediately, WJ begins to shout until someone arrives. His requests are often minor and he could have waited.

   The staff isn't certain how much WJ knows about his surgery, but his response is "I'm glad it wasn't cancer. Maybe this happened to slow me down." He usually terminates such discussions by stating that he has to rest and suggests that the attending staff care for other patients "who are sicker" than he is.
   B. From the information given:
      1. List the possible stressors before and during hospitalization.
      2. Describe WJ's present coping mechanisms.
      3. While providing nursing care for WJ, identify stressors that the staff may experience.
      4. Write informative nursing notes regarding WJ's behavior.

SELF-TEST

1. State the purpose of a psychiatric assessment or determination of a person's mental health status.
2. List data obtained during a psychiatric assessment.
3. What is the term that describes overproductivity of talk characterized by verbal skipping of one idea to another?

4. Giving much unnecessary detail while speaking is referred to as what trait?

5. State the term that describes emitting the same verbal or motor response repeatedly to verbal stimuli.

6. What is the term for a sudden stoppage in the spontaneous flow of thought or speech for no apparent external or environmental reason?

7. Differentiate among the following thought processes:
Delusion of grandeur
Nihilistic delusion
Hallucination
Depersonalization
Obsession

8. Describe the following six levels or orientation and consciousness:
Confusion
Clouding of consciousness
Stupor
Delirium
Dream state
Coma

9. Explain the phrase *neurovegetative changes.*

10. State the purposes of assessment in addition to the evaluation of one's mental status.

11. State the criteria for charting psychiatric nurses' notes:

REFERENCES

American Psychiatric Association: A Psychiatric Glossary, 5th ed. Washington, DC, American Psychiatric Press, 1980

Barry PD: Psychosocial Nursing Assessment and Intervention. Philadelphia, JB Lippincott, 1984

Bell R, Hall, R: The mental status examination. Am Fam Practitioner: Nov 1977

Burgess AW: Psychiatric Nursing in the Hospital and the Community, 3rd ed. Englewood Cliffs, Prentice–Hall, 1981

Haber J et al: Comprehensive Psychiatric Nursing, 2nd ed. New York, McGraw–Hill, 1982

Harris E, Payne W: Mental status assessment. Am J Nurs: Aug, 1981

Kolb L: Modern Clinical Psychiatry. Philadelphia, WB Saunders, 1977

Lancaster J: Adult Psychiatric Nursing. Garden City, NJ, Medical Examination Publishing, 1980

Lucus MJ, Folstein MF: Nursing assessment of mental disorders on a general medical unit. J Psych Nurs: May 1980

Murray RB, Zentner JP: Nursing Assessment and Health Promotion Through the Life Span, 2nd ed. Englewood Cliffs, NJ, Prentice-Hall, 1979

Murray RB, Huelkskoetter MM: Psychiatric Mental Health Nursing: Giving Emotional Care. Englewood Cliffs, NJ, Prentice–Hall, 1983

Pasquali E et al: Mental Health Nursing: A bio-psycho-cultural Approach. St. Louis, CV Mosby, 1981

Reynolds, J, Logsden J: Assessing your patient's mental status. Nursing 79: Aug, 1979

Robinson L: Psychiatric Nursing as a Human Experience. Philadelphia, WB Saunders, 1983

Small, SM: Outline for Psychiatric Examination. East Hanover, Sandoz Pharmaceuticals, 1980

Snyder J, Wilson M: 10 Areas to Cover Any Psychological Assessment, Am J Nurs: Feb, 1977

Stuart G, Sundeen S: Principles and Practice of Psychiatric Nursing, 2nd ed. St. Louis, CV Mosby, 1983

Urdang L: Mosby's Medical and Nursing Dictionary. St. Louis, CV Mosby, 1983

Wilson HS, Kneisl C: Psychiatric Nursing, 2nd ed. Menlo Park, Addison–Wesley, 1983

12

COPING WITH ANXIETY

LEARNING OBJECTIVES

1. Define anxiety.
2. Differentiate between anxiety and fear.
3. Define the following terms:
   Signal anxiety
   Anxiety trait
   Anxiety state
   Free-floating anxiety
   Acute anxiety
   Chronic anxiety
4. Discuss factors that contribute to the development of anxiety disorders.
5. List the common symptoms of anxiety.
6. Compare the levels of anxiety.
7. Define phobic disorders.
8. Describe post-traumatic stress disorder.
9. Explain the supportive role of the nurse in dealing with anxiety.
10. Formulate a nursing care plan for a patient with a generalized anxiety disorder.

A STUDENT nurse had just completed the fundamentals course and was scheduled to begin her clinical laboratory experience. Her assignment was to care for a middle-aged patient with chronic obstructive pulmonary disease (COPD). The evening before her laboratory experience she was unable to sleep. In the early morning as she dressed for clinical laboratory she experienced dizziness, frequency of urination, abdominal cramping, and an increased heartbeat. When she arrived at the hospital and met with her instructor, the student nurse looked rather pale and was extremely quiet. During preconference the student shared her feelings and concerns with other students who were on the same clinical unit. With the help of the instructor, the student was able to discuss her "nervous" feelings and explore the reason for such a physiologic and emotional reaction. She was experiencing symptoms of anxiety or apprehension about the unknown (*i.e.,* her first clinical laboratory experience).

Have you ever experienced a "lump in your throat," sweaty palms, dizziness, frequency of urination, diarrhea, insomnia, restlessness, or the inability to concentrate for some unknown reason? These are but a few of the symptoms of anxiety that are felt by each of us at one time or another because we live in a fast-paced, stressful society.

The concept of anxiety was first introduced to psychological theory by Freud. He referred to it as a danger signal a person exhibits in response to the perception of physical pain or danger. The term *anxiety* is used to describe feelings of uncertainty, uneasiness, apprehension, or tension that a person experiences in response to an unknown object or situation. A "fight" or "flight" decision is made by the person in an attempt to over-come conflict, stress, trauma, or frustration.

Walker, in *Everybody's Guide to Emotional Well-being,* refers to anx-iety as "butterflies and nuisance," which can be constructive when pres-ent in a moderate degree because it increases one's alertness and ability to perform in a positive manner. Anxiety also can be a painful reaction to internal conflict as the conflict lingers and produces physical and emo-tional symptoms. People who exhibit symptoms of increased anxiety when unable to cope with existing conflict or frustration may develop an anxiety disorder.

Fear differs from anxiety in that it is the body's physiologic and emo-tional response to a known or recognized danger. A person whose car stalls on the railroad crossing experiences fear of injury or death while the train rapidly approaches on the track. The patient who undergoes an emer-gency exploratory surgery may be afraid of the surgery and develop symp-toms of anxiety because he is uncertain what the outcome will be.

TYPES AND SEVERITY OF ANXIETY

Types of anxiety are described as signal anxiety, anxiety trait, anxiety state, and free-floating anxiety. *Signal anxiety* is a response (anxiety) to an anticipated event. A mother who normally is relaxed exhibits tachy-cardia, dizziness, and insomnia when her child attends school for the first time; this is signal anxiety.

An *anxiety trait* is a component of one's personality that has been present over a long period of time and is measurable by observing the person's physiologic, emotional, and cognitive behavior. The person who responds to various nonstressful situations with anxiety is said to have an anxiety trait. For example, a 25-year-old secretary frequently complains of blurred vision, dizziness, headaches, and insomnia in a relatively stress-free job.

An *anxiety state* occurs as the result of a stressful situation in which the person loses control of his emotions. A mother who is told her son has been injured in a football game and has been taken to the emergecy room may exhibit an anxiety state by becoming hysterical, complaining of tightness in the chest, and insisting on seeing her injured son.

Free-floating anxiety is anxiety that is always present and accom-panied by a feeling of dread. The person may exhibit ritualistic and avoid-ance behavior (phobic behavior). A woman who is unable to sleep at night because she is certain someone will break into her home goes through a ritualistic behavior of checking all the windows and doors several times. She also avoids going out after dark because she fears coming home to a dark, empty home.

Severity of anxiety is described as normal, acute, chronic, and panic. Normal anxiety is anxiety that is present in a small degree, can motivate people, and is necessary for survival. Acute anxiety interferes with one's ability to think and is referred to as extreme nervousness. It usually occurs suddenly and lasts a short period of time. Chronic anxiety may be present over a period of months or years. The person appears to be stable but exhibits tremulous motor activity and rigid posture. Panic anxiety is a severe form of anxiety that causes disintegration of the personality, resulting in the inability to function normally. These categories of anxiety states are discussed under the classification of anxiety disorders later in this chapter.

ETIOLOGY

Theorists have classified causes of anxiety as stress, childhood conflicts, faulty learning, and social or cultural factors. Selye has written several books regarding the affect of stress on the body known as the stress adaptation syndrome or the general adaptation syndrome(GAS). Stress causes wear and tear on the body and requires some type of response or change in a person. These responses may be seen as adaptive or healing (positive) or maladaptive (negative), resulting in exhaustion and disintegration of the mind or body or both.

Stressors (factors that cause stress), can be physical, social, economical, chemical, psychological, or developmental, and can be classified as helpful (promoting positive change) or harmful (promoting negative change). A middle-aged man who receives an unexpected job promotion and an increase in salary (considered to be a positive stressor) can experience as much anxiety as a young woman who faces divorce proceedings (a negative stressor). Both persons may describe feelings of uncertainty about the future, uneasiness about the changes taking place in their lives, or tension that is present as they attempt to cope with or adapt to these changes. Initially, they will experience shock or an alarm reaction followed by a phase of increased resistance or adaptation to the stressors as they attempt to use various defense mechanisms. A state of adjustment and healing or of exhaustion and disintegration will then occur.

Freud states that unconscious conflicts of childhood, such as fear of losing a parent's love or attention, fear of losing security, competition with a parent of the same sex, resentment and anger, or the fear of being considered a "bad person," all may provide anxiety in childhood, adolescence, or early adulthood. An example of the development of a phobic disorder because of a threatened loss of security is given later in this chapter.

Response to a stressful event is often the result of learned or conditioned behavior. If a person, experiences too many life changes over a short period of time, he does not have enough time to adjust or condition himself to each change and may exhibit negative or maladaptive behavior.

Two people can react to the same stressful event with opposite responses. For example, college roommates both receive probationary notices because of failure to complete a required college course successfully. One student makes an appointment to discuss her grades with her advisor, whereas the other student is unable to sleep, complains of a headache, light-headedness, and shortness of breath. The first student has learned to be responsible for her actions and is seeking help, thereby showing a positive response to the stress of probationary action. The second student is exhibiting signs of anxiety. She is displaying a negative response to the stress of probationary action. As a child she may have had limited opportunity to condition herself to stress, her parents may have fostered dependency by making decisions for her, or this may be her first experience with what she considers to be a failure.

Theorists who believe social or cultural factors cause anxiety state that as a person's personality develops, his impression of self may be negative (low self-concept). He experiences difficulty adapting to everyday social problems owing to this low self-concept and inadequate coping mechanisms. The stressful stimuli of modern society pose a psychological threat for such a person and can result in the development of maladaptive behavior and the onset of an anxiety disorder. For example, a 19-year-old male who had difficulty maintaining a "C" average in high school and did not "fit in" with the crowd works as a delivery boy for a pizza company. As he makes a delivery he receives a traffic ticket for driving with a faulty muffler. The police officer informs him that if he has the defective muffler replaced within 24 hours he will not be fined. The young man makes an appointment to have his car fixed; however, his boss tells him he cannot allow him to take time off. The young man becomes tense, experiences feelings of dizziness, tachycardia, and shortness of breath as he responds to his employer's comment. Owing to inadequate coping mechanisms, he is unable to consider alternative options, such as asking the employer to use the company car for one day or suggesting that he change work schedules with another employee. His low self-concept prevents him from pointing out to his employer that he has been a faithful employee with a good work record, whose request should receive a special consideration owing to the nature of his problem. Unless this young man develops a positive self-concept and adequate coping mechanisms, he will continue to experience difficulty dealing with the stress of daily social or cultural problems.

CLINICAL SYMPTOMS

Clinical symptoms of anxiety are too numerous to list in detail. They are generally classified as physiologic, psychological or emotional, and intellectual or cognitive responses to stress. Some of the more common physiologic symptoms exhibited are

Elevated pulse and blood pressure

Dyspnea or hyperventilation

Diaphoresis

Vertigo or light-headedness

Blurred vision

Anorexia, nausea and vomiting

Frequency of urination

Headache

Insomnia or sleep disturbance

Weakness or muscle tension

Tightness in the chest

Sweaty palms

Psychological or emotional responses to anxiety include the following behaviors:

Restlessness

Withdrawal

Depression

Irritability

Crying

Lack of interest or apathy

Hypercriticism

Feelings of worthlessness

Intellectual or cognitive responses to anxiety include:

Decreased interest

Inability to concentrate

Nonresponsiveness to external stimuli

Decrease in productivity

Preoccupation

Forgetfulness

Symptoms of anxiety range from a state of euphoria to panic. A brief description of the four levels of anxiety follows.

LEVEL 0: EUPHORIA. This is an exaggerated feeling of well-being that is not directly proportionate to a specific circumstance or situation. Euphoria generally precedes the onset of level 1, mild anxiety.

LEVEL 1: MILD ANXIETY. This is an increased alertness to one's inner feelings or the environment. During this level the person has an increased ability to learn. Feelings or restlessness also may be present during this stage. The person experiences an inner "drivenness" and is unable to relax. He may or may not be able to identify the cause of this restlessness.

LEVEL 2: MODERATE ANXIETY. During this stage, a narrowing of the ability to perceive occurs. The person is able to focus or concentrate on only one specific thing. Pacing, voice tremors, increased rate of verbalization or talking, and physiologic changes such as those described earlier occur.

LEVEL 3: SEVERE ANXIETY. The ability to perceive is reduced, and focus is on small or scattered details. Inappropriate verbalization, or the inability to communicate clearly, occurs at this time owing to increased anxiety and decreased intellectual thought processes. Lack of determination or the ability to perform occurs as the person experiences feelings of purposelessness. Questions such as "What's the use?" or "Why bother?" may be voiced. Physiologic responses also occur at this time.

LEVEL 4: ANXIETY, PANIC STATE. There is complete disruption of the ability to perceive. Disintegration of the personality occurs as the individual becomes immobilized, experiences difficulty verbalizing and the inability to focus on reality. Physiological, emotional and intellectual changes occur.

Anxiety disorders are more prevalent during adolescence and young adulthood but may begin during childhood.

CLASSIFICATION OF ANXIETY DISORDERS

The term *neurosis* no longer is used as a separate DSM-III classification, although it is used as a descriptive term to differentiate clinical symptoms exhibited by people.

Neurosis is considered to be an emotional disturbance in which the person experiences increased subjective psychological pain or discomfort. As a result of stress the person handles anxiety or internal conflict in a maladaptive way, such as by developing a phobia or by experiencing a state of panic. Phobic disorder and anxiety disorder are two examples of the new DSM-III classification that still may be termed phobic neurosis and anxiety neurosis by some clinicians.

Neurosis is differentiated from psychosis in the following ways:

NEUROTIC BEHAVIOR	PSYCHOTIC BEHAVIOR
Reality oriented	Out of contact with reality or denies reality
Demonstrates socially acceptable behavior	Demonstrates bizarre, inappropriate behavior (as described in the chapters on schizophrenic disorders and manic–depressive psychosis)
Interacts with the real environment	Creates a new world or environment and withdraws from reality in an effort to seek security in the newly created world
Does not exhibit maladaptive behavior (e.g., hallucinations or delusions)	Exhibits maladaptive behaviors (e.g., delusions, hallucinations, and autism)
Uses coping mechanisms in an attempt to decrease anxiety (primary gain)	Coping mechanisms are ineffective, resulting in disintegration of one's personality

Primary gain is defined as the relief from emotional conflict and freedom from anxiety that a person achieves by means of the use of defense or coping mechanisms. A patient refuses to talk about her mastectomy because she becomes "anxious" when the surgery is discussed. She is using the defense mechanism of suppression to decrease her anxiety.

Secondary gain is any external gain derived from an illness, for example, attention, disability benefits, monetary gain, or the release from responsibliity. For example, a 25-year-old man injured his back while lifting crates at work a year ago. He asks the company physician to place him on sick leave to collect disability benefits because he feels that he has never recovered from the injury.

Subclassifications of anxiety disorders are phobic disorders (phobic neuroses), anxiety states (anxiety neuroses) and post-traumatic stress disorder.

Phobic Disorders (Phobic Neurosis)

Phobia is described as "an irrational fear" of an object, activity, or situation that is out of proportion to the stimulus and results in avoidance of the identified object, activity, or situation. The person has unconsciously displaced the original internal source of fear or anxiety, such as an unpleasant childhood experience, to an external source. Avoidance of the object or situation allows the person to remain free of anxiety.

Rowe (1984) cites that 2% to 3% of those persons who receive psychiatric care have phobias. This does not include occasional excessive fears seen in young children between ages 3 and 4. Confrontation with the phobic stimulus may result in one of the four degrees of anxiety discussed earlier in this chapter. Some categories of phobia include agoraphobia with or without panic attacks, social phobia, and simple phobia.

AGORAPHOBIA. This is described as a fear of being alone or in open or public places such as crowds, or tunnels, from which escape might be difficult. The person may or may not experience feelings or panic initially. As fear increases, they dominate the person's life and the person may become housebound and incapacitated. This disorder is seen more frequently in women.

SOCIAL PHOBIA. This is a compelling desire to avoid situations in which a person may be criticized by others. The person experiences persistent, irrational fear of criticism, humiliation, or embarrassment. The person does realize that the fear is excessive or disporportionate to the activity or situation. Social phobia rarely is incapacitating but may cause considerable inconvenience. The abuse of alcohol and drugs may occur as the person with social phobia attempts to reduce anxiety.

SIMPLE PHOBIA. This is the clinical category assigned to all other phobic reactions and is termed a residual category. Phobic objects are often animals, or situations (e.g., heights and closed spaces).

There are approximately 700 identified phobias. Some of the more common ones are

Acrophobia—fear of heights

Androphobia—fear of men

Astraphobia—fear of storms, lightning, thunder

Ceraunophobia   fear of thunder

Claustrophobia—fear of enclosed places

Hematophobia—fear of blood

Hydrophobia—fear of water

Iatrophobia—fear of doctors

Nyctophobia—fear of night

Ochlophobia—fear of crowds

Pyrophobia—fear of fire

Zoophobia—fear of animals

Reactions by student nurses caring for patient with phobic symptoms include comments such as "Why do people have such fears?", "How do fears develop?", "Can't the patient tell her fear is silly? Elevators can't hurt you," and "How did she survive, never leaving her house in five years? It must be terrible to experience so much fear that it controls your life!"

Phobic Disorder: Clinical Example

MS, 19 years old, was attending a movie when she began to perspire pro-fusely, tremble, breathe rapidly, and feel nauseated. She left the movie before it ended. Her symptoms became more common when she was around a group of people. As a result of these feelings, MS began to avoid crowds and her daily activity consisted of going to work and returning home immediately after work. Within a month MS became housebound. She attempted to relieve her anxiety by using alcohol to relax but did not experience any relief. MS was encouraged by her family to seek psychiatric help. Counseling revealed that she had been "lost" in a crowd as a child while attending a circus and had been separated from her parents for several hours. Recently she had moved into an apartment. The therapist explored her feelings about moving away from home. Memories of being separated from her parents as a child were identified as the underlying cause of her phobic reaction.

Anxiety States (Anxiety Neuroses)

Panic disorder, generalized anxiety disorder, and obsessive–compulsive disorder (obsessive–compulsive neurosis) are included in the subclassification of an anxiety neurosis.

PANIC DISORDER. The diagnostic criteria for this category include at least three anxiety (panic) attacks within a 3-week period that are not the result of severe physical exertion, a life-threatening situation, or exposure to a phobic stimulus. The person experiences sudden, overwhelming anxiety that produces a feeling of terror, with physiologic changes described earlier.

According to the DSM-III at least 4 of the following symptoms must be present to diagnose an anxiety or panic attack:

Dyspnea or shortness of breath

Palpitations

Chest pain or discomfort

Choking or smothering sensation

Vertigo or unsteady feelings

Diaphoresis

Feelings of unreality

Trembling or shaking

Syncope

Hot and cold flashes

Tingling in hands or feet (paresthesia)

Fear of losing control or dying

The above symptoms occur in the absence of a physical or mental disorder and are not associated with the phobic disorder, agoraphobia.

The onset of panic disorder generally is seen in late adolescence or early adult life. It may be an acute disorder lasting several weeks or months, reoccur several times, or become a chronic condition. Symptoms of panic disorder are seen more frequently in women than in men.

Panic Disorder: Clinical Example

MJ, a 21-year-old woman who lived in New York, just recently had become engaged to a Marine stationed in California. On three separate occasions, two weeks following her engagement, MJ had experienced episodes of dizziness, fainting, fatigue, chest pain, and choking sensations while at work. At the suggestion of her employer, she scheduled an appointment with her family physician to discuss her physical symptoms. After a negative physical examination, the family physician asked MJ if she was excited about her engagement. She hesitated at first, then stated that she loved her fiancé but was reluctant to leave her job, friends, and family to move to California. MJ was able to relate the onset of her symptoms to the time of her engagement. The family physician helped MJ to explore feelings of ambivalence about her engagement and suggested that she seek the help of a therapist. After several weeks of counseling, the panic attacks subsided and she was able to discuss her feelings with her fiancé.

GENERALIZED ANXIETY DISORDER. This disorder is characterized by at least one month's duration of generalized anxiety in the absence of panic attacks, disorders, depression, or other psychiatric disorders.

The DSM-III classifies the symptoms according to four categories. They include

Motor tension, such as muscle aches, inability to relax, fidgeting, restlessness, and being easily startled

Autonomic hyperactivity, including cold and clammy hands, dry mouth, dizziness, frequent urination, flushing, increased pulse rate while resting, and upset stomach

Apprehensive expectation, including symptoms such as anxiety, worry or fear

Vigilance and scanning, a state in which the person is hyperactive, easily distracted, has difficulty concentrating, experiences insomnia, and is irritable or impatient

The person experiencing a generalized anxiety disorder may be mildly depressed. Symptoms rarely interfere with social or occupational functioning.

Generalized Anxiety Disorder: Clinical Example

A 50-year-old woman was admitted to the psychiatric hospital for treatment of a generalized anxiety disorder. As the student nurse completed the initial assessment form, she noted that the patient was quite restless, sitting on the edge of her bed and fidgeting with her gown. She constantly rearranged her personal items on the bedside stand. Complaints of dizziness, an upset stomach, insomnia, and frequency of urination were noted. She appeared to be easily distracted as various people walked into the room to care for another patient and was rather impatient with the student nurse as she took the admitting vital signs. The patient's hands were cold and clammy and the radial pulse was 120 while the patient sat on the edge of her bed.

During clinical postconference the student nurse shared her feelings of irritation about the patient. She also stated that the patient's anxiety was "infectious" and that she found herself becoming tense although she tried to remain calm during the admission procedure. Another student stated that she would have given the patient a sedative first to allow her to settle down and then would have attempted to carry out the initial assessment. The group discussed interpersonal reactions with persons who exhibit clinical symptoms of generalized anxiety and how easy it would be to avoid such behavior deliberately.

OBSESSIVE–COMPULSIVE DISORDER (OBSESSIVE–COMPULSIVE NEUROSIS). This disorder is characterized by two main clinical features, namely, recurrent obsessions or compulsions (or a combination of both).

An *obsession* is a persistant, painful, intrusive thought, emotion, or urge that one is unable to suppress or ignore. Common obsessive thoughts include topics such as religion, sexuality, violence, and contamination.

We have all experienced recurrent thoughts at one time or another. Lines of a song or poem may invade one's thoughts and continually run through one's mind. "I just can't seem to get this name off my mind", or "His words keep coming back to haunt me" are statements made by persons experiencing recurrent thoughts. The difference is that obsessions are not produced voluntarily. They are considered senseless or repugnant, and they can not be eliminated by logic or reasoning. A repetitive thought of killing one's mate is an example of a violent obsession.

A *compulsion* is the performance of a repetitious, uncontrollable but seemingly purposeful act to prevent some future event or situation. Resistance to the act increases anxiety. Yielding to the compulsion decreases anxiety (primary gain). The person is aware of the senselessness of the behavior and does not derive pleasure from performing the act. Examples include repetitive touching, counting, checking, and handwashing; such actions are not uncommon in children and adolescents.

Some people perform various rituals in the same sequence and these have become a part of their daily routine. Washing clothes on Monday, ironing on Tuesday, shopping for groceries on Wednesday, and so forth, is an example of a weekly ritual. Getting up at the same hour each morning and following the same routine of showering, eating breakfast, and dressing is considered a daily routine. Leaving the house and returning to see if the gas burner is turned off or the door is locked is obsessive–compulsive behavior; however, normally it is not done to decrease anxiety and is not considered uncontrollable behavior.

The DSM-III lists features such as depression, phobic avoidance and impaired social or role functioning as being present in patients with an obsessive–compulsive disorder.

Obsessive–Compulsive Disorder: Clinical Example

AY, a 56-year-old patient, was observed performing the following ritualistic behavior continuously. The only time she would interrupt the activity was to go to the patient's dining room for meals, attend to personal hygiene at the insistence of the staff, and to sleep. AY would begin by standing at the nurses' station for a few moments, mumbling incoherently at the staff, and then continue by starting on a ritualistic pathway. As she left the nurses' station she would walk ten steps to the right, touch the wall with her right hand, flicker the light switch, and then proceed to her next objective approximately twenty steps away. There she would touch another wall, do a 360° turn, and again mumble a few incoherent words. She then headed back to the nurses' station, repeating the behavior on the opposite side of the room. If there were any intrusions during this ritualistic performance, AY would exhibit signs of extreme anxiety. Needless to say, this behavior dominated her life and interfered with her role and social functioning.

Students who observed AY were amazed at the energy she possessed since she never seemed to tire. They were hesitant to approach her during this ritualistic activity because they were uncertain what she might do. One student stated,"I know this sounds foolish, but I'm afraid she might get upset and become hostile toward me." Another student said she felt foolish trying to walk with AY as she attempted to show AY she wanted to help her and be with her. A third student observed that the behavior was accepted by other patients on the unit and that no one seemed to interrupt AY.

Post-traumatic Stress Disorder (Traumatic Neurosis)

The DSM-III reserves this category for persons who experience a psychological traumatic event that is considered to be outside the realm of usual human experience. Examples include rape or assault, military combat, natural disasters, serious physical injury as a result of a catastrophic event such as a fire, and torture. Vietnam War veterans have been one of the largest groups of persons to exhibit symptoms of this disorder.

Diagnostic criteria are as follows:

The existence of an identifiable stressor that would cause almost anyone to exhibit symptoms of distress (i.e., rape or torture).

Reliving the traumatic event by experiencing recurrent and intrusive recollections of each detail, recurrent dreams or nightmares, or suddenly responding as if the traumatic event were reoccurring.

Exhibiting a reduced involvement with or minimal responsiveness to external stimuli for some time after the original traumatic event. The person shows a markedly decreased interest in significant activities, experiences feelings of detachment or estrangement from others, or is unable to feel emotions of any type. He has difficulty relating to others.

At least two of the following symptoms did not exist prior to the traumatic event: hyperalertness or startle response, insomnia, guilt feelings about having survived the experience, guilt feelings about behavior that was required to survive, difficulty concentrating or impaired memory, avoidance of any activity that might cause the person to recall the traumatic event, and experiencing intense symptoms when exposed to any event that resembles the original traumatic event.

These symptoms may occur immediately after the traumatic event, soon after, or emerge years later. The diagnosis of acute subtype is used if the onset of symptoms is within 6 months of the trauma and they do not last more than 6 months. The diagnosis chronic or delayed subtype is used if symptoms occur more than 6 months after the trauma or last over 6 months. Impaired role and social functioning may occur, as well as interference with occupational and recreational functioning. Low self-concept and suicidal ideation or thoughts may occur, along with substance abuse because the individual has difficulty coping with the recollections of the traumatic experience.

Post-traumatic Stress Disorder: Clinical Examples

KW, a 35-year-old accountant, and his 5-year-old son were visiting his wife's family in Chicago when an electrical storm occurred during the early morning hours. KW awakened about 3:00 AM when he heard the loud crackling sound of fire in the hallway outside his second-floor bedroom.

He attempted to reach his son, who was also sleeping on the second floor, but was driven back by the intense heat and smoke. KW managed to escape from the second story by climbing down an outdoor television antenna. He immediately attempted to enter the front door of the house in another effort to reach his son and in-laws who where calling for help. He was unable to climb the stairway, which was engulfed in fire. When the fire department arrived, the firemen were able to revive KW's mother-in-law but her husband and grandson had been burned severely and died of smoke inhalation. KW's wife arrived shortly after she received the news of the fire. As she and her husband slept in their motel room, he began to have nightmares about the fire and yelled out several times in his sleep. These nightmares recurred nightly for several months and began to interfere with KW's daily life. He repeatedly told his wife that he should have died instead of their son and his father-in-law. KW eventually was seen by a counselor, who was able to help him explore his feelings of guilt about having survived the fire.

Two student nurses had the opportunity to care for a Vietnam War veteran who was hospitalized for emergency surgery. During the initial assessment the patient revealed that he had tried marijuana and other drugs to help him forget some of the experiences he had had. He also stated he had expected a warm welcome when he returned to the United States but was shocked to find he was considered a murderer. His wife, who was present during the interview, stated that she learned very quickly not to awaken him from a deep sleep as he was "on guard" all the time and had "thrown a few punches." He also talked in his sleep frequently. The patient was somewhat bitter when he related that he had been unable to find a job since his discharge from the service. He stated, "Not only do I have horrible nightmares about Vietnam, but I am beginning to question my future as a human being."

The students stated that they felt helpless as they listened to the patient's feelings of rejection, hopelessness about the future, and anger toward those people who labeled him a murderer. During postconference they explored various interventions to help decrease the patient's anxiety and increase his self-esteem.

Atypical Anxiety Disorder

The atypical category is a catchall for persons who exhibit signs of an anxiety disorder but do not meet criteria for any of the previously described conditions listed in this classification.

TREATMENT OF ANXIETY DISORDERS

Learning to cope with and decrease anxiety by identifying the underlying conflict or frustration and by verbalizing concerns is a goal in the treatment of anxiety. Various techniques are used; the selection of a specific therapy depends on the particular situation.

Relaxation therapies or techniques have become quite popular because they can be used as therapeutic interventions in a variety of situations. Examples of relaxation techniques include:

1. *Visual imagery:* Use of relaxation along with the creation of a mental image. This technique has been used effectively to reduce anxiety exprienced by cancer patients. As the patient relaxes he engages in a fantasy in which he visualizes the identified cause of anxiety, such as pain due to cancer or the cancer itself. A person who has an unresolved conflict, such as not attending the funeral of a loved one, could utilize this technique in an attempt to work through guilt feelings or unresolved grief.

2. *Change of pace or scenery:* Helps to remove oneself from the source or cause of stress. A walk in the woods or along the beach, listening to music, caring for a pet, or engaging in a hobby are examples of ways to change pace or scenery in an attempt to decrease anxiety.

3. *Exercise or massage:* Exercise can be a release or outlet for pent-up tension or anxiety. Massage is soothing and helps to relax one's muscles. Expectant mothers who practice the Lamaze technique for prepared childbirth use effleurage, or a massage of the abdominal muscles during uterine contractions, to promote relaxation.

4. *Transcendental meditation:* Four components of this relaxation technique include a quiet environment, a passive state of mind, a comfortable position, and the ability to focus on a specific word or object. Physiologic, psychological, and spiritual relaxation occur.

5. *Biofeedback:* The person is able to monitor various physiologic processes by auditory or visual signals. This technique has proven effective in the management of conditions such as migraine headaches, essential hypertension, and pain that is the result of increased stress and anxiety.

6. *Systematic desensitization:* Simply stated, this technique refers to the exposure of a person to a fear-producing situation in a systematized manner to decrease a phobic disorder. A behavioral therapist usually works with the person.

7. *Relaxation exercise:* Various methods are used to help people to learn to relax. The common steps to relaxation include taking a deep breath and exhaling (similar to the cleansing or relaxing breath of Lamaze technique), tensing and then relaxing individual muscles, starting with the head and progressing to the toes, and finally relaxing all parts of the body simultaneously. Some methods suggest that the person imagine a peaceful scene before doing the exercise.

8. *Therapeutic touch or "laying on of hands":* This technique is controversial and has not been accepted completely by the helping profes-

sions. Vivid examples are cited in the Bible, and faith healers use this technique.

9. *Hypnosis:* Some behavioral therapists use hypnosis to enhance relaxation or imagery. People have been taught self-hypnosis to decrease anxiety.

Other techniques used to treat anxiety include behavioral modification, psychoanalysis, group therapy, family therapy, insight psychotherapy, and environmental modification. These are discussed in Chapter 5.

Minor tranquilizers or anitanxiety agents (e.g., Valium, Serax, or Tranxene) may be prescribed; however, many therapists feel that these agents should be for short-term use only. Sedative-hypnotics (e.g., Placidyl or Doriden) may be prescribed to alleviate insomnia. Antidepressants (e.g., Elavil or Asendin) may be used when depression is seen as an associated feature in an anxiety disorder.

NURSING INTERVENTION

People who exhibit signs of acute anxiety or a panic state may harm themselves or others and need to be supervised closely until the anxiety is decreased. The person may need to be placed in a protective environment such as a general hospital, mental health center, or psychiatric hospital.

The person may be in severe distress or immobilized, or he may be engaged in purposeless, disorganized, or aggressive activity. Feelings of intense awe, dread, or terror may occur. The patient may state he fears that he is "losing control."

After the patient is examined, a nursing care plan is initiated to correspond with the physician's or psychiatrist's treatment plan for an acute anxiety attack or panic state.

During the panic state the nursing interventions include:

1. Staying with the patient at all times.

2. Remaining calm. The patient will sense any anxiety exhibited by the nurse.

3. Speaking in short, simple sentences.

4. Displaying firmness to provide external controls for the patient.

5. Keeping the patient in a quiet environment to minimize external stimuli. The patient is unable to screen such stimuli and may become overwhelmed.

6. Providing protective care because the patient may harm himself or others. The patient's behavior also may elicit responses from other patients, who are unable to tolerate his anxiety state.

7. Attempting to channel the patient's behavior by engaging him in physical activities that provide an outlet for tension or frustration.

8. Administering anti-anxiety medication to decrease anxiety.

Persons who exhibit symptoms of mild to moderate levels of anxiety may be treated as outpatients. If the anxiety does not interfere with the patient's ability to function, he generally is seen as an outpatient.

Nursing interventions for mild-to-moderate anxiety levels include assessment of the patient's anxiety level, reducing anxiety, providing protective care, encouraging verbalization of anxiety, meeting basic human needs and setting realistic goals for patient care.

The nurse provides supportive care by

1. Recognizing the patient's anxiety. Help him identify the anxiety and describe his feelings.

2. Reassuring the patient

3. Accepting the patient unconditionally. Do not pass judgment or respond emotionally to the patient's behavior.

4. Listening to the patient's concerns. Be available but respect the patient's need for personal space.

5. Protecting the patient's defenses (e.g., ritualistic behavior). Any attempt to stop such behavior increases anxiety because he has no other defenses.

6. Encouraging verbalization of feelings. Answer questions directly.

7. Allowing the patient time to respond to nursing interventions. Set realistic goals for improvement. Allow the patient to set the pace.

8. Exploring alternative coping mechanisms to decrease present anxiety to a manageable level. Assist the patient in learning to cope with anxiety.

9. Identifying the patient's development stage and helping the patient to work through unmet developmental tasks.

10. Exploring one's own feelings

11. Administering treatments or medications to reduce anxiety or other discomfort

Hospitalization of the patient with an anxiety disorder may be short-term and intensive. Outpatient follow-up care usually is recommended to continue with supportive therapeutic care. Discharge planning will include an evaluation of the patient's present status, recommendations for outpatient referral, and instructions regarding drug therapy if a maintenance dose is necessary. The patient should be instructed about whom to contact if anxiety increases and panic or a crisis occurs.

The following are examples of nursing diagnoses and nursing interventions for patients with anxiety disorders:

NURSING DIAGNOSES	NURSING INTERVENTIONS
Anxiety	Assess the patient's level of anxiety. Nursing interventions for the panic state and mild to moderate anxiety were covered in depth earlier in this chapter. Assess for suicidal ideation.
Ineffective individual coping; obsessive–compulsive, ritualistic behavior	Remove patient from any situation that stimulates or increases behavior. Observe for signs of increasing anxiety and intervene before the patient resorts to ritualistic behavior. Establish trust and one-to-one relationship. Anticipate needs. Seek out and spend time with the patient. Discuss thoughts and behavior with the patient. Explore conflicts in relation to ritualistic behavior. Allow time for rituals. Set priorities and time for other tasks to be done (i.e., eating, chores, and personal hygiene). Protect the patient from ridicule. Encourage the patient to explore and develop new interests outside self. Seek opportunities to communicate your expectation of the patient's recovery. Encourage the patient to participate in planning activities after allowing time for ritualistic behavior to decrease. Support any positive decisions made by the patient. Plan diversional activities.
Alteration in thought process: Inability to concentrate	Encourage patient to share feelings. Speak concisely and clearly. Reassure the patient. Be readily available. Keep decision making and competitive situations to a minimum.
Ineffective individual coping: Demanding, manipulative behavior such as crying and talking excessively because of anxiety	Interpret behavior as a need for attention or pleas for help. Be alert to what the patient is trying to say and help the patient communicate more clearly. Anticipate needs. Don't give false, generalized reassurance such as "everything will be fine" or "there's nothing to worry about".

NURSING DIAGNOSES	NURSING INTERVENTIONS
Dysrhythm of sleep–rest activity: Insomnia due to anxiety	Recognize signs of increasing agitation. Decrease environmental stimuli that could be upsetting to the patient. Offer relaxing nursing measures such as back-rubs and warm bath. Teach relaxation exercises. Limit rest periods during the day.
Ineffective individual coping: Numerous somatic complaints due to anxiety	Avoid reinforcing physical complaints (e.g., taking vital signs frequently increases preoccupation with symptoms). Present reality regarding physical condition. Encourage participation in activities that provide distraction and an outlet for tension or anxiety and increase self-esteem. Identify activities that the patient enjoys and encourage participation to decrease the patient's self-absorbing thoughts.

SUMMARY

Anxiety is defined as feelings of uncertainty, uneasiness, apprehension or tension that a person experiences in response to an unknown object or situation. It is differentiated from fear, which is the body's physiologic and emotional response to a known or recognized danger. Clinical symptoms of anxiety may be manifested in physiologic, emotional, or intellectual (cognitive) responses. The types, severity, levels, and etiology of anxiety were discussed. A differention of neutotic and psychotic behavior was presented. The clinical symptoms of the DSM-III classifications of anxiety disorders were discussed, including phobic disorders, anxiety states, post-traumatic stress disorders, and atypical anxiety disorders. Treatment of anxiety disorders, focusing on relaxation techniques, various types of psychotherapy, behavioral and environmental modification, and psychotropic drug therapy, was included. Nursing diagnoses and interventions focusing on anxiety, ineffective individual coping, alteration in thought process and dysrhythm of sleep–rest activity were discussed.

LEARNING ACTIVITIES

I. Clinical activities
   A. Care for a patient exhibiting clinical symptoms of anxiety.
   B. Describe symptoms of anxiety exhibited by the patient.
   C. Identify the level of anxiety being experienced by the patient.

   D. Identify coping mechanisms used in an attempt to decrease anxiety.
   E. Identify any situation or event that increases the patient's anxiety.
   F. Discuss the nursing interventions used to decrease the patient's anxiety.
II. Case study: Generalized anxiety disorder

   A 24-year-old female patient was admitted to the hospital with complaints of dyspnea, chest pain, rapid pulse, and a feeling of "something stuck in her throat." The tentative diagnosis was acute respiratory infection.
   While caring for the patient, the student nurse was able to assess the patient's behavior and discussed various aspects of the woman's home life. The patient related feelings of a low self-concept and stated that she felt depressed at times as she attempted to work full-time and care for an invalid mother who lived with her. Nonverbal behavior included fingering the sheets as she talked, clearing her throat frequently, and shaking her right foot as she sat in the chair with her legs crossed.

   1. Identify the symptoms of a generalized anxiety disorder exhibited by the patient.
   2. Develop a nursing care plan listing the nursing diagnosis and nursing interventions appropriate for this patient.
III. Independent activities
   A. Select a television program that portrays stressful situations and discuss the reactions of the various actors and actresses.
   B. In a clinical agency emergency room, identify various stressful situations and discuss specific interventions that were employed to reduce stress.
   C. Describe your nonverbal behaviors and physical symptoms experienced in your last stressful situation. How do you usually cope with situations? What changes could you make to cope more effectively?

SELF-TEST

   1. List examples of responses to stress in each of the following categories:
   Physiologic responses
   Psychological or emotional responses
   Intellectual or cognitive responses

   2. Differentiate among the levels of anxiety:
   Euphoria
   Mild anxiety
   Moderate anxiety

Severe anxiety
Anxiety, panic state

3. List three causative factors (etiology) of anxiety and cite an example of each causative factor.

4. Define the following terms:
Signal anxiety
Anxiety trait
Anxiety state
Free-floating anxiety

5. Differentaite between a panic disorder and a generalized anxiety disorder.

6. Define obsession and state an example.

7. State an example of compulsive behavior and explain the purpose that it serves.

8. Define phobia and list three examples.

9. Explain why Vietnam War veterans may develop a post-traumatic stress disorder.

REFERENCES

Basic Systems: Anxiety recognition and intervention: Programmed instruction. Am J Nurs: Sept, 1965

Bayer M: The multipurpose room: A way-out outlet of staff and clients. J Psych Nurs: Oct, 1980

Benson H: The Relaxation Response. Boston, Little, Brown, & Co, 1975

Billings CV: Providing better emergency care when behaviors bar the way. Nursing 82: May, 1982

Brallier L: Successfully Managing Stress. Los Altos, CA, National Nursing Review, 1982

Brown B: Stress and the Art of Biofeedback. New York, Harper & Row, 1977

Burgess A: Psychiatric Nursing in the Hospital and the Community. 3rd ed. Englewood Cliffs, NJ, Prentice–Hall, 1981

Ciuca et al: When a disaster happens, how do you meet emotional needs? Am J Nurs: Mar, 1977

Cox T: Stress. Baltimore, University Park Press, 1978

Dean P: The neurotic process: An overview and its application to nursing. J Psych Nurs: Oct, 1979

Donahue: Anxiety Attacks: Causes and Cures. Vogue: March, 1982

Donlon P, Rockwell D: Psychiatric Disorders: Diagnosis and Treatment. Bowie, IN, Robert Brady Co, 1982

Elliott SM: Denial as an effective mechanism to allay anxiety following a stressful event. J Psych Nurs: Oct, 1980

Faan WE, Goshen, CE: The Language of Mental Health, 2nd ed. St. Louis, CV Mosby, 1977

Freedman, Kaplan, Sadock: Comprehensive Textbook of Psychiatry. Baltimore, Williams & Wilkins, 1975

Haber J et al: Comprehensive Psychiatric Nursing. New York, McGraw–Hill, 1982

Hagerty BD: Obsessive–compulsive behavior: An overview of four psychological frameworks. J Psych Nurs: Jan, 1981

Hopping, B: Physiological response to stress. Nurs Forum XIX, (3): 1980

Introduction to Psychiatric Nursing (film). Philadelphia, JB Lippincott Audiovisual Program, 1977

Knowles RD: Dealing with feelings: Overcoming guilt and worry. Am J Nurs: Sept, 1981

Kolb L: Modern Clinical Psychiatry. Philadelphia, WB Saunders, 1977

Lancaster J: Adult Psychiatric Nursing. Garden City NJ, Medical Examination Publishing, 1980

Mereness D, Taylor C: Essentials of Psychiatric Nursing. St. Louis, CV Mosby, 1982

Murray R, Huelskoetter MM: Psychiatric/Mental Health Nursing: Giving Emotional Care. Englewood Cliffs, NJ, Prentice–Hall, 1983

Peplau HE: Interpersonal Relations in Nursing. New York, GP Putnam & Sons, 1952

Rector C: The Concept of Anxiety and Nursing Intervention (film). Atlanta, GA, Colonial

Roberts S: Behavioral Concepts and Nursing Throughout the Lifespan. Englewood Cliffs, Prentice-Hall, Inc, 1978

Robinson L: Psychiatric Nursing As a Human Experience. Philadephia, WB Saunders, 1983

Rowe CJ: An Outline of Psychiatry. Dubuque, William Brown, 1984

Schultz J, Dark S: Manual of Psychiatric Nursing Care Plans. Boston, Little, Brown & Co, 1982

Seyle H: Stress Without Distress. New York, The New American Library, 1974

Seyle H: The Stress of Life. New York, McGraw–Hill, 1956

Sills G, Wise D: Anxiety concept and manifestation (film). American Journal of Nursing Company

Smith N, Seyle H: Reducing the negative effects of stress. Am J Nurs: Nov, 1979

Stress: A Blue Print for Health (pamphlet). Chicago, Blue Cross Association, 1974

Stuart G, Sundeen S: Principles and Practice of Psychiatric Nursing. St. Louis, CV Mosby, 1983

Walker JI: Everybody's Guide to Emotional Well-Being. San Francisco Harbor Publishing, 1982

Walsh MJ: An affair of the heart. Nursing 78: Sept. 1978

Weekes C: The reassuring truth about anxiety attacks. New Woman Magazine: Apr, 1983

Williams T(ed): Post-traumatic stress disorder in Vietnam veterans. Am J Nurs: Nov, 1982

Wilson H, Kneisl C: Psychiatric Nursing. Menlo Park, Addison–Wesley, 1983

13

MALADAPTIVE ADJUSTMENT

TO IDENTIFIABLE STRESS

Learning Objectives

1. Define adjustment disorder.
2. Describe the subtypes of adjustment disorder according to DSM-III.
3. Cite examples of adjustment disorders during
   Childhood
   Adolescence
   Young adulthood
   Middle adulthood
   Later maturity or adulthood
4. Describe the treatment approach for a person experiencing an adjustment disorder.

A N adjustment disorder is a classification differentiated from other disorders in that the maladaptive reaction is in response to an identifiable event or situation that is stress producing and is not the result of or part of a mental disorder. The reaction generally occurs within 3 months after the onset of the stressor, manifests itself as impaired social or occupational functioning, and is exaggerated beyond the normal reaction to an identified stressor. Remission of the reaction generally occurs as the stressor diminishes or disappears.

The DSM-III lists 8 subtypes that describe an adjustment reaction to a single or multiple psychosocial stressors. The behavioral manifestations include adjustment disorder with:

1. Depressed mood (includes tearfulness and hopelessness)

2. Anxious mood (includes nervousness, worry, and jitteriness)

3. Mixed emotional features (includes combinations of depression, anxiety, or other emotions)

4. Disturbance of conduct (includes violation of rights of others or age-appropriate societal norms and rules)

5. Mixed disturbance of emotions and conduct

6. Work or academic inhibition (occurs in a person whose previous work or academic record was adequate)

7. Withdrawal (such as social withdrawal without significant anxious or depressed moods)

8. Atypical features (unable to code in any of the specific categories)

The DSM-III also describes or rates the severity of psychosocial stressors that have a significant impact on the development of an adjustment disorder. They are rated as minimal, mild, moderate, severe, extreme, catastrophic, or unspecified. The rating is based on how the "average" person who is in similar circumstances with similar sociocultural values would react to a specific stressor. The rating takes into consideration 1) the amount of change caused by the stressor; 2) the degree to which the event is desired and under control of the person; and 3) the number of stressors present (DSM-III, 1980, p. 26). Types of stressors considered include natural or man-made disasters; unwanted pregnancy; physical illness or injury; developmental (*e.g.,* puberty, adolescence, or menopause); legal (*e.g.,* being arrested or incarcerated); financial problems; living circumstances (*e.g.,* change in residence or immigration); occupational (*e.g.,* unemployment or retirement); conjugal (*e.g.,* separation or death of a spouse); parenting (*e.g.,* becoming a parent); and interpersonal problems (relating to one's friends, neighbors, or associates). A review of Erikson's eight developmental stages or Havinghurst's six periods of development is suggested to help one to identify anticipated transitions and resulting conflicts or stressors that can occur at various times in life.

Young children are considered quite vulnerable to stressors because of limited coping abilities and the fact that they are dependent on their environment. Vacationing with the family, starting school, or changing teachers are considered minimal-to-mild stressors, whereas the divorce of parents, hospitalization, death of a peer, or a geographical move could be considered severe stressors. Examples of extreme stress in children include repeated physical or sexual abuse, or the death of a parent.

Adolescence has received attention as one of the most difficult adjustment periods. Breaking up with a steady significant other, being "cut" from a sport, death of a peer, or leaving home for the first time are examples of stressors experienced during adolescence, any of which may result in adjustment disorders. When the adolescent receives support during this developmental period, the likelihood of the onset of additional emotional disturbances would be lessened.

During adulthood, young adults (ages 20–40) face a number of new experiences and changes in life-style. Decision making generally focuses on education, employment, marriage, and social responsibilities. Dropping out of college, breaking an engagement, the death of a close friend, losing a job, the death of a child, or beginning employment are examples of stressors that may be difficult for a young adult to face. Middle adulthood (ages 41–64) generally focuses on rearing teenage children, adjusting to physiologic changes of middle age, relating to one's significant other as a person, and caring for aging parents. Such persons are generally productive and creative for themselves and others. Psychosocial stressors that could lead to adjustment disorders at this time include placing one's parents in a nursing home, experiencing the death of a spouse or child, experiencing the "empty nest" syndrome as grown children leave home, a major financial loss, or recognizing the fact that both marriage partners have drifted apart and suddenly have nothing in common. Later, maturity or adulthood (ages 65 and older) is a period of time when one may experience decreasing physical health and strength, retirement from work, or the death of a spouse or significant other. Such situations could produce stress resulting in depression, anxiety, withdrawal, or other features associated with an adjustment disorder.

TREATMENT AND NURSING INTERVENTION

Early detection of symptoms and identification of stressors play an important part in the treatment of adjustment disorders. An assessment by a member of the health team may be all that is necessary to help the patient or significant others identify the source of stress, appropriate coping mechanisms, and situational supports. (Crisis intervention is discussed in a separate chapter.)

The stressor should be evaluated to determine whether it is a time-limited situation that will diminish or disappear; the person should be encouraged to explore any exaggerated responses or impairment of social or occupational behavior owing to stress; and previous and alternative methods of adaptation to the identified stressor should be explored. Previous coping mechanisms may be strengthened as a result of such action.

Behaviors generally seen when major life changes or the culmination of several smaller stressors result in an adjustment disorder include the inability to handle the current situation emotionally, feelings of being overwhelmed, difficulty adapting to change, loss of control during the situation, or difficulty effecting problem-solving strategies.

Short-term goals during hospitalization generally focus on establishing rapport; identifying difficulties associated with the current life change or stress; decreasing feelings such as fear, anxiety, or depression; and helping the patient meet basic human needs.

Adjustment Disorder With Depressed Mood

The following is a clinical example of an adjustment disorder with depressed mood. AL, a 58-year-old housewife, was seen in the physician's office with symptoms of depression. During the interview she stated that she and her husband had moved from New York to Florida 6 months ago after his early retirement as an executive with a major department store. Although she did not want to leave her family and friends behind, she agreed to move because her husband wanted to play golf, go boating, and enjoy other year-round activities. Since the move she has become housebound because of a lack of friends and activities to attend. Although her husband was enjoying his retirement, she felt "lost, lonely, and isolated." When asked what she would like to do, the woman said, "Move back to all my family and friends in New York." She was exhibiting symptoms of an adjustment disorder owing to an unwanted move from her friends and family. The following are examples of nursing diagnoses and nursing interventions for AL.

NURSING DIAGNOSES	NURSING INTERVENTIONS
Anxiety due to change in environment by moving away from family and friends	Assess the patient's level of anxiety. Listen to the patient's concerns. Encourage verbalization of feelings. Explore past and present coping mechanisms to decrease the present anxiety to a manageable level. Administer prescribed medication to reduce anxiety or feelings of depression.
Ineffective individual coping related to depression in response to moving	Accept the patient. Assess the degree of depression and suicidal ideation (see chapter on suicidal behavior). Display empathy. Encourage ventilation of feelings regarding change of environment. Explore methods of coping with the change of environment including communication with family, socialization, and establishment of independence. Assist with grief work pertaining to loss, that is, move from family and friends.
Ineffective individual coping due to an unwanted relocation resulting in loneliness	Explore the reason for feelings of loneliness. Seek out the patient and spend time with him on a regularly scheduled basis. Assess the developmental level of the patient by referring to Erikson's, Havinghurst's, or Piaget's theories of personality development. Encourage verbalization of feelings. Promote age-appropriate independent thinking and actions whenever possible. Explore ways to increase socialization and decrease feelings of loneliness. Encourage involvement in group activities.

Summary

Adjustment disorders may occur in children as well as adults and are the result of an identifiable event or situation that is stress producing but not the result or part of a mental disorder. The DSM-III criteria and seven subtypes of adjustment disorders are described in this chapter, as are the classification and examples of psychosocial stressors affecting children and adults. Early detection of symptoms and identification of stressors were stressed as integral parts of the treatment plan. Behaviors generally seen in major life changes or during the culmination of several small stressors were discussed. Short-term goals during hospitalization were stated. Examples of nursing diagnoses and nursing interventions for an adult with an adjustment disorder with depressed mood because of moving away from family and friends were cited.

LEARNING ACTIVITIES

I. Clinical activities
  A. Care for a patient with an adjustment disorder.
     1. Identify the source(s) and duration of stressor(s) experienced by the patient.
     2. Assess the patient's past and present coping mechanisms.
     3. Identify positive coping mechanisms and situational supports (refer to Chapter 9 for additional information).
     4. Develop short-term goals appropriate for this patient.
     5. State nursing diagnoses and interventions based on the patient's behavioral symptoms.
     6. Discuss those stressors and appropriate supportive nursing interventions during clinical conference.
  B. Identify in your clinical facility a list of agencies available as support systems to persons who exhibit symptoms of adjustment disorders.
II. Independent activities
  A. Contact a support agency to arrange an observational visit or volunteer your services for a day.
  B. With the help of your fellow classmates, arrange a Community Resources Day during which speakers share information about their helping agencies (i.e., Salvation Army, Meals-on-Wheels, Legal Aid Society, and Public Health).

SELF-TEST

1. State the characteristics of an adjustment disorder.

2. Describe behavioral manifestations that may occur during an adjustment disorder.

3. State stressors in each of the following developmental levels that may occur during an adjustment disorder:
    Childhood
    Adolescence
    Young adulthood
    Middle adulthood
    Later maturity or adulthood

4. List nursing interventions appropriate for a 60-year-old male who has been forced by his employer to take an "early retirement" and exhibits symptoms of anxiety and depression.

REFERENCES

Barker P: Basic Child Psychiatry, 4th ed. Baltimore, University Park Press, 1983

Carpenito LJ: Nursing Diagnoses: Application to Clinical Practice. Philadelphia, JB Lippincott, 1983

Haber J et al: Comprehensive Psychiatric Nursing, 2nd ed. New York, McGraw–Hill, 1982

Kolb L: Modern Clinical Psychiatry. Philadelphia, WB Saunders, 1977

Kozier B, Erb G: Fundamentals of Nursing: Concepts and Procedures. Menlo Park, Addison–Wesley, 1979

Murray R et al: The Nursing Process in Later Maturity. Englewood Cliffs, Prentice–Hall, 1980

Murray R, Huelskoetter MM: Psychiatric/Mental Health Nursing: Giving Emotional Care. Englewood Cliffs, Prentice–Hall, 1983

Robinson L: Psychiatric Nursing As a Human Experience. Philadelphia, WB Saunders, 1983

Rowe CJ: An Outline of Psychiatry. Dubuque, William Brown, 1980

Schultz JM, Dark SL: Manual of Psychiatric Nursing Care Plans. Boston, Little, Brown & Co, 1982

Stevenson JS: Issues and Crisis During Middlescence. New York, Appleton–Century, 1977

14

PSYCHOLOGICAL FACTORS

AFFECTING PHYSICAL

CONDITION

The sorrow which has no vent in tears
may make other organs weep.

Henry Maudsley

LEARNING OBJECTIVES

1. Explain the following theories:
   Emotional specificity theory
   Organ specificity theory
   Familial theory
   Learning therory

2. Describe type A behavior or personality.

3. Explain the Social Readjustment Rating Scale.

4. Briefly describe the etiology of the following illnesses:
   Peptic ulcer disease
   Dermatitis
   Arthritis
   Asthma
   Essential hypertension
   Migraine headache

5. Describe the pathology of a psychophysiologic disorder.

6. Explain why traditional medical treatment is necessary for patients who have disorders such as peptic ulcer disease or essential hypertension.

7. Define holistic health care.

8. Develop a nursing care plan for a patient with the diagnosis of essential hypertension.

THE quote that opens this chapter vividly but simply states the effect of stress or emotional conflict on the body. Seyle's general adaptation syndrome states that if a person is unable to regain equilibrium or homeostasis following the "fight-or flight" reaction to stress, he experiences the stage of exhaustion. Physical deterioration and death can occur as a result of continued stress in the presence of a weakened physical condition.

Why a person develops a physical illness such as an ulcer, essential hypertension or low back pain, rather than exhibiting symptoms of an obsessive–compulsive disorder or an acute anxiety attack, is not answered by the concept of stress. The person may be unable to express feelings such as anger or frustration, cope with stress, or resolve a psychological conflict. As the person represses or buries such stressors, they cause chronic tension, produce tissue damage, and surface as a physical illness. This process is called *physiological regression* (similar to the childish behavior exhibited by an adult who regresses in an attempt to decrease anxiety).

The DSM-III has changed this classification to that of psychological factors affecting physical condition (previously called psychophysiologic or psychosomatic disorders). The term *psychophysiologic disorder* still is commonly used. According to the DSM-III criteria, this diagnosis is intended for any physical condition caused by or influenced by psychological factors. Diagnostic criteria include:

1. Psychological factors either cause or exacerbate (make worse) a physical condition. For example, stress can produce symptoms of an ulcer, arthritis or low back pain. It also can cause a person with an existing condition, such as an ulcer, to become acutely ill.

2. The psychological factors are meaningful environmental stimuli. A man who is told that his wife has died in an auto accident or a young couple who have had an intense argument experience psychologically meaningful environmental stimuli that will have an effect on their physical conditions.

3. The physical condition has an organic pathology that can be identified, (*e.g.,* an ulcer, colitis or arthritis), or the physical condition exhibits a pathophysiologic process (*e.g.,* a migraine headache, vomiting, asthmatic attack or diarrhea).

ETIOLOGY

Theories commonly cited to explain the onset of psychophysiologic disorders include the emotional specificity theory, the organic specificity theory, the familial theory, and the learning theory.

Emotional Specificity Theory

Shapiro and Crider (1969) investigated the effect of different emotions on physiologic functioning. They found anger and hostility to be underlying factors in the presence of essential hypertension (high blood pressure in the absence of a physiologic cause). Once the underlying anger or hostility was released, the symptoms diminished.

Friedman and Rosenman (1974) researched the type A behavior or personality, characterized by an excessive competitive drive, impatience, aggressiveness, and a sense of urgency. These people were found to have higher levels of serum triglycerides, cholesterol, adrenalin, and steroids than the more relaxed type B personalities. Because these substances have an adverse effect on the heart, causing the person to be at risk, they concluded that a person with type A personality was more susceptible to the development of coronary heart disease.

Another theorist, Franz Alexander (1950), lists seven basic psychophysiologic disorders that may be due to emotional conflict. These are asthma, peptic ulcer, ulcerative colitis, hypertension, thyrotoxicosis, neurodermatitis, and rheumatoid arthritis. He proposes that specific emotions cause a particular illness; for example, inhibited rage may cause hypertension, and the need to be loved may cause an ulcer.

Organ Specificity Theory

Lacey, Bateman, and Van Lehn (1953) studied characteristic physiologic response patterns that they believed to be present since childhood. They concluded that a person responds to stress primarily with one specific organ or system; thereby showing susceptibility to the development of a specific disease. For example, whenever faced with an emotional conflict, a 25-year-old secretary would experience the sudden onset of midepigastric pain. The pain would persist until the conflict was resolved. She has the potential to develop an ulcer if she continues to experience frequent episodes of stress. Other persons may be prone to low back pain, asthmatic attacks, or skin rashes, depending on their susceptible organ or system.

Familial Theory

Proponents of the familial theory feel that dynamic family relationships influence the development of a psychophysiologic disorder.

A family therapist, Salvador Minuchin, believes that role modeling is an important factor in personality development. He identified the "psychosomatogenic family"as a group of individuals who develop physiologic symptoms rather than face or resolve conflict. Children of such families observe the coping mechanisms of their parents and other family members and develop similar behaviors when the need arises, to avoid conflict and experience positive reinforcement.

Learning Theory

According to this theory, a person learns to produce a physiologic response to achieve a reward, attention, or some other type of reinforcement.

Lancaster (1980) states that the following dynamics occur during the development of a learned response:

The learning is of an unconscious nature.

There was a reward or reinforcement in the past when the person experienced specific physiologic symptoms.

Such reinforcements can be positive or negative. Negative reinforcement is considered better than no reinforcement at all.

The person is not able to give up the disorder willfully.

For example, a child stays home from school when he is ill and receives attention from his mother as she reads to him, fixes his favorite meals, and monitors his vital signs. As a result of this experience, he unconsciously learns to produce physiologic symptoms of a migraine headache or an upset stomach as he feels the need for attention. This behavior may continue throughout his life as he attempts to satisfy unmet needs.

THE SOCIAL READJUSTMENT RATING SCALE

Holmes and Rahe (1967), along with a group of other scientists, developed the social readjustment rating scale. This scale ranks 43 critical life events according to the severity of their impact on a person. Each event has a point value; the death of a spouse is considered to be the most significant critical life event, and minor violations of the law the least significant of the 43 events. The point value of events a person experiences for a single year are totaled, thus indicating the severity of environmental stressors and the potential for the onset of a physical illness.

The rating scale is scored as follows:

150–199 point value places the person at a mild risk for a health change in the next 2 years (25%–37% chance).

200–299 point value indicates that the person is at a moderate risk for a health change within the next 2 years (50% chance).

300–or greater point value indicates that the person is at a major risk for a health change within the next 2 years (79%–90% chance).

THE SOCIAL READJUSTMENT RATING SCALE*

Life Event	Mean Value
1. Death of spouse	100
2. Divorce	73
3. Marital separation	65
4. Jail term	63
5. Death of close family member	63
6. Personal injury or illness	53
7. Marriage	50
8. Fired at work	47
9. Marital reconciliation	45
10. Retirement	45
11. Change in health of family member	44
12. Pregnancy	40
13. Sex difficulties	39
14. Gain of new family member	39
15. Business readjustment	39
16. Change in financial state	38
17. Death of close friend	37
18. Change to different line of work	36
19. Change in number of arguments with spouse	35
20. Mortgage or loan for major purchase (home, etc)	31
21. Foreclosure of mortgage or loan	30
22. Change in responsibilities at work	29
23. Son or daughter leaving home	29

Life Event	Mean Value
24. Trouble with in-laws	29
25. Outstanding personal achievement	28
26. Wife begins or stops work	26
27. Begin or end school	26
28. Change in living conditions	25
29. Revision of personal habits	24
30. Trouble with boss	23
31. Change in work hours or conditions	20
32. Change in residence	20
33. Change in schools	20
34. Change in recreation	19
35. Change in church activities	19
36. Change in social activities	18
37. Mortgage or loan for lesser purchase (car, TV, etc)	17
38. Change in sleeping habits	16
39. Change in number of family get-togethers	15
40. Change in eating habits	15
41. Vacation	13
42. Christmas	12
43. Minor violations of the law	11

*From Holmes TH, Rahe RH: The social readjustment rating scale. J Psychosom Res 11:213–218, 1967

One method of classifying physical disorders that are caused by psychological factors is to discuss the more common system responses to stress, such as the circulatory or respiratory system.

THE GASTROINTESTINAL SYSTEM AND STRESS

The most commonly seen condition of the gastrointestinal (GI) tract related to stress is peptic ulcer disease. The person with a peptic ulcer appears to have a conflict regarding dependency and independency needs. Although the person appears to be aggressive, ambitious, and independent, the desire to be fed, loved, and cared for is always present. Conflict also may be experienced whenever suppressed feelings of resentment, anger, guilt, fear, or helplessness emerge. The desire for oral gratification is said to stimulate an excessive secretion of hydrochloric acid, causing the development of an ulcer. Peptic ulcer disease also can be caused by a combination of environmental, inherited, and physiologic factors.

Other commonly seen GI disorders include irritable bowel syndrome (IBS), gastritis, obesity, and chronic diarrhea or constipation. People also may exhibit pathophysiologic processes such as nausea and vomiting, belching, and heartburn, all as a result of stress.

Irritable Bowel Syndrome: Clinical Example

BS, a 30-year-old housewife and mother of two children (ages 5 and 3), is a perfectionist. She continually cleans up after the children and is known as a spotless housekeeper. Her husband, who is a traveling salesman, is home on weekends. BS's mother died when she was 13 years old, and her father remarried. She sees him once or twice a year. Whenever the children are unruly, forget to clean up after playing with their toys, or spill something, BS becomes upset and experiences abdominal cramping and frequent soft stools or diarrhea. The last episode occurred when her husband had to cancel a weekend trip home. BS had planned on a relaxing weekend with her husband and children. She developed severe abdominal pain, accompanied by diarrhea and rectal bleeding. Her symptoms could be attributed to a dependency–independency conflict. She is filling the roles of both mother and father independently and has no one to relate to or meet her dependency needs when her husband is gone. Her need to be loved and cared for is not being met because of the absence of her husband and father and death of her mother.

Peptic Ulcer Disease: Clinical Example

JC, a 35-year-old accountant, is married and has four children. His parents were divorced when he was a year old, and consequently he did not spend much time with his father. His mother had to work to provide for herself and two other children. Because JC was the oldest of three children, his mother relied on him to babysit the children and help with chores around the house. He was expected to work after school and to save for his college expenses. After graduation from college, JC married and worked as an accountant for a progressive firm. His job required much detailed work and included meeting several deadlines set by his employer. JC began to experience epigastric pain, as well as nausea and vomiting as more demands were made by his employer. As his symptoms became progressively worse, JC was seen by his attending physician, who diagnosed the presence of a peptic ulcer. His disorder may be because as a child he was given adult responsibilities, was forced to be independent, and did not receive the love and attention he required. He repressed his feelings, became an accountant, and again met with numerous demands by his employer. His emotional conflict has surfaced as an ulcer.

One student who had cared for a patient with the diagnosis of peptic ulcer disease questioned why the person became a "workaholic" and subjected himself to so much stress. A student commented, "No amount of money is worth all the headaches he has. No wonder he has an ulcer." Another student asked why a female patient with ulcerative colitis did not seek help rather than put up with the symptoms for 5 years.

THE INTEGUMENTARY SYSTEM AND STRESS

Persons who exhibit dermatologic responses to stress may blush, become pale, perspire excessively, experience generalized itching, develop a rash, or lose hair (alopecia). The onset of pruritus is thought to be the result of a hostile, dependent relationship in which the person has an inordinate need for affection. Lack of touching in childhood also may contribute to the cause of such a disorder. Approximately 75% of all people with pruritus experience emotional reactions, such as anger, guilt, tension, anxiety, or fear. Symptoms of intense itching and scratching may be considered the inward and therefore masochistic result of such feelings.

Dermatitis: Clinical Example

A 37-year-old woman, mother of three teenaged boys, had recently obtained a legal separation from her husband. As she attempted to make decisions about housing and employment, the boys began to argue frequently and disobey their mother. One morning, as the mother prepared to go to work, she developed a generalized skin rash and hives. When the itching became unbearable, the woman was seen by her family physician, who explained that stress was the underlying cause of her condition. He prescribed an antianxiety agent, medication for the skin rash and hives, and recommended family counseling.

THE MUSCULOSKELETAL SYSTEM AND STRESS

Muscular tension, backaches, muscle strain, low back pain, tremors, and involuntary tics are all examples of the response of the musculoskeletal system to stress.

According to some theorists, rheumatoid arthritis may be considered an example of hostility or anxiety released through a bodily function. The personality profile of an arthritic patient includes characteristics such as perfectionistic, self-sacrificing, shy, sensitive, conscientious, having exaggerated sense of responsibility, and being unable to handle aggressive feelings. This inability to deal with aggression may be due to a relationship with domineering, stern, or unreasonable parents who promote dependency. The arthritic patient may be unable to express anger, and, as anxiety or hostility increases, activity is impaired owing to muscular contraction and an underlying inflammatory process of the joints.

Low Back Pain Because of Stress: Clinical Example

PW, a 45-year-old schoolteacher, has experienced periodic bouts of low back pain for several years. Although he has been immobolized and confined to bed in the past, he has not sought medical advice or treatment. PW's wife was admitted to the hospital for a complete medical examination and possible breast biopsy. His schedule consisted of going to work early, visiting his wife after work and assuming housekeeping responsibilities while she was hospitalized. The day of surgery, PW spent the entire time at the hospital waiting for the report of his wife's biopsy. That evening he and his wife were informed that she did have cancer of the breast and were given several options to consider. As PW visited with his wife, he suddenly experienced symptoms of low back pain. He went home and the next morning was unable to get out of bed because of severe muscle spasms. As a result of his physical symptoms, PW was taken to the emergency room by ambulance and was admitted to the hospital with the diagnosis of acute low back pain. A complete physical exam and x-rays revealed no pathologic cause of symptoms. The attending physician explored PW's feelings about his wife's physical condition. He explained that anxiety about his wife's illness was probably the cause of the severe muscle spasms and low back pain.

The student nurse who cared for PW had difficulty communicating with him. She stated, "I feel so helpless. His wife is dying and he's here in the hospital. What can I say to him? There really isn't anything physically wrong with him." Postclinical conference focused on the patient's inability to express feelings of fear and anxiety. Students suggested that encouraging verbalization of feelings would be an appropriate nursing intervention. Within a few days the student who cared for PW stated that "He cried while I was making his bed. He is very angry with God and his wife because she has cancer." PW was able to express his normal feelings of grief, and as his symptoms subsided, he was discharged.

THE RESPIRATORY SYSTEM AND STRESS

Comments such as "what breathtaking scenery," "it took my breath away," and "I was so scared I lost my breath" are examples of respiratory reaction to internal and external stimuli. A person may exhibit rapid respirations, wheezing, breathlessness, hyperventilation, or an asthmatic attack. Anxiety, stress, emotional trauma, and allergic reactions can precipitate such respiratory responses.

Asthma is considered to be the leading cuase of chronic illness among persons under 17 years of age. Underlying causes of asthma have been identified as fear of rejection, fear of potential or actual separation, ambivalence toward the mother, inability to cope with the environment, and feelings of helplessness or depression. Characteristics of the asthmatic personality include immature coping abilities, extreme sensitivity, excessive dependency on the mother, and the intense desire to please others.

Asthmatic attacks have been described as a conditioned response in which a person is suppressing a cry for mother because of fear of rejection or separation. Asthmatics seldom cry or shed tears and have difficulty with communication.

There appears to be some conflict regarding the etiology of asthmatic attacks. A few theorists have stated that no specific cause has been proven. They consider hypersensitivity to allergens to be the precipitating cause but do concede that emotional upset can aggravate asthma.

Asthmatic Attack: Clinical Example

A 23-year-old pregnant woman was admitted to the general hospital during her fourth month of pregnancy with symptoms of status asthmaticus. When she was transferred from the intensive care unit to the medical service, a student nurse was assigned to help with the transfer procedure and administer nursing care. As the student completed an assessment, she noticed that the young woman was quite courteous and wanted to "do everything just right so she wouldn't upset the nurses." The following day, as the student was caring for the patient, the patient's mother telephoned to see how she was feeling. Later in the day the patient confided in the student that her mother was caring for a younger child at home. She stated, "My mother is always telling me how to raise my daughter. I never seem to do the right thing. Sometimes I almost hate her when she criticizes the way I do housework. I wish just once she'd tell me I'm a good mother!" When the student asked the patient how frequently she had asthmatic attacks, she stated, "They seem to occur whenever my mother and I disagree on things."

In clinical postconference, the student nurse stated, "I'm surprised that a 24-year-old woman is so dependent on her mother. Doesn't she realize what these attacks can do to her unborn child?" Other statements made: "What about her relationship with her husband?", "She reminds me of a little girl who wants to please her mother", "How long will these attacks continue?" and "What can be done to help her overcome these attacks?"

CARDIOVASCULAR SYSTEM AND STRESS

A recent newspaper article reported "Stress of divorce a health hazard." The author, Jane E. Brody, a reporter for the New York Times, stated that divorce can cause longer lasting emotional and physical illness than any other life stress. She quoted James Lynch, psychologist at the University of Maryland, as stating "friendship and love involve physiologically cost-free communication. For the bereaved and the divorced, however, communication takes place at a great physiologic cost. They may actually talk themselves into high blood pressure."

Circulatory responses to stress include palpitations, tension or migraine headaches, cardiac arrhythmias, angina, tachycardia, essential hypertension, and myocardial infarction.

Essential hypertension, defined as the sustained elevation of blood pressure at 140/90 or higher in the absence of any organ pathology, is seen frequently in our society as a result of disruptive social conditions, job stress, poverty, and emotional stress. Persons who repress their emotions, especially rage, are unable to vent feelings of anger, aggression, or guilt. They possess chronic, inhibited aggressive impulses. The reaction–formation defense mechanism is in operation since the person appears to be easygoing, helpful, considerate, and gentle, although he harbors feelings of guilt or anger. Such persons are hesitant to form close interpersonal relationships, may feel that they are not in control, and lack the ability to resolve conflicts.

Migraine headaches are also a common cardiovascular response to stress affecting approximately 15 to 25 million people yearly. The person who develops migraine headaches is described as perfectionistic, compulsive, and hard-working. The environment in which he lives and works is conducive to anxiety, emotional tension, frustration, and fatigue.

When a person is under stress, for example experiencing intense anger, vasoconstriction occurs. As the stress subsides and relaxation occurs, blood vessels dilate and an increased blood flow results, producing pressure on surrounding interstitial tissue. Some people experience sharp, throbbing pain that is described as unilateral but may become generalized. Photophobia, nausea, blurred vision, dysplopia, and vomiting may occur. Migraines occur after the stress subsides.

Migraine Headache: Clinical Example

SK, a 45-year-old mother of three grown children and telephone operator, just recently has obtained a divorce after 14 years of marriage to her second husband. Her first husband had been killed in an auto accident, and, after 2 years of attempting to support three children alone, SK remarried. Although her second husband was kind and considerate to her children, he was never able to develop a positive interpersonal relationship with the middle child, an eight-year-old girl. As the girl grew older, she developed behavioral problems and attempted to run away from home on two separate occasions. SK's relationship with her husband and daughter became quite stressed. Her job as a telephone operator was quite frustrating at times, producing tension and anxiety as well as causing fatigue. As SK attempted to adapt to the stress she encountered at work and at home, she began to experience severe prefrontal headaches, which often were accompanied by feelings of nausea, vomiting and blurred vision. When SK was unable to tolerate the headaches any longer, she consulted a physician, who conducted a thorough physical examination. As the doctor completed the examination, he asked SK about her family life and relationship with her children and second husband. She confided in the doctor that her first marriage had been "perfect" and that she wanted this second marriage to be "just like the first." SK also stated that her daughter had been "daddy's little girl" and that she had hoped her second husband would be able to continue the relationship. She then commented that although she was a hard-working, industrious person, she felt that she had failed at trying to "recreate the family life in her first marriage."

Essential Hypertension: Clinical Example

JB, a 54-year-old executive, was seen by the company's attending physician for his annual physical examination. As the office nurse assessed him, she noted that his face was flushed, his blood pressure was 160/110, and he stated that he only had 30 minutes until he had to attend an executive meeting. After his physical examination was completed, the physician instructed JB to return to his office twice a week to have his blood pressure monitored and placed him on antihypertensive medication. The next few weeks JB returned faithfully as directed, continuing to present symptoms of hypertension. Although the nurse continued to stress preventive measures, JB did not change his lifestyle. Approximately four months later JB was admitted to the intensive care unit of the local community hospital with the diagnosis of a cerebral vascular attack. As a result of this condition JB is a right-sided hemiplegic, with expressive aphasia. He has had to retire early and presently is engaged in a rehabilitative program.

A student nurse caring for JB commented, "He could be my father. He's so young to spend the rest of his life as a disabled person." After reading the history and admission forms, the same student stated, "Why didn't he follow his doctor's advice to prevent this attack? Didn't he care what happened?" JB eventually answered this question, stating, "I didn't think this would happen to me. I never lost my temper when I was upset. Maybe I should have said what I thought rather than worry about hurting the other guy's feelings."

In summary, psychophysiological disorders such as those described involve a single organ system, are under the control of the autonomic nervous system, exhibit structural change, and can become life-threatening. The symptoms are real as they are experienced by the patient. Not all people who exhibit the disorders discussed in this chapter have psychological problems. Some of the conditions can occur as a direct result of physiologic stress, without the influence of emotional factors. Hair loss can occur as a natural aging process, or in someone undergoing chemotherapy for cancer. Hyperventilation can be intentionally induced by a swimmer just before leaving the starting block. Emotional responses to physical illness, such as the grieving process, loneliness, helplessness, hopelessness, and dependency are discussed separately.

The following is a list of diagnosed psychophysiologic disorders and the emotional components identified by student nurses during clinical rotation in the general hospital. The focus was to identify the psychological needs of assigned patients.

MEDICAL DIAGNOSES	EMOTIONAL COMPONENTS
Acute exfoliative dermatitis (62-year-old man)	Anger stage of the grieving process regarding wife's recent diagnosis of multiple sclerosis was revealed during interview. Fear and anxiety regarding the outcome of her illness also were identified. The onset of dermatitis occurred when his wife was initially diagnosed. No previous history of dermatitis was noted.
Gastric ulcer (50-year-old woman)	The initial interview revealed the patient's fear of cancer and unresolved grief (anger stage) regarding the death of her parents. Both parents had died of cancer at an early age. She also conveyed feelings of a dependency–independency conflict as she discussed her feelings of loneliness. She had lived alone near her parents and enjoyed a close family relationship. The ulcer developed approximately 1 year after the death of her mother.
Gastritis and acute esophagitis (60-year-old woman)	Frequent hospitalizations occurred within the past year to avoid family problems. The patient revealed that her husband was a workaholic who never showed much affection. She resented his commitment to his job and neglect of the family. Feelings of helplessness and depression were identified during the interview. The patient stated that the only place she could relax was in the hospital.
Tachycardia and chest pain (60-year-old man)	This patient's sister had died as a result of a myocardial infarct 2 weeks before his hospitalization. They had been quite close. Symptoms of acute anxiety were identified during the interview, as well as signs of the depressed stage of the grieving process. The patient discussed his fear of his own death. He was certain he would not leave the hospital alive. (He was discharged 2 weeks later.)

MEDICAL DIAGNOSES	EMOTIONAL COMPONENTS
Bronchial asthma (24-year-old man)	Extreme apprehension was noted on the admission notes. This patient was married to an older woman with a physical handicap, who was totally dependent on him. During the interview he stated "I am 24 years old, feel like 50, and look at least 35." Assessment revealed symptoms of anxiety, depression, and a poor self-concept.
Acute duodenal ulcer (25-year-old man)	The initial interview revealed intense anger at being unemployed. The patient also stated that he was experiencing poor interpersonal relationships with his stepmother and significant other as a result of his unemployment. He felt they were nonsupportive of his decision to sue his former employer for job discrimination.
Sinusitis, chronic (16-year-old girl)	During the initial interview this young patient stated she was "allergic to people and things." She stated she had not attended school for 3 years owing to severe allergy attacks and sinusitis. When questioned further about the onset of her "chronic" illness, the patient revealed that her father died unexpectedly at that time. She stated "I never even got a chance to tell him I loved him." The anger stage of unresolved grief was identified by the student nurse.
Acute low back pain (35-year-old woman)	The admission notes on this patient revealed sporadic bouts of low back pain for approximately 10 years. As the student interviewed the patient, she revealed that she had been divorced less than a year when her father died of cancer. She moved in with her mother, who was a very domineering person. Symptoms of anxiety and the anger stage of the grieving process were identified by the student nurse.

TREATMENT OF PSYCHOLOGICAL FACTORS AFFECTING PHYSICAL CONDITION

The medical problem is treated before focusing on the emotional needs exhibited by the patient. Treatment is an individualized approach that considers the following factors:

1. Severity of clinical symptoms, both physical and psychological (*i.e.,* life-threatening structural changes requiring immediate medical attention or psychiatric care)

2. Type of psychophysiologic reaction including presenting symptoms (*i.e.,* elevated blood pressure, tachycardia, skin rash, or gastric pain)

3. Emotional component of illness (*i.e.,* anxiety, anger, depression or dependency needs)

4. Insight regarding illness displayed by patient (*i.e.,* awareness of stressors or conflict causing physical illness)

Many patients are admitted to the general hospital and receive traditional medical treatment such as bed rest, diet as tolerated, moist heat, antacids, and pain medication. Antianxiety agents, antidepressants, or sedative–hypnotic agents also may be prescribed. A decision may be made to refer the patient for counseling or psychiatric care. Referrals may be made for follow-up care by community counseling services after the patient is discharged.

Other treatments that may be prescribed include biofeedback for hypertension, irregular pulse, low back pain, tension, or migraine headache. The person is taught to relax so that he can control his body processes in response to stress. Electrodes are connected to the hands, forehead, and chest as the person reclines in a comfortable chair. Heart rate, muscle tone, and brain waves are monitored. These factors influence a signal light that glows more intensely when the patient becomes tense. When the person relaxes the glow diminishes. As a result of this conditioning process, the person is able to use biofeedback to relax and control physiologic responses to stress or anxiety.

Friedman and Rosenman list several drills that a client with type A behavior can follow to decrease stress. Rephrased they include exercises such as

1. Ask yourself why you are always rushing.

2. Ask yourself if the urgent task you do now will matter in 5 or 10 years.

3. Tell youself that work is never finished completely.

4. Set aside time for yourself; no one else will.

5. When you feel stress or tension as you work, stop to relax; the task will be there to complete later; *you* may not be.

Suggestions by Friedman and Rosenman to decrease feelings of hostility are summarized as follows:

1. Tell youself that everyone has feelings of hostility; these are normal.

2. Attempt to lessen your sensitivity to hostility or anger expressed by others.

3. Do not hesitate to tell others you appreciate their help. A simple "thank you" will do.

4. Smile. External appearances need to be changed before changing internal emotions.

Relaxation techniques and behavior modification are described in detail in Chapters 12 and 5.

NURSING INTERVENTIONS

Nursing interventions should use the holistic health care approach by treating the patient's physical, psychological, and spiritual needs. Assessment of the patient includes collection of data regarding:

1. Unmet psychological and physical needs
2. Present coping mechanisms
3. Present self-concept
4. Available support systems
5. Developmental level
6. Strengths that the patient demonstrates
7. Insight regarding illness

These data can be used to develop an individualized nursing care plan to meet the patient's needs. When providing traditional medical treatment, give detailed explanations regarding the importance of taking medications, adhering to a specific diet, and following through with treatments like physical therapy. Patient education should emphasize the importance of following medical treatment and reducing stress to prevent any further structural change.

The patient's role in the holistic approach is to attempt to identify any stressor(s) related to the present physical condition, discuss ways to modify or eliminate these stressor(s), and then state specific changes that can be made. Implementation of change by the patient is attempted with minimal supervision of the nurse. For example, a patient with peptic ulcer disease identifies the fact that he has dependency needs or is angry but has been unable to reveal his feelings in the past. He states that his supervisor expects too much of him and gives him unrealistic deadlines requiring long work hours. Once the stressors are identified, the patient is assisted in citing specific ways to modify or eliminate them, such as working fewer hours, setting priorities at work regarding deadlines, and discussing his feelings with his supervisor. Identified strengths are emphasized at this time to assist the patient in modifying or eliminating stressor(s).

Other therapeutic interventions that may be considered individually include

1. Separating the person from a specific stressor; for example, visiting may be restricted if a family member causes emotional conflict. Inde-

pendent housing may be considered as a long-term goal to reduce conflict and promote independence.

2. Assisting the patient to identify positive or alternative coping mechanisms.

3. Assisting the patient in identifying support systems, such as a minister, close friend, family member, or professional counselor.

4. Reviewing developmental tasks with the patient and exploring ways to handle difficult or unmet tasks successfully.

5. Teaching the person relaxation techniques or exercises.

6. Assisting with referrals for counseling, biofeedback technique, and other options.

7. Administering prescribed medication for physical or psychological needs.

SUMMARY

Etiology and diagnostic criteria pertaining to the DMS-III classification of psychological factors affecting physical condition were discussed. Four theories described were the emotional specificity theory, organ specificity theory, familial theory, and learning theory. Holmes and Rahe's social readjustment rating scale was explained, including its use as an indicator of the onset of a physical illness within 2 years after exposure to various environmental stressors. Physical conditions considered secondary to or the result of psychological factors were presented according to system responses to stress. Clinical examples cited include peptic ulcer disease, IBS, dermatitis, low back pain, asthma, essential hypertension, and migraine headache. Information also was presented about identification of psychological needs of hospitalized patient by student nurses. Traditional medical treatment, as well as treatment of psychological needs, was described such as biofeedback and drills to decrease stress by Friedman and Rosenman. Nursing interventions were presented, focusing on holistic health care. The need for individualized nursing care plans was emphasized as well as for patient education and participation in the holistic approach.

LEARNING ACTIVITIES

I. Clinical activities
   A. Care for a patient with a psychophysiologic disorder.
   B. Identify the psychological factor(s) affecting the patient's physical condition.

    C. Assess the patient's self-concept by having the patient identify personal likes and dislikes about his personality. Which list is longer?

    D. Assess the patient's stressors during this hospitalization and ability to cope.

    E. Have the patient identify present support systems. Is he using them?

    F. Evaluate the patient's insight regarding the cause or contributing factor to the illness.

    G. Evaluate the nursing care plan written for your assigned patient. Is it appropriate? State any changes that should be made.

II. Independent activity

    A. Investigate community resources available to assist people with alternative ways to adapt to stress (*e.g.,* biofeedback, exercise groups, hypnosis, meditation, relaxation therapy, relaxation tapes).

    B. Examine your own coping abilities.

        1. Identify at lease one stressful situation in your life. How did you cope?

        2. How do you physiologically respond to stress?

    C. Evaluate the following impacts on an individual who has experienced a myocardial infarction:

        1. Emotional impact (initial reaction to diagnosis)

        2. Social impact (Does the patient feel he will be able to continue to socialize?)

        3. Sexual impact (Does the patient feel the diagnosis affects his sexuality?)

        4. Somatic impact (how he views his body)

        5. Occupational impact (ability to function in present occupation)

    D. What support groups are present in the community to help people through stressful periods?

SELF-TEST

1. Explain the rationale for the title (changes in physical condition due to psychological factors) of this classification of disorders.

2. State how Seyle's general adaption syndrome applies to the onset of a psychophysiological disorder.

3. Explain Minuchin's theory regarding the "psychomatogenic family."

4. List four emotional reactions that can lead to the development of a physical illness.

5. State the underlying conflict that can lead to the development of peptic ulcer disease.

6. List three examples of dermatologic responses to stress.

7. Describe the personality of a person who may exhibit rheumatoid arthritis as a response to stress.

8. State the dynamics involved in an asthmatic client's response to stress.

9. Describe the personality profile of a person who has clinical symptoms of essential hypertension.

10. Give an example of reaction–formation.

11. Describe the personality of a person who is prone to migraine headaches.

12. State three methods of medical treatment for patients with psychological factors affecting physical conditions.

13. Describe four areas of assessment when caring for patients with physical disorders resulting from stress.

14. Discuss the patient's role in the treatment plan.

15. Discuss four nursing interventions for patients with physiologic responses to stress.

16. Explain how Holmes and Rahe's social readjustment rating scale could be used when planning nursing interventions for a patient exhibiting symptoms of a psychophysiologic disorder.

REFERENCES

Alexander F: Psychosomatic Medicine: Its Principles and Applications. New York, Norton Press, 1950

American Psychiatric Association: A Psychiatric Glossary. Washington DC, American Psychiatric Association, 1980

Billings C: Emotional first aid. Am J Nurs: Nov, 1980

Burgess A: Psychiatric Nursing in the Hospital and the Community, 3rd ed. New Jersey, Prentice–Hall, 1981

Campsey J: Psychophysiological illness. J Psych Nurs: Nov, 1979

Freedman, Kaplan, Sadock: Comprehensive Textbook of Psychiatry. Baltimore, Wilkins & Wilkins, 1975

Friedman M, Rosenman R: Type A Behavior and Your Heart. New York, Knopf, 1974

Haber J, et al: Comprehensive Psychiatric Nursing. New York, Mc-Graw–Hill, 1982

Hopping B. Physiological response to stress: A nursing concern. Nurs Forum: Mar, 1980

Kolb L: Modern Clinical Psychiatry. Philadelphia, WB Saunders, 1977

Kreck-Frank R: Psychosomatic problems in the people's republic of China. J Psych Nurs: December, 1980

Lacey J, Bateman D, Van Lekn R: Autonomic response specificity. Psychosomatic Medicine, XV: 1953

Lancaster J: Adult Psychiatric Nursing. New York, Medical Examination Publishing, 1980

Lewis CW: Body image and obesity. J Psych Nurs: Jan, 1978

Mereness D, Taylor C: Essentials of Psychiatric Nursing, 11th ed. St. Louis, CV Mosby Co, 1982

Pasquali E, Alesi E, Arnold H et al: Mental Health Nursing: A Bio-Psycho-Cultural Approach. St. Louis, CV Mosby, 1981

Robinson L: Psychological Aspects of the Care of Hospitalized Patients. Philadelphia, FA Davis, 1984

Robinson L: Psychiatric Nursing As a Human Experience. Philadelphia, WB Saunders, 1983

Schultz J, Dark S: Manual of Psychiatric Nursing Care Plans. Boston, Little, Brown & Co, 1982

Seyle H: The Stress of Life. New York, McGraw–Hill, 1956

Shapiro D, Crider A: Psychophysiological approaches in social psychology. In: The Handbook of Social Psychology, 2nd ed. Reading, Addison–Wesley, 1969

Shontz F: The Psychological Aspects of Physical Illness and Disability. New York, MacMillan, 1975

Walker JI: Everybody's Guide to Emotional Well-Being. San Francisco, Harbour Publishing, 1982

Walsh MJ: An affair of the heart. Nursing 78: Sept, 1978

Wilson H, Kneisl C: Psychiatric Nursing. 2nd ed. Menlo Park, Addison–Wesley, 1983

15

ALTERED PHYSIOLOGIC

CONDITIONS

DUE TO ANXIETY

LEARNING OBJECTIVES

1. Define somatoform disorders.
2. Describe the subclassification of somatoform disorders.
3. Differentiate malingering from conversion disorder.
4. Define "la belle indifference."
5. Define primary gain.
6. Differentiate between primary and secondary gain.
7. Define psychalgia.
8. Discuss nursing interventions for a patient with a somatoform disorder.

ACCORDING to the DSM-III classification, somatoform disorders differ from psychological factors affecting physical conditions in that somatoform disorders are reflected in disordered physiologic complaints or symptoms, are not under voluntary control, and do not demonstrate organic findings. Faan and Goshen (1977) state "the patient converts his psychological distress into complaints pertaining to different parts of the body (for example, complaining of palpitation or pain instead of fear) (p. 43).

This classification is subclassified into five categories:

1. Somatization disorder or Briquet's syndrome

2. Conversion disorder

3. Psychogenic pain disorder

4. Hypochondriasis

5. Atypical somatoform disorder

SOMATIZATION DISORDER

A somatization disorder is a free-floating anxiety disorder in which a person expresses emotional turmoil or conflict through a physical system, usually with a loss or alteration of physical functioning. Such a loss or alteration of physical functioning is not under voluntary control and is not explained as a known physical disorder. The onset generally begins before age 30 and is considered to be a chronic illness in persons who demonstrate a dramatic, confusing, or complicated medical history, since they seek repeated medical attention. The physical symptoms or complaints that occur in the absence of any medical explanation govern the person's life by influencing him to take medication, to alter his life-style, or to see a physician.

The following organ system symptoms occur in somatization disorder (Donlon, 1982):

ORGAN SYSTEM	EXAMPLES OF SYMPTOMS
Gastrointestinal (GI) symptoms	Abdominal pain, food intolerance, diarrhea
Pseudoneurologic or conversion symptoms	Paralysis, weakness, blindness, difficulty swallowing
Psychosexual symptoms	Pain during intercourse, lack of sexual pleasure, sexual indifference
Gynecologic or female reproductive symptoms	Painful menses, excessive bleeding, hyperemesis gravidarium,
Pain	Back or joint pain
Cardiopulmonary symptoms	Chest pain, dizziness, palpitations

The person with a somatization disorder must complain of at least 14 (female) or 12 (male) symptoms from a list of 37 identified symptoms similar to those listed.

Anxiety and depression frequently are seen, and the patient may make frequent threats or attempts at suicide. He also may exhibit antisocial behavior or experience occupational, interpersonal, or marital difficulties. Because the patient constantly seeks medical attention, he frequently submits to unnecessary surgery.

CONVERSION DISORDER

As described by Faan and Goshen (1977, p. 43), a conversion disorder is a psychological condition in which an anxiety-provoking impulse is converted unconsciously into functional symptoms, for example, anesthesia, paralysis, or dyskinesia. Although the disturbance is not under voluntary control, the symptoms occur in organs under voluntary control, serve to meet the immediate needs of the patient, and are associated with a secondary gain.

Patients with conversion disorder benefit by primary and secondary gain. *Primary gain* is obtaining relief from anxiety by keeping an internal need or conflict out of awareness. *Secondary gain* is any other benefit or support from the environment that a person obtains as a result of being sick. Examples of secondary gain are attention, love, financial reward, and sympathy.

Conversion disorders can be seen clinically as motor symptoms or sensory disturbances. Examples include muscular weakness, analgesia, or a diminished ability to feel pain.

The term *la belle indifference* is used to describe patient reactions such as indifference to the symptoms and displaying no anxiety. This is because the anxiety has been relieved by the conversion disorder.

Malingering should be differentiated from conversion disorder. *Malingering* is a conscious effort to simulate or feign the symptoms of an illness to avoid an unpleasant situation. It is done for a selfish gain. An example is a person complaining of back injury following an auto accident to sue for financial gain.

Age of onset for conversion disorder is usually adolescence or early adulthood but may occur for the first time during middle age or in later maturity. Such a disorder frequently impairs normal activities and may promote the development of a chronic sick role. Examples of conversion disorder inlude the sudden onset of blindness, paralysis, deafness, or numbness that has no physiologic basis.

PSYCHOGENIC PAIN DISORDER (PSYCHALGIA)

The following criteria generally are used when assessing a person complaining of severe prolonged pain:

Are physical findings related to the pain?

Are findings caused by any mental or physical disorder?

Is the pain out of proportion to a complaint with physical findings?

Is there evidence of psychological causes?

The DSM-III criteria state that the severe prolonged pain is the predominant disturbance or complaint presented by the person; the pain is inconsistent owing to a lack of proof of organic pathology; and the pain is due to psychological factors; no other mental disorder is the cause.

Although psychalgia may occur at any stage of life, it is more frequently seen in adolescence or early adulthood and occurs more frequently in women. The pain may subside because of appropriate intervention or may persist over a period of several months or years if reinforced.

HYPOCHONDRIASIS

Hypochondriasis is a term used to describe persons who present with unrealistic or exaggerated physical complaints. They become preoccupied with the fear of developing or already having a disease or illness in spite of medical reassurance that such an illness does not exist. Minor clinical symptoms are of great concern to the person and often result in an impairment of social or occupational functioning. Preoccupations generally focus on bodily functions or minor physical abnormalities. Such a person is commonly referred to as a "professional patient" who shops for doctors because he feels he does not get proper medical attention. These people often elicit feelings of frustration and anger from health care providers.

This disorder usually is accompanied by anxiety, depression, and compulsive personality traits. It generally occurs in adolescence and usually becomes chronic, causing impaired social or occupational functioning. The person may adopt an invalid's life-style and actually may become bedridden.

ATYPICAL SOMATOFORM DISORDER

The category of atypical somatoform disorder is used when physical symptoms or complaints are unexplainable by demonstrable organic findings or a known pathophysiologic mechanism. The disorder apparently is linked to psychological factors.

TREATMENT OF SOMATOFORM DISORDERS

Treatment for persons with somatoform disorders is considered both challenging and frustrating owing to the chronicity of these disorders. Before having the patient pursue psychiatric care, establish trust with the patient and eliminate any physical disease. A person who frequently complains of being ill may be unable to convince a member of the health team when an illness does occur.

The person and the family should be told after a thorough, essentially negative physical examination that the patient has no life threatening or severe illness, although he does continue to exhibit symptoms. Antidepressants may be prescribed, as well as low-dosage psychotropic drugs (*e.g.,* Thorazine or Mellaril). These drugs are effective in the treatment of moderate to marked depression with variable degrees of anxiety.

Psychotherapy directed at emotional support is the most common form of therapy. Modification of the environment may be necessary, as well as the use of behavior modification. Psychotropic drugs, usually antianxiety agents, are used because patients often report anxiety secondary to their major concerns.

NURSING INTERVENTIONS

Health care givers must remember that physical symptoms are quite real to the hypochondriacal patient, as well as to the person with a conversion disorder, psychogenic pain, or somatization disorder. Nurses must be aware of verbal and nonverbal responses to the patient so that they do not appear judgmental.

Patients with somatoform disorders do not produce their symptoms intentionally. Nurses should avoid reinforcing complaints by ignoring the symptoms but never the patient. They should assess the patient's physical condition carefully, refer physical complaints to the medical staff, and attempt to understand the purpose that blindness, deafness, itching, paralyses, numbness, or whatever the complaint may serve. The person may be using such complaints to avoid certain responsibilities (*i.e.*, educational, vocational, or familial), to receive attention, to manipulate others, to handle conflict, or to meet dependency needs.

Common behaviors or problems the hypochondriacal patient may exhibit include 1) denial of any emotional problem; 2) self-preoccupation; 3) difficulty expressing self and feelings; 4) numerous somatic complaints; 5) reliance on medications; 5) history of repeated visits to physicians, visits to emergency rooms, admissions to hospitals, or surgeries; 6) anxiety; or 7) ritualistic behaviors. Patients with conversion reactions generally experience feelings of guilt, anxiety or frustration; physical limitations due to paralysis, blindness, and so forth; low self-esteem; or difficulty dealing with anger, frustration, or conflict.

Examples of nursing diagnoses and nursing interventions of persons with somatoform disorder follow:

NURSING DIAGNOSES	NURSING INTERVENTIONS
Ineffective individual coping, exhibited by numerous unfounded somatic complaints due to stress and anxiety	Establish rapport. Assess the patient's insight regarding the reason for somatic complaints. Help the patient to identify stressors in life situations. Refer complaints to medical staff for evaluation. Minimize the amount of time and attention spent on the discussion of physical complaints. Present reality when possible (*i.e.*, "Your x-rays do not show any lesions in your right lung.") Encourage verbalization about feelings rather than physical complaints. If no serious illness exists, limit the amount of time spent in room to avoid reinforcement of the sick role. Explore alternative ways of coping with stress and anxiety such as relaxation techniques. Focus on realistic goals for self. Include significant others in the conversation (if able).
Disturbance in self-concept: Low self-image	Assess the patient's level of self-concept. Encourage verbalization of feelings regarding self-image. Have the patient list positive traits or attributes. Give positive recognition or feedback whenever he discusses issues other than somatic complaints.

Conversion Disorder: Clinical Example

PK, a 21-year-old college senior, was first-string quarterback of the football team for 2 years until a new freshman student was recruited by the coaches. The new player had been an all-state quarterback his junior and senior year in high school and had received a significant amount of publicity for his accomplishments. PK was suddenly under great stress because of the competitive nature of the young quarterback and found himself doubting his ability to retain his position as the starting player for the team. The day of tryouts, PK suddenly developed an unexplained paralysis of his passing arm and was unable to participate in the competitive bid for first-string quarterback. After an extensive physical examination, the physician explained to PK that he was exhibiting clinical behavior of a conversion disorder due to increased stress and anxiety.

Hypochondriasis: Clinical Example

MC, a 35-year-old mother of two children, came to the physician's office with complaints of a headache, vertigo, and occasional irregular heartbeat. She was certain that she had heart touble. Her history revealed repeated visits to the same physician the past 6 months with vague physical complaints that could not be attributed to any physical disorder. Before that time, she had visited five other area doctors and presented numerous somatic complaints that "kept her from going to work" due to the fear of having a heart attack. Her present employer insisted that she obtain a physician's statement indicating that she was unable to work due to a specific physical disorder or she would not be compensated for any future absenteeism. The examining physician was unable to substantiate any cause for MC's recurring physical complaints and recommended that she receive counseling for her hypochondriacal condition.

Nursing interventions for persons such as PK and MC should center on treating them as whole persons, that is, assessing their expectations of self and teaching them how to cope in a more direct, mature manner. Communication skills and assertive behavior should be explored and reinforced to discourage a patient's assumption of the sick role.

SUMMARY

Somatoform disorders may take the form of somatization, conversion, psychogenic pain, hypochondriasis, or an atypical somatoform disorder. A brief summary of each is presented herein, including the DSM-III criteria. Terminology including malingering, la belle indifference, primary gain, secondary gain and psychalgia, were discussed. Treatment and nursing interventions were explained, including the establishment of trust, assessment of the patient by the nurse, the importance of a physical examination, referral of physical complaints to the medical staff, the use of psychotropic drugs (*e.g.,* antidepressants, antianxiety agents, and tranquilizers), and the importance of psychotherapy. Examples of nursing diagnoses and nursing interventions focused on ineffective individual coping as exhibited by numerous unfounded somatic complaints due to stress and anxiety and disturbance in self-concept or a low self-image. Clinical examples of conversion disorder and hypochondriasis were given.

LEARNING ACTIVITIES

I. Clinical activities
   A. Care for a patient with the diagnosis of somatoform disorder.
   B. Identify the subclassification according to the clinical symptoms.
   C. Evaluate the patient's insight into his or her condition.
   D. Evaluate the treatment plan. Is it appropriate? How would you improve it?
   E. Write a process recording of your interaction with the patient.
II. Somatoform disorder: Conversion reaction
   MJ, 32 years old, married and an art instructor, is admitted to the medical unit with the complaint of numbness and loss of strength on her left side, affecting both her arm and leg. She denies any history of injury.
   During the interview she tells you that she is having marital problems. History reveals that 3 years before admission, she received psychiatric help for increased anxiety due to a poor sexual relationship with her husband.
   At present both she and her husband are working, and, because of social responsibilities, they are unable to spend much time together. MJ has become friends with a male teacher and is worried that her husband will think she is unfaithful. She states that shortly after her husband learned about her relationship with this man, she began experiencing symptoms of numbness and weakness.
   A. What purpose do the numbness and loss of strength serve?
   B. Develop a nursing care plan for MJ.

SELF-TEST

1. Define the following terms:
   Somatoform disorder
   Malingering
   La belle indifference
   Primary gain
   Secondary gain
   Psychalgia

2. Give examples of a secondary gain.
3. Differentiate between hypochondriasis and somatization disorder.
4. State the diagnostic criteria for psychogenic pain disorder.
5. Explain why the treatment of somatoform disorders is frustrating.
6. List nursing interventions for the following:
   Ineffective individual coping as exhibited by unfounded somatic complaints due to stress and anxiety
   Disturbance in self-concept: Low self-image

REFERENCES

Carpenito LJ: Nursing Diagnoses: Application to Clinical Practitioner. Philadelphia, JB Lippincott, 1983

Donlon P, Rockwell D: Psychiatric Disorders Diagnosis and Treatment. Bowie, IN, Robert Brady, 1982

Faan WE, Goshen CE: The Language of Mental Health, 2nd ed. St. Louis, CV Mosby, 1977

Freedman, Kaplan, Sadock: Comprehensive Textbook of Psychiatry. Baltimore, Wilkins & Wilkins, 1975

Gluck MM: Group Therapy in a Pain Management Program. J Psych Nurs: Nov, 1980

Haber J et al: Comprehensive Psychiatric Nursing, 2nd ed. New York, McGraw–Hill, 1982

Kolb L: Modern Clinical Psychiatry. Philadelphia, WB Saunders, 1977

Lancaster J: Adult Psychiatric Nursing. New York, Medical Examination Publishing, 1980

Lego S: The American Handbook of Psychiatric Nursing. Philadelphia, JB Lippincott, 1984

Munford PR: Conversion disorders. Psychiatr Clin North Am: Aug, 1978

Murray RB, Huelskoetter MM: Psychiatric/Mental Health Nursing: Giving Emotional Care. Englewood Cliffs, Prentice–Hall, 1983

Pasquali A, Arnold D: Mental Health Nursing: A Bio-Psycho-Cultural Approach. St. Louis, CV Mosby, 1981

Robinson L: Psychiatric Nursing As a Human Experience. Philadelphia, WB Saunders, 1983

Rowe CJ: An Outline of Psychiatry. Dubuque, William Brown 1980

Schultz J, Dark S: Manual of Psychiatric Nursing Care Plans. Boston, Little, Brown & Co, 1982

Stuart GW, Sundeen SJ: Principles and Practice of Psychiatric Nursing, 2nd ed. St. Louis, CV Mosby 1983

Wilson HS, Kneisl CR: Psychiatric Nursing, 2nd ed. Menlo Park, Addison-Wesley Publishing, 1983

16

MALADAPTIVE COPING

BY DISSOCIATIVE

BEHAVIOR

LEARNING OBJECTIVES

1. Define the term *dissociative disorders.*
2. Describe the clinical types of psychogenic amnesia.
3. Differentiate between fugue and amnesia.
4. Explain the term *multiple personality.*
5. Discuss nursing interventions for patients who are diagnosed as having disso- ciative disorders and state the rationale for each.

AMNESIA, fugue, multiple personality, or depersonalization disor- ders are rare conditions identified as dissociative disorders, Persons afflicted with these disorders handle psychosocial stressors, anxiety, or dangerous situations by "purposeful forgetting." There is a sudden, temporary alteration in one's consciousness, identity, or motor behavior in the absence of psychotic symptoms, organic brain damage, or alcohol- ism. The person is unable to recall a cluster of related mental events. Per- sons subject to the development of dissociative disorders are said to be self-centered and immature, often with a history of an emotional distur- bance earlier in life. The previous DSM-II classification was hysterical neu- roses, dissociative type. A summary of each of these subclassifications follows.

PSYCHOGENIC AMNESIA

Psychogenic amnesia is a disorder described as a sudden inability to recall an extensive amount of important personal information because of phys- ical or psychological trauma. It is not the result of an organic mental dis- order. Examples of predisposing factors include an intolerable life situa- tion, unacceptability of certain impulses or acts, or a threat of physical injury or death. Amnesia can be described as

1. Circumscribed or localized (occurring a few hours after a traumatic experience or major event)

2. Selective (inability to recall part of the events of a specific time)

3. Generalized (inability to recall one's entire life events)

4. Continuous (inability to recall events after a specific event up to and including the present)

Clinical features include perplexity, disorientation, and purposeless wandering. Although the person may experience a mild or severely impaired ability to function, it is usually temporary because rapid recov- ery generally occurs. This condition is seen rarely but is more common during natural disasters or wartime.

Suggested treatment measures include hypnosis or narcoanalysis. Narcoanalysis is the injection of barbiturates before therapy, during which the patient's fantasies or memories are explored.

Psychogenic Amnesia: Clinical Example

JC, a 35-year-old business executive, was flying to Reno, Nevada in his private plane when it crash landed in the mountains. Two days later he was found by a rescue team wandering down a mountain road. When he was called by name, JC did not respond. He told the rescuers that he could not remember who he was or what he was doing on the mountainside. After an assessment by the emergency squad, he was found exhibiting symptoms of generalized psychogenic amnesia.

PSYCHOGENIC FUGUE

Fugue differs from psychogenic amnesia in that the person suddenly and unexpectedly leaves home or work and is unable to recall the past. Assumption of a new identity, partial or complete, usually occurs after relocation to another geographic area when the person is unable to recall his identity. Fugue is a rare occurrence that may be seen in wartime during extreme stress, conflict or a natural disaster, and may last days or months. Excessive use of alcohol may contribute to the development of this rare disorder.

Rapid recovery usually occurs, but the person generally must receive psychiatric care.

MULTIPLE PERSONALITY

Sybil and *The Three Faces of Eve* are both popular media representations of multiple personality in which the person is dominated by at least one of two or more definitive personalities at one time. Emergence of various personalities occurs suddenly and often is associated with psychosocial stress and conflict. When two or more subpersonalities exist, each is aware of the others to varying degrees. One personality can interact with the external environment at any given moment; however, one or any number of the other personalities actively perceives all that is occurring. The individual personalities are generally quite discrepant and frequently appear to be opposites. Each is complex and integrated with its own unique behavior patterns and social relationships. For example, a shy middle-aged bachelor may present himself as a gigolo on weekends.

This diagnosis may occur in early childhood or later but rarely is diagnosed until adolescence. The degree of impairment may vary from moderate to severe, depending on the persistence, number and nature of the various subpersonalities. This disorder can be difficult to identify unless the person is observed closely.

Psychiatric treatment of these rare complex personalities is quite challenging and requires the services of an experienced psychiatrist. Intermittent periods of hospitalization may be appropriate while attempting to integrate the personalities. If legal issues are raised, the person is referred to a forensic expert.

DEPERSONALIZATION DISORDER

The person who exhibits symptoms of this disorder experiences a strange alteration in the perception or experience of the self associated often with a sense of unreality. This temporary loss of one's own reality includes feelings of being in a "dreamlike state," "out of the body," "mechanical," or bizarre in appearance. Predisposing factors include fatigue, meditation, hypnosis, anxiety, physical pain, severe stress, and depression.

Clinical diagnosis includes documentation of frequent prolonged episodes that impair occupational and social functioning. Dizziness, depression, anxiety, fear of "going insane," and a disturbance in the subjective sense of time are common associated features. Adolescents and young adults are more likely to experience this disorder; it is considered rare after age 40.

Although prognosis of an acute onset is good, the person may need to be removed from a threatening situation or environment to prevent the development of a chronic disorder.

Treatment similar to that listed for a conversion disorder is suggested. (see Chap. 15). Psychoanalysis is also effective.

NURSING INTERVENTIONS

Although care of patients with dissociative disorders is administered by psychiatrists or law enforcement officers to establish identity, nursing intervention may occur in such settings as the emergency room, a crisis center, or in patient settings.

A thorough physical assessment should be done to eliminate organic causes (*e.g.,* a brain tumor). A psychosocial assessment is used to identify behavioral changes such as degree of orientation, level of anxiety, depth of depression, degree of impaired social and occupational functioning, and amount of amnesia present, if any. Environmental manipulation may reduce anxiety and make the patient feel safe and secure. People who experience feelings of being "mechanical" or in a "dreamlike state" may require assistance with their activities of daily living (ADL). Family counseling may be necessary to help family members learn new ways to deal with the patient. The following are examples of nursing diagnoses and nursing interventions for patients with dissociative disorders.

NURSING DIAGNOSES	NURSING INTERVENTIONS
Alteration in thought process because of amnesia	Establish rapport and trust. Identify amount or degree of amnesia present. Present reality by stating as much factual information as possible (*i.e.*, "Today is Monday, February 4, 1986," or "Your name is James Smith and you are in Memorial Hospital.")
Anxiety due to amnesia	Decrease feelings of anxiety by encouraging verbalization of feelings. Present reality. Provide a safe, protective environment. Identify positive coping mechanisms. Explore alternative coping mechanisms or techniques such as relaxation exercises (see Chap. 12). Medicate with antianxiety agents as prescribed. Refer to social service for environmental manipulation if necessary.
Self-care deficit because of feelings of depersonalization	Assess cause and degree of impaired self-care. Provide assistance as necessary to perform ADL. Encourage verbalization of feelings regarding depersonalization. Present reality if the patient discusses feelings of being in a "dreamlike state."

SUMMARY

Dissociative disorders are subclassified as 1) psychogenic amnesia, 2) psychogenic fugue, 3) multiple personality, and 4) depersonalization disorders. A summary of each disorder was presented, focusing on precipitating factors, clinical features, and suggested psychiatric treatment. Nursing interventions were discussed, including physical and psychosocial assessment. Areas of psychosocial assessment suggested identification of degree of orientation, level of anxiety, depth of depression, degree of impaired social and occupational functioning, and amount of amnesia present. The purpose of environmental manipulation was discussed. Examples of the following nursing diagnoses and nursing interventions for each were given: alteration in thought process due to amnesia; anxiety due to amnesia; and self-care deficit due to feelings of depersonalization.

LEARNING ACTIVITIES

I. Clinical activities

    A. Identify examples of dissociative disorders in your clinical agency. If no disorders are present, interview the personnel to obtain information pertaining to patients previously hospitalized with symptoms of dissociative disorders.

    B. Role play psychogenic amnesia in the presence of your clinical peers. Discuss feelings experienced by those participating in the role-play situation and the reactions of those observing.

II. Situation for discussion: Dissociative disorder

MJ, a 52-year-old treasurer of a large accounting firm, is suspected of having embezzled money for several years. An audit of the books occurs that substantiates the employer's suspicions. MJ is relieved of his duties and is scheduled to appear at a court hearing regarding his employer's charges. The day of the court hearing MJ is interrogated by the attorney representing his employer. MJ states that he cannot remember anything that happened during the time he worked as treasurer of the firm. The judge postpones the hearing pending the results of psychiatric testing. The tentative diagnosis is psychogenic amnesia.

    A. Describe the clinical symptoms of MJ.

    B. Discuss your role as a psychiatric nurse when caring for MJ during his psychiatric evaluation.

III. Independent activities

    A. Read an article or book on multiple personality, for example, *Sybil* or *The Three Faces of Eve.*

    B. Interview a local law enforcement person about the protocol followed when handling a patient exhibiting symptoms of amnesia of fugue.

SELF-TEST

1. Define psychogenic amnesia.

2. The inability to recall part of the events of a specific time is which type of amnesia?

3. The inability to recall one's previous life is _____ amnesia.

4. _____ amnesia occurs within a few hours after a traumatic experience.

5. State a situation in which psychogenic fugue may occur.

6. Define multiple personality.

7. Describe depersonalization disorder.

8. State nursing interventions for
   Alteration in thought process due to amnesia
   Anxiety due to amnesia
   Self-care deficit due to feelings of depersonalization

REFERENCES

Donlon P, Rockwell D: Psychiatric Disorders: Diagnosis, and Treatment. Bowie, IN, Robert Brady Co, 1982

Faan E, Goshen E: The Language of Mental Health, 2nd ed. St. Louis, CV Mosby, 1977

Freedman, Kaplan, Sadock: Comprehensive Textbook of Psychiatry. Baltimore, Williams & Wilkins, 1975

Haber R et al: Comprehensive Psychiatric Nursing, 2nd ed. New York, McGraw–Hill, 1982

Kolb L: Modern Clinical Psychiatry. Philadelphia, WB Saunders, 1977

Lancaster J: Adult Psychiatric Nursing. New York, Medical Examination Publishing Co., 1980

Manfreda L, Krampitz SD: Psychiatric Nursing. Philadelphia, FA Davis, 1977

Murray RB, Huelskoetter MM: Psychiatric/Mental Health Nursing: Giving Emotional Care. Englewood Cliffs, Prentice–Hall, 1983

Robinson L: Psychiatric Nursing As a Human Experience. Philadelphia, WB Saunders, 1983

Rowe CJ: An Outline of Psychiatry. Dubuque, William C Brown, 1980

Schreiber FR: Sybil. Chicago, Regnery, 1973

Schultz M, Dark L: Manual of Psychiatric Care Plans. Boston, Little, Brown & Co., 1982

Stevenson RL: The Strange Case of Dr. Jekyll and Mr. Hyde and Other Famous Tales. New York, Dodd, Mead, 1961

Stuart GW, Sundeen SJ: Principles and Practice of Psychiatric Nursing, 2nd ed. St. Louis, CV Mosby, 1983

Thigpen CH, Cleckley HM: The Three Faces of Eve. New York, McGraw–Hill, 1957

Toffler A: Future Shock. New York, Random House, 1970

Wilson H, Kneisl C: Psychiatric Nursing, 2nd ed. Menlo Park, Addison Wesley, 1983

17

MALADAPTIVE BEHAVIOR

RESULTING IN

PERSONALITY DISORDERS

LEARNING OBJECTIVES

1. Define personality disorder.
2. List the common characteristics shared by the various categories of personality disorders.
3. Describe the possible etiologic factors in the development of a personality disorder.
4. State the 12 DSM-III categories of personality disorder.
5. Identify the correct category of a personality disorder when specific clinical symptoms are given.
6. State appropriate nursing interventions for the following behaviors:
   Acting out
   Manipulation
   Dependency
   Impaired verbal communication
   Sensory perceptual alteration resulting in paranoid ideation
   Ineffective individual coping
7. Develop a nursing care plan for a patient diagnosed with a passive–aggressive personality disorder.

D URING the process of personality development, the person establishes certain traits which enable him to observe, interact with, and think about the environment and himself. If he develops a positive self-concept, body-image, and sense of self-worth and is able to relate to others openly and honestly, he is said to have characterisitcs of a healthy personality. Should the person develop inflexible, maladaptive behaviors (*e.g.,* manipulation, hostility, lying, poor judgment, and alienation) that interfere with social or occupational functioning, he exhibits signs and symptoms of a personality disorder.

Personality disorder is described as a nonpsychotic illness characterized by maladaptive behavior, which the person utilizes to fulfill his or her needs and bring satisfaction to self. These behaviors begin during childhood or adolescence as a way of coping and remain throughout most of adulthood, becoming less obvious during middle or old age. As a result of inability to relate to the environment, the person acts out his conflicts socially. Emotional, economic, social, or occupational problems are often seen as a result of such conflicts.

Characteristics of a personality disorder are as follows:

1. The person denies the maladaptive behaviors he exhibits; they have become a way of life for him.

2. The maladaptive behaviors are inflexible.

3. Minor stress is poorly tolerated, resulting in increased inability to cope.

4. Ego functioning is intact but may be defective; therefore, it may not control impulsive actions of the id.

5. The person is in contact with reality although he has difficulty dealing with it.

6. Disturbance of mood, such as anxiety or depression, may be present.

7. Psychiatric help rarely is sought because the person is unaware or denies that his behavior is maladaptive.

Older terms used to describe personality disorder include character neurosis, psychopath, and character disorder.

Before the development of the DSM-III, the classification of personality disorder also included alcoholism, drug abuse, and sexual deviancy. There are now 12 diagnoses grouped into three clusters or descriptive categories. Persons who exhibit paranoid, schizoid, and schizotypal personality disorders are considered "odd" or eccentric in the vernacular. The second cluster of disorders, histrionic, narcissistic, antisocial, and borderline are considered to be emotional, erratic, or dramatic in behavior. Anxious or fearful behaviors are often present in the third cluster, which includes avoidant, compulsive, and passive–aggressive personality disorders. A residual category (labeled atypical, mixed or other personality disorder) is used for conditions not included in the original 12.

ETIOLOGY OF PERSONALITY DISORDERS

Theorists state the following etiologic factors in the development of personality disorders:

1. The person is biologically predisposed or more subject to the development of the disorder. Examples of biologic predispositions include improper nutrition, neurologic defects, and genetic predisposition.

2. Childhood experiences foster the development of maladaptive behavior.

   Receiving reward for behavior such as a temper tantrum encourages acting out (i.e., the parent gives in to a child's wishes rather than setting limits to stop the behavior).

   Creativity is not encouraged in the child; therefore, the child does not have the opportunity to express himself or to learn to relate to others. The ability to be creative would provide a child with the opportunity to develop a positive self-concept and sense of self-worth.

   Rigid upbringing during childhood also has a negative effect on the development of a child's personality because it discourages experimentation and promotes the development of low self-esteem. It may also cause feelings of hostility and alienation in the child–parent relationship.

Fostering dependency discourages personality development and allows the child to become a conformist rather than an independent being with an opportunity to develop a positive self-concept.

A child identifies with parents or authority figures who display socially undesirable behavior. As a result of this identification process, the child imitates behavior that he believes to be acceptable by others. Such behavior frequently puts him in direct conflict with society.

3. Socially deviant persons have defective egos through which they are unable to control their impulsive behavior.

4. A weak superego results in the incomplete development of or lack of a conscience. Persons with immature superegos feel no guilt or remorse for socially unacceptable behavior.

5. The drive for prestige, power, and possessions can result in exploitative, manipulative behavior. Such is the case in prostitution, embezzlement, and gambling.

6. Urban societies, such as inner cities, are characterized by a low degree of social interaction, thereby fostering the development of deviant behavior.

CLINICAL TYPES OF PERSONALITY DISORDERS

The following are categories of personality disorders.

PARANOID PERSONALITY DISORDER

Theorists believe that the person who develops a paranoid personality has chronic hostility that is projected onto others. This hostility develops in childhood owing to poor interpersonal family relationships. As a result, the person who has experienced much loneliness becomes unwarrantedly suspicious and mistrusts people. He may suspect attempts to trick or harm him, question the loyalty of others, display pathologic jealousy, observe the environment for any signs of threat, display secretiveness, become hypersensitive, or display excessive feelings of self-importance. The person also may appear to be unemotional, lack a sense of humor, and lack the ability to relax. Features such as delusions and hallucinations may be absent. Interpersonal relationships are poor, especially when relating to authority figures or co-workers. This disorder is seen more frequently in men.

Reactions by student nurses to patients with unwarranted thoughts of suspicion include feelings of frustration, helplessness, anger, or disgust. If the patient exhibits signs of hostility, the nurse may fear aggressive behavior.

Paranoid Personality: Clinical Example

JJ, a 29-year-old school teacher, has been having difficulty interacting with the other teachers at work. He has become quite suspicious of their actions and argues with them during faculty meetings. They notice that he tends to exaggerate and trusts no one to help him with his faculty responsibilities. He also appears to be quite guarded and secretive. His tenseness is noted when he counterattacks any suggestions that relate to his job. He appears quite serious and "cold" during conversations with other faculty members.

SCHIZOID PERSONALITY DISORDER

Synonyms for someone with a schizoid personality include introvert, "loner," and "lone wolf" because the person has no desire for social involvement.

The clinical symptoms include shyness; indifference to criticism, praise, or the feelings of others; inability to form social relationships; absence of warm, tender feelings; aloofness or isolation; and excessive daydreaming.

The person displaying schizoid personality traits is unable to express feelings of hostility or aggressiveness. He focuses attention on objects such as books and cars rather than people. He may function well in situations of social isolation; (*e.g.,* truck driver, artist, muscian, or poet).

Schizoid Personality: Clinical Example

HG, a 22-year-old truck driver, was admitted to the general hospital for injuries received in an auto–truck accident. While being treated in the emergency room, the nurse noted that HG was emotionally cold as he described the accident. He showed no concern for the driver of the car involved in the accident. When asked if he had any relatives or friends that he wanted to be notified, HG stated, "I don't have any friends or relatives." As he continued to recuperate from his injuries, the nurse noted no change in his emotional reaction to hospitalization. The day of his discharge, HG was indifferent to the citation he received from the state highway patrol.

Nurses who care for persons like HG find it extremely difficult to establish any type of therapeutic relationship because of the patient's reserved, withdrawn, or seclusive behavior.

ANTISOCIAL PERSONALITY DISORDER

Synonyms for this personality disorder include sociopathic, psychopathic, and semantic disorder.

Several theories have been proposed to explain the development of the antisocial personality, although the exact cause is not really known. They are as follows:

1. Genetic or hereditary factors interfere with the development of positive interpersonal relationships during childhood. The child therefore does not learn to respect the rights of others. He may become self-indulgent and expect special favors from others, but does not display appreciation or reciprocal behavior.

2. Brain damage or trauma can precipitate the development of antisocial behavior.

3. Low socioeconomic status encourages the development of an antisocial personality. People may turn to maladaptive behaviors, such as stealing, lying, and cheating, just to survive.

4. Faulty family relationships in a broken home inhibit normal personality development during childhood.

5. Parents unconsciously foster antisocial behavior in children during developmental years. If parents are too involved in their own personal problems or life-styles and neglect to spend time with the child or be available when help is needed, the child learns to "fend for himself." Any behavior that will result in a secondary gain of attention, security, or love is tried. If desirable results are obtained, the child continues to use the maladaptive behavior to meet his needs.

Antisocial behavior is usually seen in persons between ages of 15 and 40. If diagnosed before age 18, the term, according to the DSM-III, is conduct disorder. Symptoms may be evident before age 15 and include behaviors such as truancy, misbehavior at school resulting in suspension or expulsion, delinquency, substance abuse, vandalism, and disobedience.

The DSM-III states that the diagnosis of an antisocial personality is reserved for people age 18 or over who exhibited signs of antisocial behavior before age 15. They also must exhibit four or more of the following clinical symptoms at age 18 or older:

1. Lack of capacity to show concern for others or to form a responsible relationship with family or friends

2. Inability to sustain a satisfying sexual relationship. Displays a history of two or more divorces or separations, promiscuous behavior, or desertion of a significant other.

3. Expects immediate gratification (the pleasure principle) and fails to accept social norms, resulting in unlawful behavior such as theft, selling drugs, prostitution, etc. Usually presents with a history of multiple arrests because of being unable to modify the maladaptive behavior

4. Impulsive actions such as moving without making specific plans for relocation or for securing a job

5. Poor occupational record owing to frequent job changes, unemployment, or chronic absenteeism

6. Inability to function as a responsible parent. The antisocial person may neglect the child's nutritional needs, health, need for shelter, or security.

7. Aggressive behavior that results in fighting or assault of strangers as well as abuse of significant others

8. Inability to remain financially stable, resulting in default of debts and not meeting financial obligations

9. Lack of respect for the truth results in repeated lying and similar behavior.

10. Reckless behavior such as speeding or driving while under the influence of alcohol

Cessation of criminal activities tends to occur around age 40. Statistics show that 80% to 90% of all crime is committed by antisocial people who are incarcerated to protect society. Statistics also show that the diagnosis is made more frequently with men.

The following information is a summary of an interview with a 21-year-old patient diagnosed as an antisocial personality.

The client revealed she had problems since she was 13 years old when she ran away from her home. Her parents had marital problems and were divorced when she was 15. At that time she became unmanageable, involved with drugs, skipped school, and eventually was placed in a juvenile home.

At age 16 she married impulsively, 3 days after meeting her first husband. The marriage lasted only a few days and ended in divorce. Between the ages of 17 and 21 the client stated that she had had five pregnancies, and married a second time. After approximately 6 months, this marriage also ended in divorce. Difficulties with the law included arrest for possession of marijuana, selling drugs, passing bad checks, stealing a car, and robbery. The client cited numerous hospitalizations in mental and penal institutions. She stated she felt good when she was either pregnant or locked up. Hospitalization made her feel secure. The client stated that her mother disliked her because she styled her hair similar to her father's haircut and had mannerisms similar to his. Although she attempted to imitate her father's appearance, she described ambivalent feelings for him.

Persons who exhibit antisocial behavior elicit a variety of responses from nursing personnel. Working with persons who are manipulative, impulsive, aggressive and do not conform to social norms may be quite challenging as well as discouraging. Although many are incarcerated, some of the persons are able to respond to treatment. Group peer therapy with strong external controls seems to be a successful treatment modality.

BORDERLINE PERSONALITY DISORDER

Latent, ambulatory, and abortive schizophrenics are examples of previous labels for this new DSM-III classification. The person has symptoms that fall between moderate neurosis and frank psychosis, yet usually remains quite stable.

Theorists state that borderline disorders may be a result of a faulty parent–child relationship, in which the child does not experience a healthy separation from mother to interact with the environment. Negative feelings are shared by parent and child who are bound together by mutual feelings of guilt. Trauma experienced at a specific stage of development, usually 18 months weakening the person's ego and ability to handle reality is another possible cause. A third theory states that the person experiences an unfulfilled need for intimacy. As a result of attempting to establish an ideal relationship, the person becomes disillusioned and experiences feelings of rage, fear of abandonment, and depression.

According to the DSM-III, clinical symptoms may include

1. Unstable interpersonal relationships
2. Impulsive, unpredictable behavior that may involve gambling, shop lifting, and sex. Such a person tends to use and can tolerate large amounts of drugs and alcohol
3. Inappropriate anger and inability to control anger
4. Disturbance in self-concept, including gender identity
5. Unstable affect that shifts from normal moods to periods of depression, dysphoria (unpleasant mood), or intense anger
6. Chronic feelings or boredom
7. Masochistic behavior (self-inflicted pain) and thoughts of suicide

Other features include feelings of overwhelming loneliness, inability to experience pleasure, and the inability to maintain an occupation. This disorder is seen more frequently in women.

The main defense mechanisms identified in the borderline personality include denial, projection, splitting, and projective identification.

Rowe (1984) describes splitting and projective identification as primitive defenses. He defines *splitting* as the inability to integrate and accept both positive and negative feelings at the same moment. The person can only handle one type of feeling at a time. This characteristic is the opposite of the feeling of ambivalence, in which a person can experience feelings of love and hate simultaneously for another person.

Projective identification is described as the ability to project uncomfortable or aggressive aspects of one's own personality onto external objects. The person is then able to protect himself from the danger or threats he perceives in the external object by attempting to control it.

Examples of uncomfortable aspects of oneself include inadequacy, helplessness, guilt, and failure.

Borderline Personality: Clinical Example

MF, 29 years old, does secretarial work on a part-time basis through a secretarial pool. During the past 3 years she has been unable to keep a steady part-time job for more than 3 months because of an unstable mood in which she exhibited inappropriate anger and impulsive behavior. The personnel director of the secretarial pool suggested MF seek counseling because of feedback from previous employers. During an intake interview, MF disclosed to the therapist her inability to establish a stable interpersonal relationship, which has resulted in periods of depression. At times she also experiences mood changes in which she becomes bored, angry, and hostile. She also reveals a poor self-image that leads to masochistic behavior (*i.e.,* pulling her hair out and biting herself) when she becomes angry.

The borderline personality is probably one of the more difficult types of behavior for the student to understand owing to the person's instability in the areas of behavior, mood, self-image, and interpersonal relationship. Various levels of disorganization occur, ranging from stable to neurotic or psychotic behavior. These symptoms are likely to make the patient less than well liked. Persons who appear bored, impulsive, and display inappropriate behavior are likely to find themselves avoided by nurses who feel inadequate or insecure in any attempt to establish a therapeutic relationship.

HISTRIONIC PERSONALITY DISORDER

The classification of a histrionic personality (also referred to as hysterical personality), is characterized by a pattern of theatrical or overly dramatic behavior. The person continually attempts to draw attention to himself and exhibits intense or exaggerated emotions to minor environmental stimuli. Temper tantrums or irrational actions also may be exhibited. Romantic fantasy occurs as result of impaired sexual adjustment or poor interpersonal relationships. Manipulative suicidal gestures may be made after the termination of a sexual relationship.

The person becomes bored with normal routines and is perceived as being vain, insincere, egocentric, flirtatious, and inconsiderate. Although he may be creative and imaginative, feelings of dependency and helplessness exist. Somatic complaints are usually present. This condition is diagnosed more frequently in women and incidence is considered more common among family members than in the general population.

Students usually react with comments such as "I have a relative who acts like that" or "One of the girls in our class is always exaggerating things. Is that what's wrong with her?" Recently one student commented that it was impossible to identify the patient's true feelings because of overly exaggerated responses when the student attempted interaction. The student felt that the patient was "pulling my leg, wanting me to believe everything she said."

PASSIVE–AGGRESSIVE PERSONALITY DISORDER

The person with a passive–aggressive disorder exhibits a "chip-on-the-shoulder" attitude. He is very dependent, lacks self-confidence, is pessimistic, and has difficulty relating to or working with authority figures. Because of a need to resent or oppose demands made on him, the patient displays behaviors such as stubbornness, procrastination, forgetfulness, tardiness, hostility, or pouting to fulfill a dependency need. This behavior is described as intentional inefficiency and usually results in social and occupational failure.

Possible causes of passive–aggressive personality include

1. Reaction to a dominant, rigid father. In an attempt to cope with stress from a poor father–child relationship, the child resorts to various maladaptive behaviors that are not overt but passive–aggressive in nature.

2. Impaired psychosexual functioning. This person is termed an "oral character" who expresses negative behavior orally to cope with stress and anxiety. This behavior is the result of unsuccessfully completing the oral stage of psychosexual development. To receive oral gratification, the adult regresses to childish behavior.

3. Fear of rejection by society when exhibiting aggressive behavior . Persons who are prone to aggressive behavior and fear rejection of others learn to express themselves in socially acceptable behavior that is subtly negative in nature.

The passive–aggressive disorder is considered the most common maladaptive behavior or psychiatric disorder. If symptoms are evident before age 18, the adolescent is diagnosed as having an oppositional disorder.

Passive–Aggressive Personality: Clinical Example

KO, a 32-year-old mother of two children and just recently divorced, has had to return to full-time work. She works as a receptionist in a medical clinic and lacks self-confidence. Because of a heavy appointment schedule, KO feels overwhelmed at times when completing all the necessary paperwork. She also feels uncomfortable with the patients, who become demanding and hostile when they have to wait for an extended period to see the doctor. After approximately 1 month of work, KO begins to misplace schedules, forgets to give messages to the personnel, and arrives late for work. When questioned about her behavior by the supervisor, KO becomes hostile and is unable to express her feelings during the interview. She is placed on probationary status for 3 months, at which time her work will be reevaluated.

People who display passive–aggressive behavior tend to "drive away" persons who initially attempt to be friendly or helpful. The comments of one student nurse reflect her reactions well. "How can I attempt to help someone who keeps pushing me away? She is never on time for our meetings, and when she does come, all I hear are pessimistic comments and self-derogatory statements."

COMPULSIVE PERSONALITY DISORDER

Individuals who are compulsive are usually preoccupied with rules and regulations, organizational and trivial detail, and are excessively devoted to their work and productivity. As a result of such devotion to work, they fail to experience pleasurable activities. Vacations are postponed indefinitely. Other features include indecisiveness; inability to express warm, tender emotions; and insistence that others do things their way. They fear making a mistake and therefore avoid making decisions. These people are perceived as being inflexible because they are unable to focus on a broad view of things. They remain preoccupied with trivial details. Depression is common. Men are affected more frequently than women.

Interpersonal relationships are affected when feelings of resentment or hurt are experienced by the significant other of the compulsive personality.

Compulsive Personality Disorder: Clinical Example

CK, a 45-year-old accountant, works approximately 70 to 80 hours per week and seldom has time to spend with his wife and three children. During the past 3 years, CK has planned summer vacations with his family but each time canceled reservations due to "urgent deadlines at work." He is so involved with his work that he leaves all family decisions to his wife, including disciplinary measures pertaining to the children. When he is at home, he insists that his wife complete errands for him regardless of her schedule and gives her detailed instructions on how to carry them out. As a result of her husband's behavior, CK's wife has begun to see a marriage counselor, hoping that she may encourage her husband to attend therapy also before their relationship disintegrates completely.

The student nurse should remember that persons such as CK are generally aloof during social interactions and therefore are difficult to approach while attempting to establish a therapeutic interaction.

DEPENDENT PERSONALITY DISORDER

The dependent person lacks self-confidence and is unable to function in an independent role. In an attempt to avoid any chance of becoming self-sufficient, the person allows others to become responsible for his life, letting them make all major decisions for him. He avoids making demands on others to avoid jeopardizing any existing dependent relationships that meet his needs. Social relationships and occupational functioning may be impaired as a result of dependent needs. According to the DSM-III, this disorder is seen more frequently in women. Intense discomfort is experienced by a dependent person who is left alone for some time.

Dependent Personality Disorder: Clinical Example

LW, a 26-year-old housewife, and her husband have relocated to a big city as a result of a job promotion for her husband. While house hunting with a real estate agent, LW is asked to describe the type of house she would like to buy and whether she has any preference for location. LW tells the real estate agent, "My husband knows what we need and where we should live. He makes all the decisions. I'm not as smart as he is when it comes to making correct choices." Once a house is located and they move in, LW lets her husband choose the color schemes for the rooms. She also asks him to select the furniture for their living room. After several weeks, LW has three job interviews for a secretarial position. When her husband arrives home from work one evening, she asks him to decide which of the three jobs she should select.

While working on a one-to-one therapeutic relationship with a female patient with a dependent personality disorder, a student nurse confided during clinical postconference that she felt "like shaking the patient" and "telling her to grow up and act her age." The student was amazed at the patient's ability to avoid taking on any responsibility. The other patients on the unit were beginning to assume responsibility for this "helpless" person.

SCHIZOTYPAL PERSONALITY DISORDER

According to the DSM-III, the schizotypal classification is used to diagnose persons whose symptoms are similar to but not severe enough to meet the criteria for schizophrenia. Diagnostic criteria include

1. Disturbance in thought process (referred to as magical thinking). Examples, according to the DSM-III, include superstitiousness, telepathy, or a "sixth sense."
2. Ideas of reference in which the person believes that casual incidents and events have a direct reference to him.

3. Social isolation (the person limits social contacts to everyday tasks).

4. Perceptual disturbance, such as recurrent illusions or depersonalization

5. Peculiarity in communication (noted as "odd" speech) but no loosening of association, as seen in the schizophrenic patient

6. Inappropriate affect that interferes with face-to-face interaction. The person is referred to as aloof or cold.

7. Paranoid ideation or suspiciousness

8. Hypersensitivity or undue anxiety to either real or imagined criticism

NARCISSISTIC PERSONALITY DISORDER

The main characteristic of a narcissistic disorder is an exaggerated or grandiose sense of self-importance. The person is egotistical and needs constant admiration or attention. When discussing his abilities or achievement, the narcissistic personality overexaggerates. He may set unrealistic goals regarding the achievement of power and wealth. Criticism or disappointment is not well received by this person, who may react with indifference, rage, shame, or humiliation. He lacks the ability to be empathetic or recognize and experience how others feel and may take advantage of others to fulfill his own needs. He may also expect special favors and act surprised or angry when people do not do what he wants.

AVOIDANT PERSONALITY DISORDER

The avoidant personality is so sensitive to rejection, humiliation, or shame that he appears devastated by the slightest amount of disapproval. Diagnostic criteria according to the DSM-III include

1. Hypersensitivity to rejection

2. Unwillingness to enter into interpersonal relationships unless given a guarantee of uncritical acceptance

3. Social withdrawal

4. Desire for affection and acceptance

5. Low self-esteem. The person may berate self–achievements and is excessively disappointed by personal failure or shortcomings.

Feelings of anxiety, anger, and depression are considered common, and social phobia may result if clinical symptoms of social withdrawal and hypersensitivity persist over a period of time. This disorder is considered quite prevalent.

ATYPICAL, MIXED, OR OTHER PERSONALITY DISORDERS

According to the DSM-III, the following guidelines are given for the use of this category

1. *Atypical personality*—Used when there is not enough information to make a specific diagnosis.
2. *Mixed personality disorder*—Reserved for the individual who exhibits features of several of the personality disorders but does not meet the criteria for any one specific category.
3. *Other personality disorders*—Used for a disorder not included in this classification (*e.g.,* masochistic personality disorder.)

TREATMENT OF PERSONALITY DISORDERS

Management of a patient displaying a specific personality disorder is very difficult because the person is basically comfortable with his personality and lacks any motivation for change. A person cannot be "sentenced" to therapy. If treatment is sought, it is generally the result of increased anxiety that disrupts social interaction, increased awareness by the person of his unsatisfactory life-style, or the result of a significant other insisting that psychiatric care be sought.

Treatment approaches include therapy that focuses on restructuring the personality, assisting the person with developmental levels and tasks, and limit setting for maladaptive behavior, such as acting out. Group therapy is used to reinforce the patient's realization that he is not unique and to discuss alternative ways to respond to stress. Reality therapy and intensive psychoanalysis also are used. Some theorists think that supportive psychotherapy is better for the borderline patient, who may be unable to endure intensive psychoanalysis.

Psychotropic drugs may be selected and prescribed for specific clinical symptoms or behaviors such as depression, paranoid thoughts, or aggression, and are individualized according to the patient's needs.

Treatment of any of the described disorders tends to be long-term and does not guarantee recovery. Many of the patients become semi-independent and have recurrent acute episodes.

NURSING INTERVENTION

The nursing care of a person who is diagnosed as having a personality disorder is directed at the specific behavior, characteristics, and symptoms that are common to the identified disorder.

Maladaptive behaviors such as acting-out, stubbornness, procrastination, over-exaggeration, manipulation, and complete dependency can elicit negative responses from nursing personnel. A friendly, accepting environment should be established in which the patient is accepted but not his maladaptive behavior. It is imperative that the nurse examine her feelings about such behavior so that she does not allow them to interfere with therapeutic nursing interventions.

The individual needs to be given an opportunity to develop ego controls such as the superego or conscience that is lacking or underdeveloped. This can be achieved by consistent limit-setting that is enforced twenty-four hours-a-day.

Examples of nursing diagnosis and nursing interventions will be discussed at this time.

NURSING DIAGNOSES	NURSING INTERVENTIONS
Ineffective coping: Hostility or acting out	Recognize signs of increasing agitation. Attempt to "talk down" the patient. Encourage verbalization of feelings to find reason for anger. Maintain a safe or spatial distance to avoid physical contact. Evaluate appropriateness of hostility. Respond positively to reasonable demands and requests. Accept the patient, but inform him when his behavior is unacceptable. Set limits and be consistent with realistic controls. Attempt to rechannel behavior by providing a safe environment for acting out hostility, providing distraction, or assigning constructive tasks. Administer p.r.n. medication to decrease anxiety. Use external controls (e.g., restraints) as a last measure.
Noncompliance: Manipulative behavior	Be aware of "power plays" or attempts to manipulate members of the staff. Identify types of manipulative behavior exhibited by the patient. Explore your own feelings regarding such behavior. Confront the patient if necessary, but without anger, disappointment, or disgust. May need to become a parental surrogate temporarily to reinforce authority. Discuss expectations with patient. Set limits and be consistent with care. Maintain consistency and continuity of approach with staff. Observe interactions with other patients to

NURSING DIAGNOSES	NURSING INTERVENTIONS
	discourage manipulative behavior. Intervene if necessary.
Self-care deficit: Dependency on staff to meet basic human needs	Evaluate patient's developmental level and ability to carry out the activities for daily lining (ADL). Identify dependency needs, physically and psychologically. Identify present coping mechanisms and support systems. Avoid assuming a parental role. Be firm when interacting with the patient. Set short-term goals with the patient to increase independence (*i.e.*, daily responsibilities related to self-care, decision making, etc).
Impaired verbal communication: Inability to develop positive interpersonal relationships	Develop trust or rapport. Establish a one-to-one relationship. Encourage expression of self-concept, including positive and negative feelings. Explore feelings regarding inability to relate positively to others.
Sensory perceptual alteration: Inability to trust others (suspicious)	Develop trust. Be honest with the patient. Be nonthreatening when interacting with patient. Convey concern and interest. Listen for expressions of anxiety, fear, or mistrust. Face but distance the patient when speaking to him. Avoid being overly friendly. Be specific and clear when presenting information to the patient. Speak in a normal tone of voice. Do not whisper when near the patient. Be selective in the use of nonverbal gestures while speaking with or near the patient. Respect the patient's need for privacy. Discuss confidentiality. Include the patient in planning treatment to allow the patient some control. Plan brief contacts with the patient. Explain procedures to the patient in detail and discuss any changes in routine. Be honest, never trick the patient into taking medication.
Ineffective individual coping owing to increased stress or anxiety	Provide a calm, quiet atmosphere to decrease excitatory environmental stimuli. Attempt to identify the source or cause of increased stress or anxiety.

(continued)

NURSING DIAGNOSES	NURSING INTERVENTIONS
	Encourage the patient to verbalize feelings. Identify previous effective coping mechanisms. Explore new coping mechanisms. Medicate with anti-anxiety agents per physician's order.

SUMMARY

A personality disorder is classified as a nonpsychotic illness. It is characterized by maladaptive behavior such as acting out, manipulation, suspiciousness, and dependency. The person may deny the maladaptive behavior because it has become a part of the personality structure. He manages to survive in the environment unless a conflict with society brings him to the attention of the law or a professional counselor. Behavioral changes are difficult to achieve because the person is basically comfortable and lacks motivation. Characteristics of a personality disorder, etiology, and the 12 clinical types were presented: paranoid, schizoid, antisocial, borderline, histrionic, passive–aggressive, compulsive, dependent, schizotypal, narcissistic, avoidant, and atypical, mixed, or other personality disorders. Examples of psychiatric treatment approaches, as well as nursing diagnoses and interventions for ineffective coping, manipulative behavior, dependency, impaired verbal communication, suspicious behavior, and ineffective individual coping were presented.

LEARNING ACTIVITIES

I. Clinical activities
   A. Identify a patient with the diagnosis of a personality disorder or with a behavioral problem such as acting out or manipulation.
   B. Establish a therapeutic relationship.
   C. Discuss the treatment program prescribed for the patient.
   D. Does the patient have insight into his or her problem?
   E. Does the patient seem to want to be helped?
   F. Is the patient cooperative? How does he relate to staff and other patients?
   G. What is the prognosis for this patient?
II. Antisocial personality: Clinical situation for discussion
   Review the summary of an interview with a 21-year-old patient diagnosed as having an antisocial personality disorder presented in this chapter. Compare her diagnosis and clinical symptoms to those of the DSM-III criteria for antisocial personality.

1. List as many clinical symptoms as possible.
2. What diagnosis should she have had prior to age 18?
3. Develop a treatment plan for this client. Consider milieu therapy, psychotherapy, and psychotropic drugs.
4. How would you describe her prognosis?

III. Independent Activity
   A. Read one of the following: *In Cold Blood* by Truman Capote, *Helter Skelter* by Vincent Bugliosi and Curt Gentry, or *"Son": A Psychopath and His Victims* by Jack Olsen. Evaluate your feelings about the characters who display antisocial behavior.
   B. View a prime time television show that presents examples of maladaptive behaviors (*e.g,* police or crime shows). Identify the following behaviors:
      1. Manipulation
      2. Acting out
      3. Hostility
      4. Lying
      5. Excessive daydreaming
      6. Impulsive actions
      7. Aggressiveness
   C. Discuss or evaluate your reactions to the following situations:
      1. A 27-year-old female is admitted to your unit for a dilation and curettage (D and C). As you read the physician's admitting history, you note that the patient is diagnosed as an antisocial personality who has a history of prostitution and using drugs. She is to be released in custody to the police department when discharged.
      2. An 80-year-old female is admitted from a nursing home with the diagnosis of pneumonia. As you making the initial assessment, the patient states "I need to go home. My husband has an eye for other women and will start to run around if I'm not there to keep him in line." Later, as you administer oral medication, the patient asks you several questions and refuses to take the medication. She states that she never saw the medication before and wants to talk to the doctor first. She also refuses to let the laboratory technician take the admitting blood sample because the technician "might hurt her."

SELF-TEST

1. Hostility and suspiciousness are exhibited by a person with a _____ personality.
2. An introverted person who is unable to form social relationships may be diagnosed as a _____ personality.

3. Projective identification and splitting are defenses exhibited by what type of personality?

4. Which personality disorder is considered the most common?

5. Name two possible causes of passive–aggressive behavior.

6. Theatrical, overly dramatized behavior, and temper tantrums are maladaptive behaviors used by the _____.

7. The compulsive personality disorder is characterized by what kinds of symptoms?

8. List three diagnostic criteria for a schizotypal personality disorder.

9. Define narcissistic behavior.

10. Describe avoidant personality disorder.

11. State the rationale for the following diagnoses:
    Atypical personality disorder
    Mixed personality disorder
    Other personality disorder

12. Persons with personality disorders seek treatment as a result of _____.

13. List three examples of treatment prescribed for personality disorders.

14. State nursing measures or interventions for the following:
    Manipulation
    Paranoid ideation
    Overly dependent behavior
    Acting out behavior

REFERENCES

Agee V: Treatment of the Violent Incorrigible Adolescent. Lexington, Ky, Heath & Co, 1979

Burgess A: Psychiatric Nursing in the Hospital and the Community, 3rd ed. Englewood Cliffs, Prentice–Hall, 1981

Dreyer S, Bailey D, Doricet W: Guide to Nursing Management of Psychiatric Patients, 2nd ed. St. Louis, CV Mosby, 1979

Haber J et al: Comprehensive Psychiatric Nursing. New York, McGraw–Hill 1982

Knowles RD: Handling anger: Responding vs. reacting. Am J Nurs: Dec, 1981

Kolb L: Modern Clinical Psychiatry. Philadelphia, WB Saunders, 1977

Kyes J, Hofling CK: Basic Psychiatric Concepts in Nursing. Philadelphia, JB Lippincott, 1980

Lancaster J: Adult Psychiatric Nursing. New York, Medical Examination Publishing Co, 1980

McMorrow M E: The manipulative patient. Am J Nurs June, 1981

Mahler M et al: Psychological Birth of the Human Infant: Symbiosis and Individuation. New York, Basic Books, 1975

Mereness D, Taylor C: Essentials of Psychiatric Nursing. St. Louis, CV Mosby, 1982

Murphy P, Schultz E: Passive–aggressive behavior in patients and staff. J Psych Nurs: Mar, 1978

Nissley B, Townes N: Guidelines for intervention in aggressive behavior. Psychiatric/Mental Health Nursing: Contemporary Readings. New York, D. Van Nostrand Company, 1978.

Pasquali E et al: Mental Health Nursing: A Bio-Psycho-Cultural Approach. St. Louis, CV Mosby, 1981

Pisarik G: Facing the violent patient. Nurs 81: Sept, 1981

Porter S: Working with a killer: Nurs 81: June, 1981

Richardson J: The manipulative patient spells trouble. Nurs 81: Jan, 1981

Robinson L: Psychiatric Nursing As a Human Experience. Philadelphia, W.B. Saunders, 1983

Rowe C J: An Outline of Psychiatry. Dubuque, William C Brown, 1984

Rzepka D: We Were No Match for 'Zorba the Greek'. Am J Nurs: Sept, 1975

Schultz J, Dark S: Manual of Psychiatric Nursing Care Plans. Boston, Little, Brown & Co, 1982

Shapiro ER: The psychodynamics and developmental psychology of a borderline patient: A review of the literature. Am J Psychiatr: Nov, 1978

Sills G, Wise D: The manipulative client (film). American Journal of Nursing

Sills G, Wise D: The suspicious client (film). American Journal of Nursing

Suprina R: Curing with kindness. Nurs 81: May, 1981

Whitman J: When a patient attacks: Strategies for self-protection when violence looms. RN: Sept, 1979

Wilson H, Kneisl C: Psychiatric Nursing, 2nd ed. Menlo Park, Addison–Wesley, 1983

18

HUMAN SEXUALITY AND

PSYCHOSEXUAL DISORDERS

In the United States, sexual behavior has a very special status, partly because of our puritanical cultural history, partly because we believe sex is very important, and partly because most people learn about sex in covert ways. Among adults, discussions of sexuality are commonly tainted with self-interest, tainted with anxiety and guilt, tainted with fears about seeming either too naive or too jaded.

Gagnon, 1977, p.3.

As evidenced by the work of Kinsey, Masters and Johnson, researchers have been given support to study the physiology, anatomy, psychology and sociology of sex. The media have been helpful in dissemenating such information by way of television talk shows and specials, seminars, newspaper articles, magazines including "Playboy" and "Psychology Today," and various textbooks on human sexuality.

A paraphrase of Walsten's foreword in Gagnon, 1977.

LEARNING OBJECTIVES

1. Define human sexuality.
2. Discuss the criteria of normal sexual behavior.
3. Describe Freud's five stages of psychosexual development.
4. Outline the development of a heterosexual personality.
5. Define each of the following classifications of psychosexual disorders:
   Gender identity disorders
   Paraphilias
   Psychosexual dysfunctions
6. State characteristics of a person witth a gender identity disorder.
7. Differentiate between transsexualism and homosexuality.
8. Define homosexual panic.
9. Describe the following paraphilias:
   Fetishism
   Transvestism
   Pedophilia
   Voyeurism
   Exhibitionism
   Sadism
   Masochism
10. Discuss nursing interventions for patients who
    Make verbal comments with sexual overtones
    Aggressively attempt to make physical contact
    Exhibit symptoms of psychosexual dysfunction due to anxiety

HUMAN sexuality is a term used to describe the result of biologic, chemical, and psychosocial influences on a person. Sexuality can be expressed verbally while talking to a significant other, it can be communicated by written form such as letters, poetry, or songs, and it can be expressed artistically. Behavioral expressions of sexuality include looking, touching, handholding, kissing, and so forth. Sexuality can be expressed in various ways during the development of an intimate interpersonal relationship.

The expression of sexuality may be influenced by cultural or ethnic factors, religious views, health status, physical attributes, age, environment, or by personal choice as a result of one's personality development. Sexuality has been defined as a desire or need for human contact, warmth, or love. "Normal" sexual behavior is described by Goldstein as a sexual act between consenting adults, lacking any type of force, and performed in a private setting in the absence of unwilling observers (1976). Abnormal and unwanted sexual behavior therefore would be considered as any act that does not meet the criteria set forth in Goldstein's definition.

Through the years various sexual practices have been viewed as "normal." The Greeks practiced homosexuality to teach young boys the attributes of manhood; Roman men openly practiced bisexual relations and frequently solicited the attention of married women. Polygamy has been practiced by various racial, religious, and cultural groups in the United States and abroad.

To work effectively with people who exhibit symptoms of psychosexual disorders, the nurse must examine any personal feelings about human sexuality. The nurse will come in contact with a variety of patient concerns regarding sexual identity or activity. The following examples may be experienced by any nurse. The mastectomy patient is concerned that her husband will no longer find her sexually attractive. A cardiac patient expresses a fear of resuming sexual activity after discharge from the hospital. Sexual intimacy is a concern of the colostomy patient who fears rejection owing a change in body image and possible repugnant odors from the stoma. The paraplegic client is afraid to ask his doctor questions about sexual activity and relates his concern to the nurse. A young man discloses his gay identity and fear of contracting the acquired immune deficiency syndrome (AIDS). The chemotherapy patient who is terminally ill requests privacy during visits by a significant other. Elderly patients of the opposite sex may ask permission to share a room in the nursing home. A teenaged girl admits to having several sexual encounters and fears having contracted a sexually transmitted disease. A middle-aged man makes sexual advances while being bathed and attempts to expose his genitals to a nurse. A young male patient asks a young nurse for her address and telephone number.

Sexuality has become a part of the nursing process in planning holistic health care. If the nurse is uncomfortable with or confused about her own sexuality, she will be unable to establish a therapeutic relationship with any of the persons just mentioned. Her role as an educator and her ability to discuss issues of sexuality will be ineffective if she is unaware of her own attitudes.

Formal sex education courses are available for those people who feel the need to explore the topic of sexuality. Masters and Johnson's books *Human Sexual Response* and *Human Sexual Inadequacy* are excellent reference sources. Other useful books are listed at the end of this chapter.

THEORIES OF SEXUAL DEVELOPMENT

Freud's theory of normal personality and sexual (psychosexual) development is helpful in understanding various sexual behaviors. His theory describes a psychobiologic process of five stages, beginning with the oral stage and ending in the genital stage.

The *oral stage* exists from birth to 18 months. During this stage, the mouth is used to attain the goal of oral gratification since the infant is able to suck, bite, talk, and kiss. Persons who are unable to complete this developmental stage may exhibit behaviors such as thumbsucking, nail-biting or hair chewing. The "mouthy" person who is vulgar or uses provocative language is also an example of a person seeking oral gratification.

During the next 18 months (ages 1½–3 yrs) the infant experiences the anal stage, focusing on the function of elimination. Freud describes the impact of strict or permissive toilet training on the personality. Strict training may result in the development of destructive, cruel behavior during this stage. Permissive training may foster the development of extroverted behavior, in which the child leads a productive life while trying to please others. This is the first time that the child must adjust behavior to the demands of others. Conflict during this stage may result in sadomasochistic behavior in adult life. Masochistic behavior (self-inflicted pain) and sadistic behavior (inflicting pain on others) are described under the section on paraphilias.

The phallic stage occurs during the next 2 to 3 years (ages 3–6 yrs). The child focuses energy on the genital area and may be rewarded or punished when this behavior is noticed by adults. Punishment may result in feelings of shame, guilt, or a sense of feeling dirty. Reward may make the child feel that sex is more important than other activities. If the child experiences a balance of both reward and punishment, the concept of sex should result in the development of appropriate sexual identity. Negative experiences may contribute to the development of a sexual disorder (*e.g.,* paraphilia).

During this stage the child also experiences the Oedipus or Electra complex. Boys are attracted to their mother (Oedipus), and girls prefer the attention of their fathers (Electra). They are envious of and feel aggressive feelings toward the parent of the same sex. Boys also experience a castration anxiety, a condition in which they fear damage to or loss of their genitals. Girls desire to possess a penis (penis envy) and become masculine. Failure to resolve these conflicts may result in difficulty with sexual identity or the development of transsexuality or homosexuality in adult life.

The latency stage occurs during prepuberty years, ages 6 though 12. There is a marked decrease in sexual urges and inactivity of sexual impulses. Homosexual or group affiliations occur during this developmental stage. Failure to progress to the genital stage may result in the development of a homosexual personality in adult life.

During the genital or final stage of psychosexual development, from puberty to young adulthood, energy is focused on the opposite sex as a love object. In puberty the person develops the capacity to love and engage in heterosexual relationships while experiencing maturation of the hormonal and genital systems. Failure to progress through this stage could result in the development of psychosexual disorders.

Mature heterosexual relationships involve a variety of modes of sexual expressions, ranging from petting to the act of intercourse. As stated earlier, value systems of various cultures may differentiate normal from deviant sexual behavior, thereby making it difficult to define psychosexual disorders.

The DSM-III classification states that various psychological factors cause the development of psychosexual disorders. These factors are identified in the following paragraphs. This classification includes gender identity disorders, paraphilias, and psychosexual dysfunctions. Homosexuality has been reclassified under the category of other psychosexual disorders but will be discussed under sexual identity disorder due to the nature of the diagnostic criteria. Previously psychosexual dysfunctions were classified under psychophysiologic disorders in DSM-III, and the paraphilias were called sexual deviations.

GENDER IDENTITY DISORDERS

Gender identity disorders are best described as the feeling of discomfort about one's own sexuality while one experiences conflict between anatomic sex and gender identity. The person has difficulty achieving normal heterosexual relations and therefore attempts to satisfy sexual needs by alternative methods. Onset of the disturbance before puberty is diagnosed as a gender identity disorder of childhood. Adults and adolescents are diagnosed as experiencing an atypical gender identity disorder.

Theorists state the following predisposing factors as possible causes for the development of gender identity disorders:

1. Lack of a father figure for the male to identify with in a broken home, or indifference by a father figure during childhood, are contributing factors toward a gender identity disorder. In either situation, the boy may identify with his mother, may develop female attitudes, and may prefer the feminine role.

Male Identity Disorder: Clinical Example

JM, age 25, has been seen in the outpatient department of the local psychiatric hospital with the complaint of increased anxiety. During the intake interview, JM states that he never knew his father. He lived with his mother and two aunts while he was growing up and never had many male playmates. He states he wasn't interested in sports and remembers being called a "sissy" and "mama's boy." He felt more comfortable staying at home learning how to sew, cook, clean house, and go grocery shopping with his mother and aunts. During high school, he was not interested in dating. He began to have feelings of sexual attraction for one of the boys in his neighborhood. This feeling disturbed him so he decided to leave home after graduation and "get away" from the boy. During the past few years, JM has experienced similar feelings for other men at work and has begun to question his identity as male. He decided to seek counseling when he began to have symptoms of tachycardia, dizziness, and chest pain.

2. Identification by a young girl with a father figure, resulting in the development of masculine attributes, is suggestive of a confused sexual role identity.

3. A female who fears her father for some reason may extend that fear to all men, resulting in the presence of "safe" relationships with members of the same sex (lesbianism).

4. Encouragement to act the role of a "boy" rather than a girl may cause confusion regarding one's sexual identity. This encouragement is usually the result of a parent who wishes that the girl had been a boy and seeks to keep her in that role. To receive love and attention and not disappoint the parent, the girl continues to assume the assigned male role and assume the attitude and behavior of the opposite sex.

5. Experiencing rape or incest during childhood may result in failure to progress through the psychosexual stages of development and failure to develop a positive gender identity.

Female Identity Disorder: Clinical Example

JC, a 17-year-old teenager, dresses and acts like a boy. Her hair is cut extremely short, and she shows no interest in wearing cosmetics, jewelry, or feminine clothing. When she was 7 years old, her father encouraged her to be active in sports such as football, soccer, and basketball. He would laughingly refer to her as "the boy daddy never had." He even bought her shirts and slacks in the boys' department of a clothing store. JC remembers hearing her father brag to family members that he'd "make a boy out of her yet." She recalls how happy her father was when she made the neighborhood baseball team when she was 11 years old. During the past several years, he has continued to encourage her to participate in sports so that she could qualify for a sports scholarship and eventually be a professional sports figure. Remarks by several classmates to JC about her physical appearance and manner of dress have caused her to feel confused about her identity. She asked the school counselor to talk with her because she had no other friends with whom she could discuss her feelings.

Homosexuality is now considered a sexual preference instead of a mental disorder *unless* the following criteria are present:

1. Heterosexual arousal is absent or weak and the person states that such feelings are interfering with establishing or maintaining a *desired* heterosexual relationship.

2. A sustained, *unwanted* pattern of homosexual arousal results in distress and the person seeks help.

If these criteria persist, the diagnosis of ego-dystonic homosexuality is made on the basis that the person desires to acquire or maintain a heterosexual relationship. Other presenting clinical symptoms may include feelings of loneliness, guilt, shame, anxiety, and depression.

Homosexuality or lesbianism is subclassified according to the following preferred sexual relationships:

1. Persons who are exclusively homosexual prefer to have sexual relations with members of the same sex.

2. Pesons who are bisexual are able to have sexual relations with either sex.

3. Persons who are heterosexual may have occasional homosexual encounters.

Homosexual panic is a term used to describe an acute reaction that occurs when a person with dormant or latent homosexual tendencies is exposed to members of the same sex in settings such as barricks, dorms, or penal institutions. The person responds with severe anxiety because of fear that homosexual actions will occur. As panic occurs, maladaptive coping mechanisms may lead to confusion and hallucinations.

Transsexualism is a subclassification of gender identity disorders that can affect both men and women. The person desires to live, dress, and act as a member of the opposite sex since he feels uncomfortable with his own anatomic sex. It is also referred to as a reversal of gender identity. Diagnostic criteria for transsexualism are as follows:

1. The person experiences discomfort and inappropriateness with his or her own anatomic sex.

2. The person desires to be rid of his or her own genitals and live as a member of the opposite sex.

3. These feelings have been present for at least 2 years.

4. No presence of genetic abnormality is noted.

5. No other mental disorder, such as schizophrenia, is present.

Various theories attempt to explain the cause of transsexualism. They suggest factors such as hormone levels, genetic traits, poor parent–child relationships, or other psychological factors.

Transsexualism: Clinical Example

KT, a 45-year-old chemist, was seen in the emergency room for an overdose of diazepam (Valium). After his condition stabilized, and the patient was admitted for furthur observation, KT confided in the nurse that he wished he had succeeded in his suicidal attempt. As the nurse attempted to explore KT's feelings, he stated, "I'm so mixed up. I don't like being a man and don't know what to do about it. I can't tell my family." He stated further that he "felt like a woman trapped in a man's body" and is attracted to men.

Persons such as KT are differentiated from homosexuals in that although transsexuals are attracted to members of the same sex, the attraction is of a heterosexual nature. KT actually feels like a woman who is attracted to men.

Responses by the student nurse concerning persons who exhibit gender identity disorders have included comments such as "I can't believe he's gay," "Why is he attracted to other men?," "He's so athletic looking that I can't believe he's homosexual," and "She acts like a man; I hope she doesn't make passes at me."

Feelings of disbelief and repugnance, as well as questions of religious and moral concern, frequently are voiced by students. These concerns need to be explored with the instructor if the student is to develop a therapeutic relationship with such patients who are seeking psychiatric help or are being seen on the medical surgical unit of a general hospital.

PARAPHILIAS

Rowe states that the classification of paraphilias identifies the person who experiences sexual arousal in response to objects or situations that are not normally arousing.

The DSM-III describes paraphilia as a disorder in which unusual or bizarre sexual acts or imagery are enacted to achieve sexual excitement. An example would be simulated bondage, in which pain is inflicted with materials such as leather straps, handcuffs, whips, and chains. Paraphiliac imagery is subclassified further as severe sexual sadism when the imagery involves a nonconsenting partner who is injured as a result of such activity. Sexual masochism describes the injury of self during imagery.

Paraphiliacs generally are not seen by mental health professionals unless their behavior has created a conflict with society. Nonconsenting partners may report such activity to the legal profession. Concerned neighbors may suspect that children are the object of sadistic sexual behavior and inform the police or the child welfare bureau of such abuse. Voyeurism, exhibitionism, and pedophilia are three subclassifications of behavior that usually result in arrest and incarceration.

A list of paraphilias follows. (This list has been compiled from several psychiatric textbooks but is not to be considered complete.)

BESTIALITY OR ZOOPHILIA. Sexual contact with animals serves as a preferred method to produce sexual excitement. It is rarely seen.

EXHIBITIONISM. An adult male obtains sexual gratification from repeatedly exposing his genitals to unsuspecting strangers, usually women and children who are involuntary observers. He has a strong need to demonstrate masculinity and potency.

FETISHISM. Sexual contact with inanimate articles (fetishes) results in sexual gratification. Most often it is a piece of clothing or footwear. Parts of the body may also take on fetishistic significance. Its occurrence is almost exclusive with men who fear rejection by members of the opposite sex.

MASOCHISM. Sexual pleasure occurs while one is experiencing emotional or physical pain. The willing recipient of erotic whipping is considered to be masochistic.

NECROPHILIA. Sexual arousal occurs while the person is using corpses to meet one's sexual needs. This disorder is classified as an atypical paraphilia.

PEDOPHILIA. The use of prepubertal children is needed to achieve sexual gratification. Pedophilia can be an actual sexual act or a fantasy.

SADISM. Sexual gratification is experienced while the person inflicts physical or emotional pain on others. Severe forms of this behavior may be present in schizophrenia.

TELEPHONE SCATOLOGIA. Sexual gratification is achieved by telephoning someone and making lewd or obscene remarks.

TRANSVESTISM. A heterosexual male achieves sexual gratification through wearing the clothing of a woman (cross-dressing). It is a learned response due to encouragement by family members. As a child, the person was considered more attractive when dressed up as a girl.

VOYEURISM. The achievement of sexual pleasure by looking at unsuspecting persons who are naked, undressing, or engaged in sexual activity. Shy and feeling inadequate in heterosexual relationships, the "peeping Tom" substitutes looking for sexual contact.

A person may experience more than one paraphiliac disorder at the same time or may exhibit clinical symptoms of other mental disorders (*e.g.,* a personality disorder or schizophrenia).

Characteristics or associated features of persons who are classified as paraphiliacs include

1. Emotional immaturity (seen in the pedophiliac or "peeping Tom" who is unable to engage in a mature heterosexual relationship owing to feelings of inadequacy.)

2. Fear of a sexual relationship that could result in rejection

3. Shyness (seen in the voyeur who views others from a distance)

4. The need to prove masculinity demonstrated by the exhibitionist

5. The need to inflict pain on another to achieve sexual satisfaction (seen in sadistic behavior)

6. The need to endure pain to achieve sexual satisfaction (experienced by the masochist)

7. Low or poor self-concept

8. Depression

Not all of these characteristics are present in each paraphiliac. Theorists state that the way a paraphiliac expresses himself sexually affords a clue to his self-concept. For example, the fetishist who has a very low self-concept chooses inaminate objects to satisfy sexual needs and therefore does not have to fear rejection by a partner.

If the nurse understands the dynamics of paraphiliac behavior and is able to separate the behavior from the person, she is prepared to handle feelings of repulsion, anger, and frustration. To give therapeutic care, the nurse needs to be nonjudgmental and display a genuine interest in the person as she deals with her own ethical and moral values.

PSYCHOSEXUAL DYSFUNCTION

The third classification of psychosexual disorders concerns the psychologically induced inability to be sexually active due to inhibitions, impaired communication between sexual partners, or psychophysiologic changes.

The most common cause of sexual dysfunction in the male is anxiety. Performance anxiety or fear of failure can result in impotence. Guilt feelings, sexual misinformation, failure to communicate with one's partner, and hidden anger are contributing factors seen in both men and women who experience sexual difficulties. This classification does not apply to sexual dysfunction that is a result of organic factors, such as the presence of a physical disorder or a medication.

Some common physical disorders that could cause difficulty with sexual activity are arteriosclerosis, liver disease, hypertension, thyroid disorder, and sexually transmitted diseases.

Medications that interfere with sexual activity have been identified as alcohol, antihypertensive drugs, cortisone, narcotic analgesics such as morphine and codeine, antihistamines, and sedatives. The presence of these conditions would need to be investigated before a diagnosis of sexual dysfunction is made.

Examples of psychosexual dysfunction include

1. A mother with a child who has leukemia is too concerned about her child to engage in sexual activity during the period that the child is ill.

2. A woman who has been raped is unable to participate in a satisfying sexual relationship because of memories and emotions related to the experience.

3. A man who experiences inhibited sexual excitement (called impotence previously) does so as a result of problems at work and the excessive use of alcohol.

4. A newly married widower experiences impaired sexual function owing to memories of his former wife.

Characteristics or associated features may include frustration, depression, anxiety, guilt, and a fear of failure in maintaining a satisfying sexual relationship.

The classification of psychosexual dysfunction includes seven categories. The psychologically induced inability to perform sexually may result in

1. Inhibited sexual desire—This diagnosis is used only if the lack of desire causes distress to the person or the person's partner. Factors such as age, health, and frequency of sexual desire and life-style are considered when one is interviewing the person seeking help.

2. Inhibited sexual excitement (also referred to as frigidity or impotence)—Diagnostic criteria include partial or complete failure to experience or maintain an erection until completion of the sexual act are included in this category. An organic cause should be ruled out before using this diagnosis. Approximately 15% of patients seeking relief from sexual dysfunctions have physical causes for impaired sexual response.

3. Inhibited female orgasm

4. Inhibited male orgasm
(These two categories are used to diagnose recurrent, persistent inhibited orgasm following an adequate phase of sexual excitement in the absence of any organic cause.)

5. Premature ejaculation—Ejaculation occurs before the person's wishes owing to the absence of reasonable voluntary control during the sexual act.

6. Functional dyspareunia—This diagnosis is used to describe recurrent, persistent genital pain in the male or female.

7. Functional vaginismus—Spasms of the musculature of the outer third of the vagina are recurrent, persistent and involuntary, thus interfering with the sexual act.

Walker (1982) states that approximately one out of ten patients seen by a physician has a sexual problem. Masters and Johnson (1970) have estimated that approximately one half of all married couples experience

sexual problems. Eighty-five percent of those people have true sexual dysfunctions not caused by an organic or physical cuase.

Walker also states that because of research done by Masters and Johnson, treatment of sexual problems is now implemented in sexual clinics.
Successful treatment has occurred in persons experiencing problems with
ejaculation and impotence, as well as painful intercourse or functional
dyspareunia. Their work also involves speaking engagements, workshops
on sexuality, and educational seminars for health care professionals.
Nurses must be aware of these various services available to persons who
exhibit symptoms of sexual disorders.

Another service available is that of patient advocacy. Jacobson, in her
article "Illness and Human Sexuality," describes a bill of seven rights to
guarantee sexual freedom and promote sexual health. These rights
include the patient's right to express his sexuality, to become the person
he or she desires to be, and to select a sex partner of choice, regardless of
the partner's sex.

Persons in the health care field need to familiarize themselves with
this type of philosophy because it provides an excellent reference when
one is handling various sexual issues. Sexual acting out may occur in the
general hospital setting as the patient attempts to test sexuality owing to
the loss of independence, low self-esteem, loss of a body part, loneliness,
fear, anxiety, or loss of control. Several examples of behavior due to these
concerns were cited earlier. Behavior frequently seen includes flirting,
deliberate exposure of the genital area, dressing in seductive attire, touching the care-giver inappropriately, using profanity or making provocative
comments. Some patients use a shock approach by blatantly discussing
promiscuous sexual activity or telling jokes that center on sexual content.

The nurse is better able to handle such behavior if she remembers that
all behavior has meaning. Reactions such as verbal chastisement, shun-
ning or ignoring the patient, or judging the patient's behavior are negative
responses that should be avoided. Exploration of feelings, evaluation of
the appropriateness of touch, and encouragement of normal sexual behavior are imperative if the nurse hopes to help the patient to express his
sexuality in a positive manner.

Treatment of Psychosexual Disorders

Treatment is individualized according to the type of disorder, underlying
causative factors, and presenting symptoms. Generalized statements will
be given in reference to the three classifications discussed.

Transsexuals have shown minimal successful response to psychotherapy or aversive therapy when attempting to resolve the conflict of gender
identity. Sex transformation or reconstructive surgery has been attempted

with a select group of patients. The treatment plan includes intensive therapy regarding the person's sexuality before surgery. To assist with sex change, hormones also are administered. Although surgery does not always relieve the clinical symptom of underlying depression, patients appear to do well postoperatively.

Homosexuals or lesbians who experience conflict regarding their gender identity may isolate themselves from society or gravitate to areas where homosexual communities exist rather than seek therapy. Others have become involved in gay liberation support groups. Those who seek therapy do so because of the inability to cope or the development of personality problems. Psychoanalysis has been successful in a significant number of persons seeking treatment.

Treatment of paraphiliacs focuses on individual or group therapy to explore feelings of sexuality, anxiety, depression, and frustration. Methods of coping are also discussed.

Behavioral therapy, group therapy, and aversive therapy all focus on altering or managing unacceptable or undesirable behaviors. In aversive therapy, negative stimuli (*e.g.,* electric shock or an emetic) are used to condition the person each time an undesirable sexual act occurs. The behavior decreases as the person wishes to avoid the punishment associated with the negative stimuli.

Environmental manipulation also has proven effective in relieving anxiety and altering undesirable behavior. Incarceration may be imposed legally in an effort to protect the public, especially children, from being victimized by persons such as pedophiles. The prisoner may then be interviewed and accepted into a special program using one or more of the therapies mentioned.

NURSING INTERVENTION

As stated earlier, the nurse must examine feelings about her own sexuality before she is able to care for patients who sexually act out or present symptoms of psychosexual disorders. Nurses are not immune to the development of gender identity disorders, unresolved Oedipal or Electra complex, or psychosexual dysfunction. Feelings of disgust, contempt, anger or fear need to be identified and explored so that they do not interfere with the development of a therapeutic relationship. This is one of the reasons patients do better with a team approach rather than with individual therapy. If the nurse is unable to be objective while giving care, she should have another member of the health team care for the patient. The quality of nursing care will depend on the nurse's ability to be nonjudgmental and her ability to understand the behavior of a patient who is sexually acting out. She needs to be supportive yet set limits, so that the patient's behavior is socially acceptable.

Nursing interventions for patients who exhibit symptoms of psychosexual disorders also include planning care to meet the basic human needs, providing a structured environment, providing protective care for the patient, exploring methods to rechannel sexually unacceptable behavior, and participation in a variety of therapies, including behavior therapy, aversive therapy, and psychotherapy. The nurse must also assume the role of patient advocate to ensure the promotion of sexual health when the opportunity occurs.

A list of nursing diagnoses and interventions for patients who exhibit symptoms of psychosexual disorders follows.

NURSING DIAGNOSES	NURSING INTERVENTIONS
Alteration in pattern of sexuality: Impulsive sexual actions resulting in physical contact	Explain to the patient that touching makes you feel uncomfortable. Ask the patient to explain his feelings at the time he acted impusively. Explore the meaning of specific behavior. Be firm but nonjudgmental when setting limits. Be consistent. Intervene in any overt acts toward other patients. Explain to the patient that he must respect the rights of others. Avoid placing the patient in activities requiring physical contact. Provide protective isolation from other patients if necessary since his overt behavior may provoke hostility.
Alteration in pattern of sexuality: Verbal comments with sexual overtones	Respond by recognizing the patient's feelings (*i.e.,* "It must be difficult to be away from your fiancée"). Allow the patient to ventilate the reason for his comment without encouraging his behavior. Explore alternative ways to channel the patient's advances to result in a more positive outcome.
Alteration in pattern of sexuality: Masturbatory behavior	Request that the patient limit his activity to a private area to avoid offending others. Intervene in any attempt by the patient to involve others in his activity. Explore the meaning behind the patient's behavior. Discuss alternative behavior with the patient.

NURSING DIAGNOSES	NURSING INTERVENTIONS
Sexual dysfunction owing to increased anxiety	Encourage verbalization of feelings. Explore reasons for increased anxiety. Assess the patient's knowledge of causes of sexual dysfunction. Inform the patient of various resources available (*e.g.,* sex education courses, clinics, counseling, therapy, and reference books). Administer any prescribed anti-anxiety agents.

SUMMARY

Psychosexual disorders are thought to be the result of a faulty psycho-biological process. This chapter presented Freud's description of five stages of normal psychosexual development, including the oral, anal, phallic, latency, and genital stages. Unresolved conflict experienced during any of these developmental stages could result in the inability to express one's human sexuality in a positive manner. The person who completes the transition through all five stages successfully develops the capacity to love and engage in a mature heterosexual relationship. The DSM-III categories of transsexualism, paraphilia, and psychosexual dysfunction were explained. Homosexuality also was discussed as a sexual preference rather than a disorder. Sexual acting out behavior of hospitalized patients as well as the responses of nursing personnel were explored. Diagnostic criteria, associated features, and treatment modalities were presented. Nursing diagnoses and interventions focusing on sexually aggressive behavior and sexual dysfunction due to increased anxiety were described.

LEARNING ACTIVITIES

   I. Clinical activities
     A. Assess your patient's sexual role satisfaction or human sexuality while giving care.
     B. Evaluate the treatment plan for appropriateness. If indicated, plan and implement nursing interventions. List any additional suggestions regarding the care of this patient.
  II. Clinical situation for discussion: Psychosexual dysfunction
     JK, a 36-year-old executive, was admitted to ICU with the diagnosis of myocardial infarction. The father of two children, JK has confided in the

nurse that he is afraid to go and resume his duties as husband and father. He also stated that he is afraid to play golf even though the attending physician assured him he would eventually be able to lead a normal life if he adhered to the doctor's orders. Following a visit by his wife, JK appeared withdrawn and apprehensive. As the nurse made evening rounds, JK complained of chest pain and stated that he thought his doctor was sending him home too early. Later that evening Mrs. K called the nurses' station and asked to talk to the head nurse. She expressed concern over her husband's withdrawal, lack of interest in visiting with her, and fear of going home. A week later JK was discharged. When he arrived home, he informed his wife that they should sleep in separate bedrooms so that he could get adequate rest. After 2 months of recuperation, JK was still unable to have sexual relations with his wife.

    A. What behavior did JK exhibit that might indicate the onset of symptoms of psychosexual dysfunction? Note that the doctor feels that JK will be able to lead a normal life.

    B. State nursing interventions that would have been appropriate to help JK to express concern about his sexual role satisfaction while he was hospitalized.

    C. What community services are available to help couples like JK and his wife understand the dynamics of their sexual relationships?

III. Independent activities

    A. Examine your feelings about your own sexuality.

    B. Discuss or evaluate your feelings in response to the following situations:

        1. A 22-year-old female college student is admitted to your unit for an emergency appendectomy. Following surgery you notice that the patient is visited by a "close friend," a female who holds the patient's hand and strokes her hair. The visitor hugs the patient quite affectionately each time upon leaving.

        2. A 29-year-old male is admitted to your unit to undergo tests before surgery for sex reassignment (transsexual surgery). You are assigned to care for this patient.

        3. A 31-year-old man is admitted for gallbladder surgery. As you prepare the patient's room for his return from surgery, you notice he has several "skin" magazines and a woman's undergarment tucked under his pillow.

    C. Refer to the works of Masters and Johnson (see bibliography) to familiarize yourself with their work.

    D. If possible, view Chernick and Chernick's videotape on "Sexuality and Communication," which describes the normal sexual response cycle and discusses sexual dysfunctions.

SELF-TEST

1. Define paraphilia.

2. Describe homosexual panic.

3. A person who desires to live, dress, and act out as a member of the opposite sex is a _____.

4. A person who achieves sexual gratification by wearing the clothing of the opposite sex is a _____.

5. List three possible causes of gender identity disorders.

6. State four characteristics of paraphiliacs.

7. Cite an example of a sexual dysfunction.

8. List three examples of treatment of paraphiliacs.

Match the following:

9. Sadism

10. An example of masochism

11. "Peeping Tom"

12. Sexual use of corpses

13. Gender identity disorder

a. Necrophilia

b. Self-inflicted pain

c. Transsexualism

d. Voyeurism

e. Erotic whipping of an unconsenting adult

14. List four nursing interventions for impulsive sexual actions that result in physical contact.

15. State the rationale for limit setting when caring for patients with psychosexual disorders.

16. List four reasons a patient may sexually act out while hospitalized for a medical or surgical problem.

REFERENCES

Benjamin H, Ihlemfeld CL: Transsexualism. Am J Nurs: Mar, 1973

Braverman SJ: Homosexuality. Am J Nurs: Apr, 1973

Brown F: Juvenile prostitution: A nursing perspective. J Psych Nurs: Dec, 1980

Burgess A: Psychiatric Nursing in the Hospital and the Community, 3rd ed. Englewood Cliffs, Prentice–Hall, 1981

Conn C: Canary: The Story of a Transsexual. Los Angeles, Nash Publishing, 1974

Conway–Rutkowski B: Getting to the cause of headaches. Am J Nurs: Oct, 1981

Gagnon JH: Human Sexualities. Glenview, Scott, Foresman & Co, 1977

Haber, J et al: Comprehensive Psychiatric Nursing. New York, McGraw–Hill, 1982

Hariton BE: The sexual fantasies of women. Psychology Today: Mar, 1973

Jacobson L: Illness and human sexuality. Nursing Outlook: Jan, 1974

Kaplan H: The New Sex Therapy. New York, Brunner/Mazel, 1974

Kolb L: Modern Clinical Psychiatry. Philadelphia, WB Saunders, 1977

Kyes J, Hofling CK: Basic Psychiatric Concepts in Nursing. Philadelphia, JB Lippincott, 1980

Lancaster J: Adult Psychiatric Nursing. New York, Medical Examination Publishing, 1980

Masters W, Johnson V: Human Sexual Inadequacy. Boston, Little, Brown & Co, 1970

Masters W, Johnson V: Human Sexual Response. Boston, Little, Brown & Co, 1966

Mereness D, Taylor C: Essentials of Psychiatric Nursing. St. Louis, CV Mosby, 1982

Rowe CJ: An Outline of Psychiatry. Dubuque, William C Brown, Publishers, 1984

Schultz J, Dark S: Manual of Psychiatric Nursing Care Plans. Boston, Little, Brown & Co, 1982

Strait J: The Transsexual Patient After Surgery. Am J Nurs: Mar, 1973

Thomas SP: Bisexuality: A sexual orientation of great diversity. J Psych Nurs: Apr, 1980

Tripp CA: The Homosexual Matrix. New York, McGraw–Hill, 1975

Walker G: Everybody's Guide to Emotional Well-Being. San Francisco, Harbor Publishing, 1982

Wilson H, Kneisl C: Psychiatric Nursing. Menlo Park, Addison–Wesley, 1983

19

INEFFECTIVE INDIVIDUAL

COPING: ALCOHOLISM

TWELVE STEPS TO DESTRUCTION

1. I stated that I could hold my liquor and was master of my own life.
2. Came to believe I was sane and rational in every respect.
3. Decided to run my own life and be fantastic in all my undertakings.
4. Made a thorough and searching inventory of my fellow man and found him lacking.
5. Admitted to no one including God and myself that there was anything wrong with me.
6. Sought through alcohol to avoid all my responsibilities and to escape from the realities of life.
7. Continued to get drunk in an attempt to remove these shortcomings.
8. Made a list of all persons that had harmed me, whether imaginary or real, and swore to get even.
9. Got revenge when ever possible, except when to do so might further injure me.
10. Continued to find fault with the world and the people in it and when I was right promptly admitted it.
11. Sought through lying, cheating, and stealing to improve myself materially at the expense of my fellow man, asking only for the means to get drunk or stay high.
12. Having a complete mental, moral, physical and financial breakdown as the result of these steps, I endeavored to drag those around me down to my level and practiced these insanities in all my affairs.

Alcoholics Anonymous

LEARNING OBJECTIVES

1. Define alcoholism.
2. State the DSM-III criteria for alcohol abuse and dependence.
3. List the more common physiologic effects of alcoholism on the following:
   Gastrointestinal tract
   Cardiovascular system
   Respiratory tract
   Reproductive system
   Central nervous system
4. State the behavioral patterns present during alcoholism as described by Liska.
5. Discuss the three general steps in the treatment of alcoholism as stated by Liska.
6. Describe the stages of alcohol withdrawal.
7. Develop a nursing care plan for a patient undergoing withdrawal due to alcoholism
8. List support groups available to the alcoholic.
9. State the purpose of
   Family group therapy
   Al-Ateen
   Al-Anon

"ALCOHOLISM" should be considered the number one major health problem in the United States" (Walker, 1982, p. 101). The following statistics about alcohol consumption are excerpted from statements by Walker (1982), Liska (1981), Barry (1984), and Altrocchi (1980):

1. Approximately 100 million Americans consume alcoholic beverages.
2. There are 9 to 10 million alcoholics or problem drinkers in the United States; more than 2 million of these alcoholics are women.
3. About 20% of hospital care expenses are due to alcohol abuse.
4. Related to or due to alcoholism: 50% of traffic accidents, 50% of homicides, 30% of rapes, 80% of robberies, 62% of child abuse cases, and 33% of suicides.
5. Alcoholism and alcohol abuse result in approximately a 15 billion dollar loss annually because of loss of work, property damage, medical expenses, overhead costs, and health and welfare services.
6. Untreated alcoholism shortens one's life span by 10 to 12 years.
7. Alcoholism is responsible for unhappy marriages, broken homes, desertion, divorce, displaced children, and impoverished families.

8. Effects of prolonged, excessive alcohol consumption include the following medical problems: Laennec's cirrhosis, pancreatitis, chronic gastritis, blood dyscrasias, infections, cardiac arrhythmia, and cerebral degeneration.

DEFINITION OF ALCOHOLISM

According to the National Council on Alcoholism, the alcoholic is powerless to stop the drinking that seriously alters his normal living pattern. Alcoholics Anonymous describes alcoholism as a physical condition associated with a mental obsession. It is considered to be one part physical, one part psychological, one part sociological, and one part alcohol.

Some major myths about alcoholism prevent alcoholics and their families from acknowledging that the condition exists. They include:

1. *Most alcoholics are skid row bums.* Only 3% to 9% of the 9 to 10 million alcoholics are on skid row. The highest rate of alcohol consumption is by "employable, family-centered persons, living in respectable neighborhoods with their spouses" (Liska, 1981, p. 159). The disease is no respecter of persons since it affects businessmen, blue-collar workers, executives, farmers salespersons, teachers, clergymen, physicians, and housewives.

2. *Very few women are alcoholics.* The ratio of men to women alcoholics was approximately 6:1 in the 1950s, whereas the ratio had risen to about 3:1 in the late 1970s.

3. *Most alcoholics are middle-aged or older.* "Studies have shown that 70% of all adolescents drink; the average age of initiation to alcohol is 12.9 years; 62% of seventh- and 80% of twelfth-graders drink . . . About 7% of the American adult population manifest the behavior of alcohol abuse and alcoholism" (Liska, 1981, p. 158).

4. *Alcoholics drink at least a pint a day.* The National Institute on alcohol abuse and alcoholism states that when, how, and why a person drinks is far more important than how much one drinks. Factors that influence alcohol abuse include the availability of alcohol, environmental and daily pressures of life, emotional instability, self-destructive tendencies, the inability to cope, genetic background resulting in a predisposition to alcoholism, unhappy childhood, cultural background (e.g., Irish and Anglo-Saxons), and the need to belong to an influential group, in which alcohol is used frequently.

5. *Alcoholics could recover if they had enough "will power."* Alcoholism is an illness that requires one treatment: total abstinence. To achieve this goal, the alcoholic needs the support of others to motivate him to have the desire to stop drinking. He also needs love and understanding about his problem.

ETIOLOGY

Why do persons who, for example, are unable to cope with environmental pressures, have an unhappy childhood, or are emotionally unstable, become alcoholics? Various theories have been stated, but none have been accepted as being absolute. Lancaster (1980) lists the following attempts to explain alcoholism:

1. Endocrine theory: Individuals with disorders or dysfunction of endocrine glands are predisposed to alcoholism.

2. Heredity theory: Children who have an alcoholic parent or parents are more likely to become alcoholics.

3. Nutritional theory: Alcoholism occurs as a result of nutritional deficiencies, such as the inability to synthesize food.

4. Metabolic theory: Metabolism increases a person's susceptibility to alcohol and predisposes one to the development of alcoholism.

Barile states that "alcoholism is viewed as a multilevel problem with no single causative factor" (Lego, 1984, p 424). She discusses the etiology of alcoholism in relation to

1. Biologic factors: "Alcoholism is either inherited in a physical trait or as a predisposition" (Lego, 1984, p. 424).

2. Psychological theories: Early childhood rejection, overprotection, or increased responsibility can produce a dependent personality. Such a person may feel rejected, anxious, guilty, depressed, or view himself as a failure. Alcohol is consumed in an attempt to reduce these feelings and may cause one to experience feelings of power and omnipotence, leading to the abuse of alcohol.

3. Social factors: Alcohol consumption is higher among Catholics, the Irish, the Anglo-Saxons, as well as being quite common among Frenchmen and men in the United States. It is considered the "manly" thing to do. Stress, anxiety, and depression are causes of increased alcoholic consumption among women.

Klewin (1977) discusses the following causative factors of alcohol abuse in teenagers:

1. Alcohol is the drug of choice among most adults. It is legal, and it is socially acceptable.

2. Advertising campaigns are aimed at youth with "soda pop wine" advertisements. Over 100 million dollars are spent yearly in such advertisement.

3. Parents indirectly sanction the use of alcohol by telling teenagers alcoholic beverages are okay but "don't touch any of those dangerous drugs like marijuana."

4. Teenagers possess more leisure time and money, and experience less parental or community supervision, especially at weekend parties.

Attempts have been made to describe the alcoholic personality. Common characteristics include the presence of increased anxiety or depression, social or sexual inadequacy, increased social pressures, a desire to lower one's inhibitions, or self-destructive tendencies. The alcoholic personality may exhibit dependency needs or avoid any type of dependent behavior in an attempt to exhibit typical masculine characteristics. Alcohol meets the hidden dependency needs of such a person (Lancaster, 1980).

Alcohol consumption early in life may lead to a high tolerance of alcohol and lead to pattern drinking over a period of years. Later in life (*i.e.,* over age 50), such tolerance decreases and problem drinking occurs. The National Council on Alcoholism, Inc., lists "13 Steps to Alcoholism." (1975). They are presented at this time:

STEP 1. The person has begun to drink alcoholic beverages. Social drinking occurs in moderation as one drinks a cocktail, a few beers, or a glass of wine occasionally. No particular drinking pattern is established.

STEP 2. The person is experiencing black outs. Drinking results in inebriation with some regularity although he feels he can stop anytime he wants to. During these drinking episodes he gets "tight," "high," or feels good, and does not remember getting intoxicated or what was said or done afterwards. He is experiencing amnesia or loss of memory.

STEP 3. Liquor becomes very important. The person stops sipping and begins gulping alcoholic beverages. Sneaking drinks may become an established behavior. He is reluctant to discuss how important liquor has become in his life. Chances of becoming an alcoholic at this step are very high if drinking does not slow down or stop.

STEP 4. The person consistently drinks too much. This behavior occurs approximately 2 years after the first blackout. At this point he cannot control the amount he drinks on any given occasion, although he is not driven to drink. He can control when he will drink again. During this period of drinking, he may become extravagant with money because liquor has helped him overcome a feeling of inferiority. This step is referred to as the basic or crucial phase of alcoholism. At this point he can stop drinking, but if he begins to make excuses to himself or anyone else, it is generally too late to stop drinking. These four steps are referred to as the early "danger signs" of alcoholism.

STEP 5. He makes excuses for drinking. "It's only beer. It relaxes me and helps me unwind," "I drive better after a few drinks," "I'm just celebrating my new promotion at work," or "It's rude to refuse a drink from the host," are a few examples made for excessive drinking. The person believes that he can handle his drinking. Guilt feelings are experienced, and the person becomes defensive, building a repertoire of alibis, excuses, or falsehoods to rationalize his behavior.

STEP 6. The person wants alcohol available at all times (especially a morning drink or "eye-opener"). Drinking is a source of energy, strength, or motivation for the day and serves a "medicinal" purpose. It also eases his conscience, lifts his ego, and reinforces his denial about abusing alcohol.

STEP 7. The person drinks alone. Solitary drinking occurs because he prefers to drink alone any time of day without listening to critical remarks of others who feel he drinks too much, or he lives in a fantasy world while drinking, distorting reality. Drinking has now become an escape from reality.

STEP 8. The person becomes antisocial while drinking. Solitary drinking can cause him to become destructive or violent in behavior while his desire to cause damage becomes intense. Such destructuve feelings may be directed toward himself or others. Alcoholism causes him to lose his inhibitions and results in the loss of control or the ability to judge his conduct. The person may react as a child or animal to meet immediate wants or needs. Realization of such behavior results in feelings of inadequacy and incompetency. The solution to such feelings is to drink more. He is now experiencing the middle stages of alcoholism. His alcoholic pattern is set, and he will follow it *unless* intervention occurs (*e.g.,* counseling or attending an alcoholic treatment program).

STEP 9. The person experiences "benders." This step begins the acute stage of compulsive drinking. He is a true alcoholic with uncontrollable behavior. This usually occurs one to three years after he began morning drinking. A "bender" is described as a period of days during which he drinks continuously and helplessly with one goal in mind: to get drunk. He no longer can control when he drinks. No thought is given to his family, friends, job, food, or shelter.

STEP 10. The person experiences a deep sense of remorse and resentment. During sober moments he feels deep remorse for his uncontrollable actions and behavior. As guilt feelings become unbearable, he drinks more and begins to blame others. The world is against him.

STEP 11. The person experiences intense anxiety. Physical deterioration shows as hands tremble, steps are shaky, and nerves are jumpy. He is experiencing "the shakes." Alcohol is the only thing that calms him so he guards his supply.

STEP 12. The person realizes that liquor controls him. This realization generally occurs after he has delirium tremens (DTs) or has talked with someone whose opinion he values, for example, a minister or psychiatrist.

STEP 13. The person may get help or give in to alcoholism. If he refuses to admit the truth to himself, his alcoholism is incurable. Severe deterioration of health, family, work, and other relationships have occurred by now. He may have lost his job, home, and family. The last five steps are considered to be the late stages of alcoholism and are referred to as compulsive drinking. Death is inevitable unless some form of intervention occurs.

DIAGNOSTIC CRITERIA FOR ALCOHOL ABUSE

"This diagnostic class [alcohol abuse] deals with behavioral changes associated with more or less regular use of substances that affect the central nervous system. These behavioral changes in almost all subcultures would be viewed as extremely undesirable" (DSM-III, 1980, p. 163). Persons may experience substance abuse or substance dependence depending upon the pathologic use of alcohol.

Alcohol abuse or dependence generally occurs between ages 20 to 40 as the social drinker abnormally increases intake of liquor and fails to adjust the drinking habit to its original and more normal pattern. He may drink episodically or continuously. *Episodic* drinking refers to periods of heavy drinking lasting for weeks or months followed by sobriety, whereas *continuous* drinking is the regular daily intake of large amounts of alcohol or regular heavy drinking limited to weekends. Such drinking over a prolonged period of time may result in alcohol withdrawal, alcohol amnesic disorder, or alcohol hallucinoses, which are considered to be organic mental disorders.

The DSM-III lists the following diagnostic criteria for alcohol abuse:

1. A pattern of pathologic alcohol use, such as
   a. The need to drink alcohol daily to function adequately
   b. The inability to cut down or stop drinking alcohol
   c. Repeated attempts to "go on the wagon" to control or reduce drinking or restricting intake to certain times of day
   d. Binge drinking, in which the person remains intoxicated for at least 2 days

    e. Occasional intake of a fifth of spirits or its equivalent in wine or beer

    f. Blackouts or amnesic periods while intoxicated

    g. Continuation of drinking alcohol in the presence of a serious physical disorder that the person knows is exacerbated by the use of alcohol

    h. Drinking of alcohol classified as nonbeverage

2. Impaired social or occupational functioning that is due to alcohol use, such as

    a. Violent behavior while intoxicated

    b. Absenteeism from work

    c. Loss of job

    d. Difficulty with the law

    e. Argumentative behavior or difficulties with family or friends as a result of excessive alcohol intake

3. Disturbance lasts at least 1 month.

Diagnostic criteria for alcohol dependence includes

1. A pattern of pathologic alcohol use as described under alcohol abuse

2. Impaired social or occupational functioning as seen in alcohol abuse

3. Withdrawal or tolerance

    a. A markedly increased tolerance for alcohol (thereby requiring more alcohol to achieve desired effects) or a markedly decreased effect when drinking regular amounts of alcohol

    b. Alcohol withdrawal when a reduction in drinking cessations occurs

    This differentiation of abuse and dependence includes all substances including alcohol, drugs, and caffeine. Tobacco is associated with dependence only. (Drug abuse and dependence are discussed in a separate chapter.)

Alcohol Abuse: Clinical Example

JY, a 55-year-old widow, drank bourbon and water daily as she attempted to perform chores such as cleaning house, doing the laundry, and cooking. Every time her 25-year-old daughter visited, she noticed that her mother was sipping one drink or another and was quite animated and talkative. One evening while JY visited her daughter, she helped herself repeatedly to wine on the bar. As the evening wore on, JY became argumentative on several topics. The following day, the daughter realized that her mother had drunk a bottle of wine while visiting. As she talked with her mother the next day, the daughter questioned JY about her drinking habits. "Yes,

I do drink frequently to get a lift. I get lonely at times," the mother replied. Following a lengthy conversation with her daughter, JY agreed to talk to her family doctor about her drinking habits.

JY was exhibiting a pattern of pathologic alcohol use, which was evident in her need to drink daily, the ingestion of a large amount of wine at her daughter's home, and her argumentative behavior while under the influence of wine.

EFFECTS OF ALCOHOL

The following is a comparison of the blood–alcohol level, approximate amount of beverage for each level, effects of alcohol, and the amount of time it takes alcohol to leave the body (Walker, 1982; Liska, 1981; and Altrocchi, 1980):

Blood Alcohol Level (%)	Approximate Amount of Beverage	Effects of Alcohol	Time Needed for Alcohol to Leave the Body
0.03	1 cocktail, 1 bottle beer, or 5½ oz wine	Slight tension Euphoria Feelings of superiority	2 hrs
0.06	2 cocktails, 3 bottles beer, or 11 oz wine	Feeling of warmth and relaxation Decreases mental efficiency Loss of normal inhibitions Loss of some motor coordination	4 hrs
0.09	3 cocktails or 5 bottles beer or 16½ oz wine	Talkative Clumsiness Exaggerated behavior	6 hrs
0.10	3–5 cocktails or 6–7 bottles beer or 20 oz–22 oz wine	Legally drunk in most states Impaired motor, mental, and speech activity Feelings of guilt are decreased.	
0.15	5–7 cocktails or 26 oz–27 oz wine	Gross intoxication Slurred speech Impaired motor coordination	10 hrs

Blood Alcohol Level (%)	Approximate Amount of Beverage	Effects of Alcohol	Time Needed for Alcohol to Leave the Body
0.20	8 cocktails	Angers easily Motor abilities severely impaired Blackout level Unable to recall events	
0.30	10 cocktails	Stupor likely Death may occur owing to deep anesthetic effect or paralysis of the respiratory center.	
0.40	13 cocktails	Coma leading to death	
0.60	20 cocktails	Severely impaired breathing and heart rate Death will probably occur.	

Physiologic effects of alcoholism are numerous. Most texts list the effects according to systems involvement. The more common effects seen include

1. Gastrointestinal (GI) tract complications, such as acute gastritis, pancreatitis, hepatitis, cirrhosis of the liver, esophageal varicies, hemorrhoids, and ascites.

2. Cardiovascular system complications, such as portal hypertension, weakened heart muscle, and heart failure. Broken blood vessels in the upper cheeks close to the nose and blood shot eyes are not uncommon.

3. Respiratory tract complications include respiratory depression and a depressed cough reflex because of the sedative effect of alcohol. The alcoholic person is susceptible to pneumonia and other respiratory infections.

4. Reproductive system complications include prostatitis, interference with voiding, and release of sexual inhibitions. Fetal alcohol syndrome during pregnancy results in abnormalities in the newborn such as heart defects, abnormally shaped heads and limbs, genital defects, and mental retardation.

5. Central nervous system depression, resulting in peripheral neuropathy, interference with nerve conduction, gait changes, and nerve palsies, is frequently seen.

The alcoholic generally has a poor nutritional status, including deficiencies of vitamins A, D, and K. Anemia, an increased susceptibility to infection, bruising, and bleeding tendencies occur as a result of a decrease in red and white blood cells and abnormal bone marrow functioning.

Liska lists the following behavioral patterns present during alcoholism (1981). These patterns are presented here:

1. Chronic absenteeism from work

2. Repeated job-related accidents

3. Overuse of reationalization or giving a variety of excuses for drinking and the use of projection and denial

4. Disruption of home, marital and family relationships

5. Frequent job changes

6. Poor job performance

7. Deterioration of health

8. Recurrent arrests for driving while under the influence of alcohol

9. Irritability and nervousness in the absence of alcohol

ASSESSMENT

During the interview process, the nurse obtains data from the patient, including interpretation of the drinking problem and attitude toward control of his alcoholism. Information regarding the patient's level of sensorium and general physical condition is pertinent. Is he inebriated, undergoing withdrawal, dehydrated, malnourished, or in any physical distress? Information regarding available support systems is also important at this time because the nursing care plan can be developed once the assessment process is completed.

TREATMENT AND NURSING INTERVENTIONS

"Nine to ten million U.S. alcoholics cannot be ignored. The pain of their alcoholism must be treated.[11] The three general steps in the difficult treatment of alcoholism are (Liska, 1981, p. 177):

1. Managing acute episodes of intoxication to save life and to overcome the immediate effects of excess alcohol.

2. Correcting the chronic health problems associated with alcoholism.

3. Changing the long-term behavior of alcoholic persons so that destructive drinking habits are not continued.

A chronic state of intoxication requires a "drying-out" period, such as withdrawal or detoxification, before treatment can begin. During withdrawal, various symptoms may develop within 12 to 48 hours after abrupt cessation of alcoholic intake. Some patients may experience withdrawal symptoms 3 to 4 days after they quit drinking. Such symptoms may last 48 hours or longer.

The first stage of withdrawal, also referred to as the tremulous stage or the shakes, is characterized by psychomotor hyperactivity with tremors, headache, an elevated pressure, nausea, loss of appetite, nervousness, flushed face, and agitation. This stage can last 36 hours to several days and may progress to the second stage of acute hallucinosis. During this second stage, the person experiences the symptoms of stage 1 as well as visual, auditory, or tactile hallucinations. Such hallucinations generally disappear in a day or two but may last several months. The most severe stage, stage 3 or the DTs, occurs within 1 to 7 days after the person's last drink and may last up to 72 hours. Relapses can occur. Symptoms include tremors, hallucinations, disorientation in person, time, and place; elevated temperature; profuse diaphoresis; severe agitation; tachycardia; delirium; and convulsions, or grand mal seizures.

Examples of nursing diagnoses and nursing interventions for the patient undergoing symptoms of alcohol withdrawal follow.

NURSING DIAGNOSES	NURSING INTERVENTIONS
Potential for injury because of convulsions or disorientation	Provide a calm, supportive, protective environment to prevent injury. Place the patient on seizure precautions including padded siderails and a padded tongue blade. Provide physical protection and restraint as necessary. Assist with ambulation. Administer anticonvulsant or sedative medication without overmedicating.
Sensory perceptual alterations: Auditory, visual, or tactile hallucinations and illusions	Provide a calm, quiet, protective environment, avoiding loud noises, abrupt movements, and dimly lit rooms because shadows increase the likelihood of visual hallucinations, illusions, and may increase the patient's fears. Reinforce reality by referring to the patient's actual surroundings during conversation. Reassure the patient that hallucinations will cease once withdrawal is completed.

(continued)

NURSING DIAGNOSES	NURSING INTERVENTIONS
Anxiety	Display a calm, empathetic, and pleasant attitude. Be readily available when the patient's behavior indicates a need for support. Encourage verbalization of feelings. Assist the patient in identifying ways of handling feelings of anxiety in ways other than by drinking (*i.e.*, relaxation techniques, tension-relieving activities, and group meetings) that provide support and motivation. Administer sedatives as prescribed to decrease anxiety.
Sleep pattern disturbance because of central nervous system agitation	Place the patient in a room in which he can be observed closely and frequently. Provide for periods of uninterrupted sleep by keeping the environment quiet. Offer a backrub. Offer a warm, nonalcoholic, noncaffeine drink to promote relaxation. Administer a prescribed hypnotic sedative. Provide protective restraints as a last resort.
Alterations in nutrition: Less than body requirements	Provide a high-protein, high-vitamin diet in small, frequent feedings. Provide a pleasant environment at mealtime. Assist with feeding as needed. Encourage mouth care before eating to increase appetite. Provide a variety of nonalcoholic, noncaffeine beverages, snacks, and fast-energy foods to decrease physical craving for alcohol.
Possible fluid volume and electrolyte deficit because of nausea and vomiting	Observe for signs of fluid and electrolyte imbalance, such as skin turgor, urine *p*H and electrolyte levels. Record intake and output. Weigh daily. Offer nonalcoholic, noncaffeine fluids frequently. Administer antiemetics as ordered to control nausea and vomiting.
Health maintenance alteration because of alcoholism	Monitor vital signs and blood pressure as indicated. Do neurologic checks as necessary. Check for signs of trauma or injury before admission. Observe for unusual signs or symptoms. Anticipate needs. Assess physical complaints.

NURSING DIAGNOSES	NURSING INTERVENTIONS
Noncompliance: Demanding, manipulative behavior	Set limits and confront manipulative behavior. Explore reasons for behavior and identify and clarify needs. Encourage ventilation of feelings. Display empathy. Communicate frequently with staff to validate impressions of manipulative behavior.
Ineffective individual coping: Use of denial, projection, and rationalization	Explain program and treatment plan. Be nonjudgmental when exploring problems related to the use of alcohol. Educate the patient about physical, psychological, social, and economic effects of alcohol.
Potential for violence: Suicidal ideation due to depression	Place on suicidal precaution. Explore feelings about depression (*i.e.*, low self-concept or guilt).

Once the patient has undergone withdrawal or detoxification, he must learn to "stay dry in a drinking world." This is not an easy task because recovery is a long-term or lifelong struggle. "Sobriety is maintained on a day-to-day basis and is dependent on the client's ability to recognize and change those living patterns that trigger drinking behavior" (Murray, 1983, p. 481). Treatment and rehabilitation often break down once the patient returns to the outside world, in which alcohol is a major part of the life-style.

During hospitalization, after withdrawal, the individualized care plan should focus on the following goals:

1. Increasing factual knowledge about alcoholism
2. Fostering interdependence on people, not alcohol
3. Encouraging the person to participate in self-determination by identifying personal strengths
4. Encouraging the patient to reestablish broken relationships
5. Encouraging the alcoholic patient to accept his own humanity
6. Allowing the person to grieve over the loss of alcohol
7. Changing or modifying one's life-style, which has contributed to drinking
8. Developing alternative approaches to coping with stressors

Various types of supportive care are available to the alcoholic person to assist him in meeting the goals just described. They include individual or group psychotherapy, family therapy, aversion therapy, the use disulfiram (Antabuse) therapy, Alcoholics Anonymous (AA), halfway houses, and industrial programs. Individual psychotherapy generally approaches the use of alcohol as a method of defending oneself from stress, frustration, or guilt feelings, as well as exploring the patient's use of denial, hostility, and feelings of depression. Group therapy is a more effective type of support for the alcoholic patient, providing the opportunity for human interaction and discussion of commonly shared problems. Family therapy serves many purposes, such as understanding the alcoholic's ability to arouse anger or provoke loss of temper and to arouse anxiety within the family unit. Helping the family to gain knowledge about alcoholism and put the knowledge into effect may also occur during family therapy since problem-solving guidance and direction are available. Aversion therapy consists of giving a drug such as emetine and then following it with alcohol. Nausea and vomiting are induced by the emetine, causing an aversion to alcohol based on the reflex association between alcohol and vomiting. Disulfiram (Antabuse) interferes with the breakdown of alcohol, causing an accumulation of acetaldehyde, a by-product of alcohol, in the body. The person who takes disulfiram (Antabuse) and drinks alcohol experiences severe nausea and vomiting, hypotension, headaches, rapid pulse and respirations, and flushed face and bloodshot eyes. This reaction will last as long as there is alcohol in the blood. Persons with serious heart disease, diabetes, epilepsy, liver impairment, or mental illness should not take Antabuse. AA is a self-help group that emphasizes both group and individual treatment approaches. "Meetings are devoted to testimonials and discussions of the problems that arise from drinking alcohol. Through mutual help and reassurance, the alcoholic gains a new sense of confidence and more successful coping abilities" (Walker, 1982, p. 111). AA promotes maturity because its members assume increasingly greater responsibility. It also helps members to gain a new self-concept and willingness to accept assistance. Halfway houses provide group living in a structured environment for recovering alcoholic patients who need a "home away from home" or who have no home. Comprehensive industrial programs for alcoholic employees have been developed in an effort to save corporations an estimated 10 billion dollars per year. Employee assistance programs include in-house alcohol counseling and AA programs.

Other services available to families of alcoholics include Al-Anon Family Groups and Al-Ateen. Al-Anon family groups help members to understand and assist the alcoholic person, whereas Al-Ateen tries to help children to understand their parents' drinking problems and to find mutual support in a group situation. The young members learn that their situations are not unique, and they cease to feel alone.

Chronic Alcoholism: Clinical Example

AK, a 54-year-old accountant, was admitted to the general hospital with symptoms of acute abdominal pain, hematemesis, and generalized edema. A thorough physical evaluation, including a neurologic examination, revealed peripheral neuropathy, an enlarged liver, hemorrhoids, ascites, and several ecchymotic areas on his upper and lower extremities. During the admitting interview, AK admitted to drinking "a six-pack or two" of beer nightly to relax after a stressful day at work. He further stated he had been drinking "on and off since his early twenties" but was always "able to handle his drinking." When asked whether he felt his drinking was affecting his health, AK stated that he did not think he was an alcoholic, just a "social drinker." Further testing revealed that AK was malnourished, anemic, and had portal hypertension from cirrhosis of the liver. When AK's attending physician suggested that he seek counseling or the support of a group such as Alcoholics Anonymous, AK denied that he had a serious drinking problem. Approximately 6 months after his discharge from the hospital, AK was readmitted with the diagnosis of hepatic coma due to chronic alcoholism. He died the following day.

SUMMARY

Alcoholism, the major health problem in the United States, affects approximately 9 to 10 million people in the United States and is considered by Alcoholics Anonymous to be a physical condition with a mental obsession. Major myths about alcoholism are described briefly herein as are various causative factors, including endocrine theory, heredity theory, nutritional theory, metabolic theory, biologic factors, psychological theory, social factors, and the alcoholic personality. The *13 Steps to Alcoholism* by the National Council on Alcoholism, were discussed, citing the early danger signs of alcoholism, the middle stages of alcoholism, and the late stages of alcoholism, or compulsive drinking. The DSM-III diagnostic criteria for alcohol abuse and dependence were listed, followed by a clinical example of alcohol abuse. The more common physiologic and behavioral effects of alcoholism were stated. The symptoms of withdrawal or detoxification following alcohol intoxication were described by stages: 1) the first stage, also referred to as the tremulous stage; 2) the second stage, characterized by hallucinations; and 3) the third stage, also known as delirium tremens or DTs. Examples of nursing diagnoses and nursing interventions focused on potential for injury, sensory perceptual alterations, anxiety, sleep pattern disturbance, alteration in nutrition, possible fluid volume and electrolyte deficit, health maintenance alteration, noncompliance, ineffective individual coping, and potential for violence. Treatment and rehabilitation measures were discussed, focusing on goals, supportive care (*e.g.,* individual, group, and family psychotherapy), aversion therapy, Antabuse therapy, and family support groups. A clinical example of chronic alcoholism was given.

LEARNING ACTIVITIES

I. Clinical activities
    A. Care for a patient with the diagnosis of alcohol abuse or alcohol dependence.
    B. Describe the patient's symptoms.
    C. Does the patient exhibit any insight into his or her problem?
    D. Does the patient express a desire to be helped?
    E. Develop a nursing care plan for this patient.
    F. Discuss supportive care for the patient after discharge.
II. Independent activities
    A. Attend an AA meeting or visit a local chapter of Al-Ateen.
    B. Obtain information about the presence or absence of industrial alcohol programs in your community.
    C. Review the "13 Steps to Alcoholism" by the National Council on Alcoholism. Discuss appropriate nursing interventions for each step to impede progress toward compulsive drinking.

SELF-TEST

1. State the definition of
    Alcohol abuse
    Alcohol dependence

2. List the realities that counter the following myths about alcoholism:
    Most alcoholics are skid row bums.
    Very few women are alcoholics.
    Most alcoholics are middle-aged or older.
    Alcoholics drink at least a pint a day.
    Alcoholics could recover if they had enough "will power."

3. Cite several theories about alcoholism.

4. Explain the causative factors of alcohol abuse in teenagers.

5. Describe the following:
    The early stages of alcoholism
    The middle stages of alcoholism
    The late stages of alcoholism

6. Explain the following DSM-III diagnostic criteria for alcohol dependence:
   A pattern of pathological alcohol use
   Impaired social or occupational functioning
   Withdrawal or tolerance

7. State the blood alcohol level with which one is considered legally drunk in most states.

8. List the more common physiologic effects of alcoholism in the
   GI tract
   Cardiovascular system
   Respiratory tract
   Reproductive system
   Central nervous system

9. Describe the nutritional status of a chronic alcoholic.

10. State behavioral patterns generally seen during alcoholism.

11. Describe the stages of alcohol withdrawal or detoxification.

12. Give nursing interventions for an alcoholic who exhibits the following:
    Potential for injury due to convulsions
    Sensory perceptual alterations
    Anxiety
    Sleep pattern disturbance
    Alterations in nutrition: less than body requirements
    Possible fluid volume and electrolyte deficit because of nausea and vomiting
    Health maintenance alteration

13. Discuss supportive care available to alcoholics.

14. Differentiate between aversion therapy and Antabuse therapy.

REFERENCES

Al-Anon: The 12 Steps and Traditions of Al-Anon Family Groups. New York, Al-Anon, 1973

Alcohol and the Adolescent: New York, National Council on Alcoholism, 1976

Altrocchi J: Abnormal Behavior. New York, Harcourt Brace Jovanich, 1980

Barry P: Psychosocial Nursing Assessment and Intervention. Philadelphia, JB Lippincott, 1984

Blane HT: The Personality of the Alcoholic. New York, Harper & Row, 1968

Bort RF: Ambulatory management in alcoholism. Am Fam Physician: May, 1977

Burkhalter P: Nursing Care of the Alcoholic and Drug Abuser. New York, McGraw–Hill, 1975

Clement J, Notaro C: Nursing intenvention in the alcohol detoxification process. Alcohol Health and Research World, 1 (2): 1975

Cohen P: How to Help the Alcoholic. New York, Public Affairs Pamphlet

Cohn L: The hidden diagnosis. Am J Nurs: Dec, 1982

Donlon PT, Rockwell DA: Psychiatric Disorders: Diagnosis and Treatment. Bowie IN, Robert J. Brady, 1982

Estes N: Counseling the Wife of an Alcoholic. Am J Nurs: July, 1974

Estes N et al: Nursing Diagnosis of the Alcoholic Person. St. Louis, CV Mosby, 1980

Goodwin D: Is Alcoholism Hereditary? London, Oxford University Press, 1976

Grienblatt M, Schnucket M (eds): Alcoholism Problems in Women and Children. New York, Grune & Stratton, 1976

Guida MA: OHNs are in the best position to help workers fight alcoholism. Occup Health Saf: May, 1976

Guide for the Family of the Alcoholic: Long Grove, Il, Kemper Insurance Companies

Haber J et al: Comprehensive Psychiatric Nursing, 2nd ed. New York, McGraw–Hill, 1982

Heineman E, Estes N: Assessing alcoholic patients. Am J Nurs: May, 1976

Hindman M: Children of alcoholic parents. Alcohol Health and Research World: Winter, 1976

Hoff EC: Alcoholism: The Hidden Addiction. New York, The Seabury Press, 1975

Jellinek EM: The Disease Concept of Alcoholism. New Haven, Hills-House Press, 1960

Johnson VE: I'll Quit Tomorrow. New York, Harper & Row, 1973

Klewin, T: Alcohol—Teenager's Drug of Choice. The Lutheran Standard: Oct 4, 1977

Klobucher J: Mother seems a little high. The Lutheran Standard: Nov, 1982

Kurose K et al: A standard care plan for alcoholism. Am J Nurs: May, 1981

Lancaster J: Adult Psychiatric Nursing. Garden City, NJ, Medical Examination Publishing, 1980

Lego S: The American Handbook of Psychiatric Nursing. Philadelphia, JB Lippincott, 1984

Lewis L: Recognizing the alcoholic. Nurs 77: May, 1977

Liska K: Drugs and the Human Body· With Implications for Society. New York, Macmillan, 1981

Marks V: Health teaching for recovering alcoholic patients. Am J Nurs: Oct, 1980

Milman DH et al: Patterns of illicit drug and alcohol use among secondary school students. J Pediatr: Aug, 1973

Milt H: Alcoholics and Alcoholism. New York, Public Affairs Pamphlet No. 426, 1974

Mitchell J, Resnik H: Emergency Response to Crisis. Bowie, Robert J. Brady Co., 1981

Murray RB, Heulskoetter M: Psychiatric Mental Health Nursing. Englewood Cliffs, Prentice–Hall, 1983

National Council on Alcoholism: The Alcoholic in the Emergency Room. New York, National Council on Alcoholism

National Council on Alcoholism: 13 Steps to Alcoholism: Which Steps Are You On? New York, National Council on Alcoholism, 1975

O'Connor R: Employee alcoholism programs: Sobering up the corporation. Corporate Fitness and Recreation: Feb/Mar 1984

Rodman MJ: Management of acute intoxification. RN: Sept 1977

Ufer L: How to recognize and care for the alcoholic patient. Nurs 77: Oct, 1977

Vaillant G: Alcoholism and drug dependence. In: The Harvard Guide to Modern Psychiatry. Cambridge, Harvard University Press, 1978

Walker JI: Everybody's Guide to Emotional Well-Being. San Francisco, Harbor Publishing, 1982

Williams A: The student and the alcoholic patient. Nurs Outlook: July, 1979

Wilson H, Kneisl C: Psychiatric Nursing, 2nd ed. Menlo Park, Addison–Wesley Publishing, 1983

Yowell S, Brose C: Working with drug abuse patients in the ER. Am J Nurs: Jan, 1977

20

INEFFECTIVE

INDIVIDUAL COPING:

SUBSTANCE ABUSE

LEARNING OBJECTIVES

1. List factors considered to be possible causes of substance abuse or dependence.
2. Define the following terminology:
   Addiction
   Psychological dependence
   Tolerance
   Physical dependence
   Multiple substance abuse
   Continuous substance abuse
   Episodic substance abuse
   Remission
3. Discuss why people abuse:
   Barbiturates
   Opioids, opiates, or narcotics
   Amphetamines
   Cannabis or marihuana
   Hallucinogens
   Deliriants
   Nicotine
4. List common medical problems associated with drug abuse.
5. Discuss treatment measures for
   Acute intoxication
   Chronic intoxication
   Detoxification
6. State the treatment principles of substance abuse as described by Marder (1972).
7. Develop a nursing care plan for a patient undergoing withdrawal because of substance abuse, including short- and long-term goals.
8. List services available to persons who abuse drugs.

Doctor Beats Drug Habit to Help Other Physicians

THE headline above was written by *Chicago Tribune* columnist, Jeff Lyon, who described the 15-year addictive behavior of a Cleveland pediatrician. The addictive behavior began when the pediatrician took diazepam (Valium) to cope with the stress of medical school. Four years later he was taking 60 mg of Valium daily, and after he received his medical degree, the pediatrician experimented by self-prescribing amphetamines and narcotic analgesics such as meperidine (Demerol) and morphine. He finally settled on diazepam (Valium), glutethimide (Doriden), chlordiazepoxide (Librium) and other drugs that made him feel

369

tranquil. His manipulative behavior enabled him to obtain large amounts of sample pills from drug companies, thus increasing his drug intake to a variety of 12 to 15 pills at a time, followed by wine. The pediatrician began experiencing blackouts and frequent depression and realized that he could die as a result of his addictive behavior; however, "it didn't matter . . . That's the trademark of a drug addict. He knows he might die, but he doesn't care." Following a 2-month detoxification treatment program, this 41-year-old pediatrician remarried and has not taken any drugs or drunk alcohol in the past 5 years. He voluntarily visits physicians who abuse drugs and shares his story with them in an attempt to let them know "you can do something about it and get well."

Although chemical dependency has had a long and continuous history, the problem of drug abuse has become a national crisis in the United States. Millions of Americans are experimenting with mood-changing or mind-altering drugs such a marihuana and cocaine. Statements such as "I was curious," "My friends dared me," "It's the thing to do," "Everyone else does it" and "It gives me a high" commonly are made by persons abusing drugs. Walker states "Drug abuse . . . has become a major problem of our society. Marihuana abuse may occur in 14% to 16% of the population; 4% to 7% abuse sedative-hypnotics" (1982, p. 113). A Gallup youth survey of 1,069 teenagers in 1981 revealed that the key problems among young people are drug use and abuse (27%), alcohol use and abuse (7%), and smoking (3%). Approximately 37% of teenagers' problems are drug related. Other problems listed in the poll included: 1) communication with parents (20%); 2) employment and money (6%); 3) peer problems (5%); 4) job disinterest (3%); 5) career uncertainty (3%); 6) immaturity (3%); 7) violence, crime, or lack of discipline in the schools (3%); 8) finding oneself (3%); 9) miscellaneous (12%); and 10) no answer (14%).

Following is a list of mood-changers categorized by George Mann, M.D., medical director at The Johnson Institute in Minneapolis, Minnesota. This list is referred to as "The Index of Addictability" and indicates the higher degrees of addictability from top to bottom (*i.e.,* heroin at the top has a high potential for addiction, whereas caffeine at the bottom has a low potential for addiction).

High	Minor tranquilizers
Heroin	"Sleeping pills"
Morphine	Codeine
Demerol	Bromides
Cocaine	Nicotine
Barbiturates	Marihuana
Amphetamines	Caffeine
Alcohol	*Low*

ETIOLOGY OF DRUG ABUSE OR DEPENDENCE

Several factors have been identified as the possible causes of an individual's response to drugs and subsequent abuse or dependence. Donlon (1982) lists such factors as:

1. The person's expectations about a drug's effect can alter the effect. Placebos are a good example of this type of response. A 25-year-old male patient hospitalized with low back pain was dependent on Demerol. The attending physician ordered "2 cc sterile water, p.r.n., for pain." The patient actually experienced pain relief following what he thought were Demerol injections.

2. Prior experience with drugs can alter one's response. "Experimental users (of marihuana) can get high on low-quality marihuana" (p. 132).

3. The setting in which a drug is taken, *i.e.,* hospital, social setting, or street use alters one's response, as does the fear of discovery.

4. Personality factors influence the selection of drugs. "People tend to be sedation seekers or sedation avoiders" (p. 132). Depressed persons tend to select sedatives to facilitate sleep, thus making it easier to become dependent on drugs that meet their needs. Type A personalities often use antianxiety drugs or sedatives to relax at the end of a stressful day. Persons with eating disorders such as anorexia nervosa or bulimia often abuse amphetamines.

5. Genetic and constitutional factors at birth may be responsible for the susceptibility to drug dependence.

6. People with personality disorders use drugs in an attempt to solve problems by escaping reality.

7. An initial attempt to self-prescribe drugs for an illness or pain may lead to the abuse of drugs. The availability of over-the-counter drugs reinforces this factor.

8. Medicine is considered to be the solution to all problems, even feelings of insecurity or inferiority. Society emphasizes that happiness is the only natural state of existence; thus, people turn to marihuana or other mind-altering drugs.

9. Peer or cultural pressure to comply with a specific way of life fosters substance abuse.

10. Parental abuse of drugs influences children. "If it's OK for mom and dad, it's OK for me."

Murray (1983) lists the following theories pertaining to drug abuse:

1. *Sociologic factors.* "The whole socializing process of adolescence seems to contribute to drug abuse. Peers and their values are particularly strong influences" (p. 487). Experimentation, curiosity, rebellion, and boredom, are just a few reasons cited by adolescents when asked why they use or abuse drugs. "Pot parties" (marihuana), make

marihuana readily accessible to adolescents. Marihuana, cocaine, and heroin frequently are dispensed at adult social gatherings.

2. *Personality type.* Although a particular addictive personality has not been identified, "many theorists consider drug abusers to be fixed at an oral or infantile level of development" (p. 488). Such a person searches for immediate gratification of needs or ways to escape tension and turns to drugs to experience feelings of euphoria or oblivion. Characteristics frequently seen in persons who abuse drugs include low self-esteem, feelings of dependency, low tolerance for frustration and anxiety, antisocial behavior, and fear. Theorists are not certain whether these characteristics were present before the addictive behavior or whether the characteristics are a result of substance abuse.

3. *Availability of drugs.* Over-the-counter drugs; prescriptions readily obtained for sleeplessness, "nervousness," anxiety, and pain relief; and medication offered on an as-needed basis during hospitalization— all are factors that make drug abuse easy. For example, EW, a 52-year-old executive, was admitted to the general hospital with symptoms of peptic ulcer disease. During the initial intake interview, the nurse asked EW to list any medication he was taking. She was surprised to find that he was taking Librax, Valium, Seconal, and Percocet. EW had seen three different doctors before being hospitalized and was given the prescriptions to treat symptoms of a peptic ulcer, hiatal hernia, acute low back pain, and insomnia. None of the physicians questioned EW about previous prescriptions, and he did not volunteer any information because he was "afraid the doctors wouldn't give me medication for my abdominal and low back pain and sleeplessness."

CLASSIFICATION OF SUBSTANCE USE DISORDERS

Various terms are used to describe persons who use and abuse drugs, although the DSM-III clearly refers to substance abuse and substance dependence (described in Chapter 19). Addiction is a term used to define a state of chronic or recurrent intoxication and is characterized by psychological and physical dependence, and tolerance. Psychological dependence or habituation implies an emotional dependence, desire, or compulsion to continue to take a drug. Tolerance refers to the person's ability to obtain a desired effect from a specific dose of a drug. As a person develops a tolerance for 10 mg of Valium, he increases his dose to 15 mg or 20 mg to obtain the effects he originally experienced when taking 10 mg of Valium. Physical dependence is manifested by the appearance of withdrawal symptoms after the person stops taking a specific drug.

"Five classes of substances are associated with both abuse and dependence: alcohol, barbiturates, or similarly acting sedatives or hypnotics, opioids, amphetamines, or similarly acting sympathomimetics, and cannabis" (DSM-III, 1980, pp. 165–166). A diagnosis of multiple-substance abuse often occurs when people mix barbiturates, sedatives, amphetamines, and alcohol. The terms *continuous, episodic, in remission,* and *unspecified* are used to subclassify substance use disorders. The term continuous refers to a regular maladaptive use of drugs for over 6 months; episodic refers to "a fairly circumscribed period of maladaptive use, with one or more similar periods in the past" (DSM-III, 1980, p. 166); in remission describes previous maladaptive use in the past; and unspecified is used to explain an unknown course or first signs of an illness. Specific diagnostic criteria will be presented as each substance is discussed.

BARBITURATES OR SIMILARLY ACTING SEDATIVE OR HYPNOTIC ABUSE

Barbiturates are widely known drugs used as sedatives to relax the central nervous system (CNS) or slow down body processes. Taken in small doses, barbiturates temporarily ease tension and induce sleep. Medically they are used to treat hypertension, peptic ulcers, epilepsy, and insomnia; as a relaxant before and during surgery; and as a sedative for use in mental and physical illness. The normal effects of barbiturates include a decrease in cardiac and respiratory rate; a lowered blood pressure; and a mild depressant action on nerves, skeletal muscles, and the heart. Overdoses of barbiturates may include symptoms of slurred speech; drowsiness, drunken appearance, staggering gait, quick temper, quarrelsome disposition, and death. When these drugs are mixed with alcohol, the person may experience confusion, lack of coordination, depression, and the possibility of a serious illness, organic damages, or death. Barbiturates are the leading cause of accidental poisoning, as well as a primary method of committing suicide. They can cause physical and psychological dependency, making barbiturate dependency one of the most difficult disorders to cure. Withdrawal can cause severe discomfort, accompanied by tonic–clonic convulsions, mental confusion, psychotic delirium, hallucinations, fever, exhaustion, and death.

Persons who abuse barbiturates usually have difficulty handling anxiety or are unable to cope with stress. Heroin users may take barbiturates to supplement heroin or use them as a substitute for heroin, whereas persons who abuse stimulants may take sedatives or barbiturates to offset the jitteriness produced by stimulants.

Examples of barbiturates and related sedatives, their street names, short-term effects of average dose, and long-term effect of chronic use or abuse are given in the table that follows on p. 374.

The DSM-III diagnostic criteria for barbiturate or similarly acting sedative or hypnotic abuse states that the person demonstrates

1. A pattern of pathologic use, including a) the inability to reduce or stop use of the drug, b) intoxication throughout the day, c) frequent drug

Trade Name	Street Name	Short-term Effects	Long-term Effects
Amytal	Blues, downers	Relaxation, sleep, slurred speech, mild intoxication, loss of inhibition, decreased alertness and muscle coordination, nystagmus, impaired judgment	Excessive sleepiness, confusion, irritability, severe withdrawal, sickness
Nembutal	Yellow jackets		
Phenobarbital	Phennies, purple hearts		
Seconal	Reds, red devils		
Tuinal	Rainbows		
Doriden	Ds		Similar to barbiturates
Noludar	Downers		
Placidyl	Dylo		
Quaaludes	Ludes	Euphoria without drowsiness	Similar to barbiturates

use, equivalent to 600 mg or more of secobarbital or to 60 mg or more of diazepam, and d) periods of amnesia for events that occurred while the person was inebriated.

2. Impaired social functioning, such as fighting, the loss of friends, absenteeism from work or loss of job, or legal problems.

3. Existence of disturbance for at least 1 month.

OPIOIDS, OPIATES, OR NARCOTICS

Opiates are narcotic drugs that relieve pain, often induce sleep, and include drugs such as heroin, which has no medical use; codeine, which is used as a cough suppressant or pain medication; and methadone, a synthetic narcotic that is a heroin substitute to help heroin addicts. Heroin accounts for approximately 90% of the narcotic dependence in the United States. Medicinal narcotics that are abused include paregoric, codeine-containing cough syrups, Demerol, methadone, and morphine.

People abuse opiates by taking them orally, inhaling them, or injecting them into the veins in an attempt to help to relieve discomforts of withdrawal symptoms or for "kicks" or to feel good. The user becomes passive and listless as the opiates depress the respiratory center of the brain, causing shallow respirations. The person also experiences reduced feelings of hunger, thirst, pain, and sexual desire. As the effects of the drugs wear off, the abuser, who becomes physically and emotionally addicted by requiring increasingly larger dosages, suffers withdrawal symptoms unless another dose of the drug is taken.

Opiates, also referred to as "white stuff," "hard stuff," and "junk," are considered to be the most addictive drugs because the body builds a tolerance and requires larger doses of it. Acute overdose is identified by symptoms of decreased, slow respirations; constricted pupils; and a rapid, weak pulse.

Opiate withdrawal symptoms begin within 12 to 16 hours after the last dose and are characterized by watery eyes, rhinitis, yawning, sneezing, and diaphoresis. Other symptoms include dilated pupils, restlessness and tremors, goose bumps, irritability, loss of appetite, muscle cramps, nausea and vomiting, and diarrhea. Symptoms subside within 5 to 10 days if no treatment occurs.

Methadone is used to decrease the severity of withdrawal and as a maintenance narcotic transferring the person's addiction to methadone, which allows him to function better in society. The cure rate among opiate addicts is extremely low, and overdose can be lethal. Experts state that it takes up to 5 years to cure an opiate addict.

The DSM-III diagnostic criteria for opioid abuse states that the person must demonstrate:

1. A pattern of pathologic use, such as intoxication throughout the day, the inability to decrease or reduce use, daily use for approximately a month, and episodes of intoxication so severe that respiration and consciousness are impaired
2. Impaired social or occupational functioning
3. Duration of disturbance that lasts at least 1 month

AMPHETAMINES AND RELATED STIMULANTS

Amphetamines ("pep pills") are drugs that directly stimulate the central nervous system and create a feeling of alertness and self-confidence in the user. They are also referred to by drug abusers as "wake-up," "speed," "eye-openers," "copilots," "truck drivers," "uppers," or "bennies." Medical use includes diet pills to reduce appetite in weight control programs (Dexedrine, Benzedrine); treatment of mild depression, fatigue, hyperkinesis or narcolepsy (amphetamines); and local anesthetic (cocaine). Caffeine and nicotine are also considered to be stimulants.

These drugs are often abused by oral ingestion, infection into veins, smoking, or inhaling increased dosages to obtain an exaggerated effect of the stimulating action. People also take these drugs for kicks, thrills, or to combat boredom; to stay awake or to allow greater physical effort; or to counteract the effects of alcohol and barbiturates. They are considered to be dangerous because they can drive a user to do things beyond his physical limits; they can cause mental fatigue, dizziness, and feelings of fear and confusion; and sudden withdrawal can lead to depression and suicide.

The heart and circulatory system also may be damaged as a result of over-production of adrenalin.

Effects of stimulants on the body include increased heart rate, elevated blood pressure, excitability, tremors of the hands, increased talkativeness, profuse diaphoresis, dry mouth, abnormal heart rhythms, headaches, pallor, diarrhea, and unclear speech. The abuser can develop a psychological dependence on stimulants and may experience delusions, auditory and visual hallucinations, or a drug psychosis that resembles schizophrenia.

Symptoms of cocaine abuse include increased pulse, increased circulation, quick, sharp reactions, rising temperature, dilated pupils, increased physical activity, shakes or tremors, restlessness, overconfidence in mental and physical abilities, feeling of well-being, loss of a sense of time, and extreme depression. Psychological dependence can occur, in which the person displays little desire to be cured. Large dosages of cocaine can produce hallucinations and feelings of persecution or paranoia. As with all injectible drugs, the abuser who "mainlines,"or shoots a drug directly into his bloodstream, risks overdosing or developing hepatitis, tetanus, or acquired immune deficiency syndrome (AIDS) because of the use of unsterile needles and poor aseptic technique. Amphetamines also may cause an unacceptable sensitivity to other medications so that treatment of an amphetamine user with other drugs may be unsafe. Repeated inhalation ("snorting") of cocaine constricts the blood vessels in the mucous membranes of the nose, causing dryness. Nasal ulcers may form, and the nasal septum can be perforated.

Long-term use of caffeine and nicotine also can cause symptoms of withdrawal. Persons who switch to decaffeinated coffee or stop drinking cola drinks may experience mild anxiety, drowsiness, or headaches. Persons who stop smoking often complain of nervousness, increase in appetite, sleep disturbances, and feelings of anxiety.

The DSM-III criteria for abuse of amphetamines and related substances are similar to that of opioid abuse.

CANNABIS OR MARIHUANA (MARIJUANA)

Marihuana is a common plant with the biological name of *Cannabis sativa.* It can act as a stimulant or depressant and is often considered to be a mild hallucinogen with some sedative properties. Although marihuana has no general medical use, researchers are studying its effect on the appetite and its use as an anticonvulsant or antidepressant. Studies have indicated that it may lower pressure in the eyeball, making it effective in the treatment of glaucoma.

Persons who abuse marihuana usually smoke it in a pipe or as a rolled cigarette ("joint") but also may take it orally in the form of capsules, tablets, on sugar cubes, or in food. Holders ("roach clips") are used to get the last puffs from marihuana butts once they become too short for conventional smoking. Slang names for marihuana include pot, tea, grass, weed, smoke, and Mary Jane.

Marihuana acts quickly, in about 15 minutes, once it enters the bloodstream and the effects last approximately 2 to 4 hours. It affects a person's mood, thinking, behavior, and judgment in different ways, and in large doses it may cause hallucinations. General physiologic symptoms include increased appetite, lowered body temperature, depression, drowsiness, unsteady gait, inability to think clearly, excitement, reduced coordination and reflexes, and impaired judgment. Users of large amounts may feel suicidal or have delusions of invulnerability, causing them to take chances.

Although marihuana is not physically addicting, it may lead to psychological dependence, thereby retarding personality growth and adjustment to adulthood. Its use also can expose the user to those using and pushing stronger drugs.

Reasons for using marihuana include the following: "getting high," escape, "to have greater personal insights," "make life more meaningful," and "expanding one's mind."

The DSM-III diagnostic criteria for cannabis or marihuana abuse are similar to those for opioid abuse.

OTHER CLASSIFICATIONS OF DRUGS

Other categories of frequently abused substances are hallucinogens, phencyclidine hydrochloride (PCP), deliriants, and tobacco. Hallucinogens and PCP are associated only with abuse because physiologic dependence has not been demonstrated. They are referred to as "mind benders" or psychedelic drugs, affecting the mind and causing changes in perception and consciousness. Examples include lysergic acid diethylamide (LSD), mescaline, dimethyltryptamine (DMT), 2,5 dimethoxy-4-methylamphetamine (STP), and psilocybin. Similar to marihuana, but stronger in effect on the body, hallucinogens are dangerous because they can lead to panic, paranoia, flashbacks, or death. Physiologic symptoms can include an increased pulse rate, blood pressure, and temperature; dilated pupils; tremors of hands and feet; cold, sweaty palms; flushed face or pallor; irregular respirations; and nausea. Effects on the central nervous system include an increased distortion of senses, loss of the ability to separate fact from fantasy, loss of sense of time, ambivalence, and the inability to reason logically.

Hallucinogens are quite unpredictable. One experience with them ("trip") may be good while the next may be disastrous. The daughter of television personality Art Linkletter leaped from her apartment in a suicidal panic brought on by LSD. Diane had an exciting career, loving family, good health, and no material worries. According to her father, no explanation could be found for her tragic death except the fact that she had taken LSD.

PCP, commonly known as "angel dust," is an extremely dangerous hallucinogen. Originally used as a surgical anesthetic, PCP was found to cause extreme agitation, stupor, hallucinations, and psychosis. Persons who experience PCP intoxication have enormous strength, experience unbelievably paranoid reactions, and literally do not know pain. They may become violent, destructive, and confused after one dose. Medical complications of PCP include vomiting, seizures, and extremely high blood pressure.

Deliriants are any chemicals that give off fumes or vapors and, when inhaled, produce symptoms similar to intoxication. The person who inhales or sniffs deliriants may become confused, excited, or experience hallucinations. Following such a "high," the person may have a loss of coordination, distorted perception of reality, and experience hallucinations and convulsions.

Dangers of inhaling deliriants include temporary blindness and damage to the lungs, brain, and liver. Deaths have occurred as a result of suffocation caused by placing plastic bags, a moistened cloth, or plastic container against one's face. Commonly abused deliriants include glue, gasoline, lighter fluid, paint thinner, varnish, shellac, nail polish remover, and aerosol-packaged products.

Nicotine, the active ingredient in tobacco, is a stimulant that elevates one's blood pressure and increases one's heartbeat. Tar, found in the smoke, contains many carcinogens. Long-term effects of tobacco dependence include emphysema, chronic bronchitis, coronary heart disease, and a variety of cancers.

Approximately 31% of adult women and 42% of adult men smoke cigarettes for stimulation, to relax or feel better, or out of habit. Regular smokers become psychologically dependent on cigarettes and find it difficult to stop smoking. Tobacco dependence generally begins in late adolescence or by early adult life and may result in tobacco withdrawal when one attempts to stop smoking. Symptoms of withdrawal include a craving for tobacco, irritability, difficulty concentrating, restlessness, anxiety, headache, drowsiness, and gastrointestinal disturbances (Lego, 1984).

Diagnostic criteria for hallucinogen and PCP abuse are similar to those of other substance abuse disorders described earlier without symptoms of psychological dependence. Criteria for tobacco dependence include:

1. Continuous smoking or use of tobacco for at least 30 days.

2. At least one of the following behaviors:

> Unsuccessful serious attempts to reduce significantly or stop the amount of tobacco on a permanent basis

The onset of tobacco withdrawal after attempts to stop smoking

The use of tobacco in the presence of a serious physical disorder such as respiratory or cardiovascular disease when the person knows the condition is exacerbated by the use of tobacco

TREATMENT

Common medical problems associated with drug abuse are

1. Malnutrition with vitamin deficiencies
2. Fluid and electrolyte imbalance
3. Constipation
4. Amenorrhea
5. Respiratory infections
6. Skin abscesses
7. Cellulitis
8. Dental caries and loss of teeth
9. Impotence
10. Hepatic dysfunction
11. Bacterial endocarditis
12. Thrombophlebitis
13. Pulmonary embolism
14. Seizures

Donlon (1982) lists treatment measures for various types of substance use disorders. Summarized, they include:

DRUG CLASSIFICATION	TREATMENT MEASURES
Barbiturates and other sedative hypnotics	Treatment of acute intoxication consists of observation and support. 1. Physical examination 2. Blood drug level 3. Blood glucose 4. "Sleep off" mild intoxication 5. Observe for several hours in emergency or other setting if stupor is present (as seen in moderate intoxication). 6. Observation for signs of trauma may include a neurologic examination and skull x-rays. 7. Assess for signs of depression and suicidal thoughts. 8. Medicate with drug such as haloperidol (Haldol) if patient is agitated or belligerent.

(continued)

DRUG CLASSIFICATION

TREATMENT MEASURES

Treatment of chronic intoxication is similar to that of acute intoxication. It also includes

1. Assessment for a variety of medical complications
2. Helping the person get treatment for his drug problem

Detoxification

1. Administer a test dose of pentobarbital orally and evaluate sensory awareness 1 hour later. The patient's response to 200 mg of pentobarbital will vary according to the degree of dependence. For example, if the patient is asleep but arousable, there is no degree of dependence; however, if there are no signs of intoxication, he is tolerant to 1000 mg or more of a barbiturate daily. If the person is awake but somnolent and exhibits symptoms of nystagmus, slurred speech, and ataxia, he is tolerant to 500 mg to 600 mg daily.
2. Stabilize the patient at the appropriate test dose using pentobarbital in equally divided doses for 2 days, during which time the patient should show symptoms of mild sedation and intoxication.
3. Adjust the dosage to allow withdrawal to occur over a 10-day period.
4. Be aware of seizure potential.
5. Refer the patient for psychotherapeutic treatment such as group and family therapy.

Opioids and Opiates

Tolerance is often exhibited by persons who use morphine or heroin repeatedly. Multiple drug abuse is common among such persons; therefore, a careful history is necessary to avoid a mixed barbiturate–opiate withdrawal, which can be fatal. Three choices of treatment include

1. Methadone substitution: This preferred method stabilizes the patient on an oral dose of methadone that suppresses opioid withdrawal symptoms. Withdrawal of methadone occurs over a period of 3 to 7 days. Insomnia may require treatment with the use of a sedative such as chloral hydrate.
2. Rapid reduction: The person is stabilized on dosages of morphine for two days to prevent symptoms of withdrawal (*i.e.*, morphine 30 mg q6hr). Withdrawal occurs within 5 to 10 days.
3. "Cold turkey": No substitution is given

DRUG CLASSIFICATION	TREATMENT MEASURES
	for abused drugs. Total abstinence must occur, although phenothiazenes may be given for sedation, antianxiety effects, and antiemetic qualities. Chloral hydrate is often given at bedtime.
	Referral to different treatment programs, for example
	1. Ex-addict programs
	2. Methadone maintenance programs or substitute addiction that allows for social rehabilitation of the addict.
	3. Morphine antagonist programs that maintain the addict on small doses and keep the patient resistant to euphoric and physiologic effects of morphine or heroin.
	4. Individual, group, or family psychotherapy
Amphetamines	The person who abuses amphetamines must be evaluated carefully for depression, anxiety neuroses, or family conflict. Treatment consists of
	1. Evaluation for the possibility of a mixed dependence
	2. Assessment for profound depression and suicidal tendencies
	3. Assessment for symptoms of insomnia, lassitude, and irritability that may persist for an extended period
	4. Referral to group therapy
Cannabis (Marihuana)	"Clinically, dependence on marihuana most closely resembles dependence on alcohol or sedative–hypnotics. The concern and controversy over marihuana are more related to sociopolitical and moral–legal issues than to pharmacologic or psychiatric issues" (Donlon, 1982, p. 159). Although marihuana does not lead to physical addiction, current research focuses on
	1. Consequences of long-term use of marihuana
	2. Effects of marihuana on physical and mental behavior and skills
	3. Chemical properties, toxicity, possible genetic damage, and effects of marihuana on the body's resistance to disease
Hallucinogens	Treatment consists of
	1. Providing protection to prevent self-harm or harm to others while experienc-

(continued)

DRUG CLASSIFICATION	TREATMENT MEASURES
	ing a mind-expanding experience. Perceptual distortions and vivid visual experiences usually occur.
	2. Medicating with diazepam (Valium) or diphenhydramine hydrochloride (Benadryl) to calm or sedate the acutely agitated patient during a "bad trip"
	3. Observing for "flashbacks," which can occur up to 18 months after the last dose of an hallucinogen has been taken. Low dosages of phenothiazines may be prescribed during this time.
PCP (Phencyclidine)	Treatment is largely supportive and symptomatic. If the patient is comatose:
	1. Intubate and do a gastric lavage.
	2. Obtain blood and urine samples for analysis.
	3. Administer ascorbic acid, which may speed excretion of the drug through acidification of the urine.
	4. Phenytoin (Dilantin) may be ordered for seizures.
	5. Observe for signs of hypertensive crisis and treat with diazoxide as necessary.
	Treatment of a confusional state consists of:
	1. Minimizing sensory stimulation and restraining as a last measure.
	2. Administering diazepam to calm the patient.

The following treatment principles of substance abuse listed by Marder (1972) should be considered by health care professionals when providing initial care:

1. Treat a patient symptomatically if the drug is unidentifiable.

2. Do not accept at face value what a patient tells you if clinical symptoms are contrary.

3. Use pharmacological antagonists sparingly.

4. Intoxicated persons should not be sent to jail or left unobserved or unattended.

5. Do not administer phenothiazines if a seizure disorder or respiratory distress is suspected.

6. Gastric lavage should not be performed if the patient has ingested petroleum products and is alert.

7. Do not use gastric lavage if the patient appears psychotic and if a drug

such as LSD or mescaline has been ingested approximately 2 hours or more before admission.

Marder also provides an extensive list of services for individuals who require treatment for substance abuse. Summarized, they include the following:

Individual psychotherapy

Group therapy

Family therapy

Encounter groups

Parent support groups

Recreational therapy

Occupational therapy

Short-term residential rehabilitation (3 mo)

Longer-term therapeutic community (6–18 mo)

Day treatment center

Reentry programs

Outpatient and after-care treatment

ASSESSMENT

The individual who abuses substances presents a variety of challenges because of fear, dependency needs, feelings of insecurity, a low self-esteem, the inability to cope, a low tolerance for frustration or anxiety, rebellion, or boredom. Persons who self-prescribe medication frequently do not admit readily to substance abuse. Defense mechanisms such as rationalization, projection, and repression commonly are used by abusive persons.

Murray (1983) lists specific information that should be obtained in all cases of suspected substance abuse. During the assessment process, which may occur in the emergency room, general hospital, psychiatric unit, or drug treatment center, questions should be directed toward:

1. Identifying the drug being used
2. Clarifying the time, kind, and dose of last use and whether this is the current usage pattern
3. Clarifying how long the person has been abusing the current drug
4. Identifying whether a multiple-drug abuse exists
5. Clarifying whether there is a history of seizures.

It is imperative that the nurse be able to recognize symptoms of drug overdose or drug withdrawal during the assessment process. Each drug reacts differently and is identified in part by behavioral and physical manifestations. Assessment measures therefore should focus on obtaining a baseline data and monitoring vital signs; observing for signs of central nervous system depression, such as irregular respirations or lowered blood pressure; recognizing signs of impending seizures or coma; assessing the person for cuts, bruises, infection, or needle tracks; assessing general nutritional status; determining the patient's level of sensorium; listening to physiologic complaints; and observing behavioral symptoms. If it is a crisis situation, data collection focuses on whatever is essential for immediate care. In a less acute situation, information gathering provides the basis for developing a care plan.

"The three major areas that must be considered in the nursing diagnosis include 1) physical problems resulting from drug dependence, 2) psychological problems that support drug dependence, and 3) sociological factors" (Murray, 1983, p. 489).

NURSING INTERVENTIONS

Attitudes of nursing personnel can influence the quality of care given to persons who abuse drugs. Nurses may view patients who overdose on drugs with disapproval, intolerance, moralistic condemnation, anger, or they may not display any emotional reaction. They need to display an accepting, nonjudgmental attitude while coping with various behaviors such as manipulation, noncompliance, aggression, or hostility. Nursing personnel need to be aware of the various signs and symptoms of abused drugs if they are to administer appropriate nursing care.

Nursing interventions include providing medical relief for symptoms such as nausea, vomiting, skin bruises, fluid and electrolyte imbalance, and withdrawal symptoms. Several examples of nursing diagnoses and nursing interventions were given in the chapter on alcoholism and apply to the drug abuser as well. They include potential for injury, sensory alterations, anxiety, sleep pattern disturbance, alterations in nutrition, possible fluid volume and electrolyte deficit, health maintenance alteration, noncompliance, ineffective individual coping, and potential for violence. The following are examples of nursing diagnoses and nursing interventions for a person who is experiencing withdrawal symptoms due to multiple drug abuse.

NURSING DIAGNOSES	NURSING INTERVENTIONS
Sensory–perceptual alteration: Delirium	Provide a safe environment. Decrease environmental stimuli by placing the patient in a partially lighted room. Avoid loud noise. Assess level of sensorium.

NURSING DIAGNOSES	NURSING INTERVENTIONS
Alteration in thought process: Hallucinations	Orient to person, time, and place. Avoid conveying to the patient the belief that the hallucinations are real. Encourage the patient to make the staff aware of the hallucinations. Be alert for signs of increased fear, anxiety, or agitation.
Anxiety related to withdrawal symptoms	Assess level of anxiety. Decrease sensory stimulation. Provide reassurance and comfort (refer to Chap. 12 for additional nursing interventions).
Potential for injury owing to altered sensorium	Assess for the causative factor of altered sensorium. Provide a safe environment by keeping the bed at lowest level at night, utilizing siderails as necessary, and restraining the patient if necessary (as a last resort). Orient to surroundings by explaining the call system, rationale for utilizing siderails, etc. Provide a night light to familiarize the patient with the surroundings.
Alterations in nutrition: Less than body requirements	Provide diet as tolerated to supply adequate nutrition for nourishment and tissue repair unless the patient is NPO. Make sure that the dietary department serves appetizing meals, including special dietary preferences. Serve dietary supplements as needed to maintain an adequate intake of vitamins, minerals, and so forth. Maintain an intake and output (I & O) if necessary.

Schultz and Dark list the following short-term goals for persons during drug withdrawal (1982, pp. 109–110):

1. The patient will be drug free.

2. Maintain homeostasis by preventing or treating physical complications.

3. Decrease feelings of fear, anxiety, or paranoia.

4. Provide a safe environment for the patient.

5. Prevent injury to the patient or others.

6. Decrease the patient's discomfort.

Murray (1983, p. 489) cites four "client-care goals" during recovery from drug dependence. These goals are

1. Withdrawal without complications

2. Return to a stable state of health

3. Learning proper health habits

4. Seeking further specialized treatment

Long-term goals listed by Schultz and Dark (p. 110) include:

1. Referral to a substance abuse treatment program

2. Developing new coping skills by nonchemical means

3. Leading a chemical-free lifestyle

4. Developing and maintaining significant interpersonal relationships

Smith (Lego, 1983) discusses the education of patients about the hazards of drug abuse by using the patient's past experiences with drugs, using the recent experience in the hospital, providing resource materials (including names of agencies and telephone numbers), and not threatening police action.

SUMMARY

The problem of drug abuse has become a national crisis in the United States. Frequently abused drugs include marihuana, sedative–hypnotics, amphetamines, barbiturates, and cocaine. Several causes of drug abuse or dependence were cited, including the person's expectations about a drug's effects, prior experience with drugs, the setting in which the drug is taken, an addictive personality, genetic and constitutional factors, personality disorders, self-prescribing of drugs, peer or cultural pressure, parental abuse of drugs, sociologic factors, and the availability of drugs. The DSM-III classifications of drugs associated with both abuse and dependence were discussed, including barbiturates and similar-acting sedatives or hypnotics, opiates or narcotics, amphetamines and related stimulants, cannabis or marihuana, hallucinogens, PCP, deliriants, and tobacco. Reasons for use of drugs, routes of administration, symptoms of physical or psychological dependence, effects of the drugs on the body, and examples of street drugs were given. Common medical problems associated with drug abuse were stated. Treatment measures for each drug classification were explained including acute intoxication, chronic intoxication, and detoxification by methadone substitution, rapid reduction, and "cold turkey." Treatment principles described by Marder (1972) were listed, as well as an extensive list of services for persons who require treatment for substance abuse. Attitudes of persons caring for persons who abuse drugs were explored. Assessment measures, nursing diagnoses, and nursing interventions were discussed, focusing on physical problems, psychological problems, and sociologic factors. Short- and long-term goals for persons during withdrawal, as well as recovery from drug addiction, were listed. Examples of methods used to educate patients about the hazards of drug abuse were given. Nursing interventions for the following nursing diagnoses were stated: sensory–perceptual alteration: delirium; alteration in thought process: hallucinations; anxiety related to withdrawal symptoms; potential for injury due to altered sensorium; and alterations in nutrition: less than body requirements.

LEARNING ACTIVITIES

I. Clinical activities
  A. Care for a patient with a history of substance abuse or dependence.
  B. Evaluate the patient's treatment plan.
  C. Does the patient display insight into his problem?
  D. Does the patient express the desire to be helped?
  E. Is the patient cooperative?
  F. Should the patient be in another hospital or treatment program?
  G. Are the patient's plans for the future realistic?
  H. Discuss supportive care for the patient after discharge.
II. Independent activities
  A. Discuss how the following possible symptoms may be related to substance abuse:
    1. Change in school or work attendance or performance
    2. Alteration of personal appearance
    3. Sudden mood or attitude changes
    4. Withdrawal from family contacts
    5. Withdrawal from responsibility
    6. Unusual patterns of behavior
    7. Unresponsive to environmental stimuli
  B. Research your local newspaper for a week, paying specific attention to articles on substance abuse:
    1. What drugs are frequently listed, if any?
    2. What age group of people is involved?
    3. Describe the circumstances in the articles pertaining to substance abuse (*i.e.,* a crime, abuse, auto accident).

SELF-TEST

1. Describe the index of addictability.
2. Describe the following theories about drug abuse or dependence.
   Sociological
   Personality

3. A term used to define a state of chronic or recurrent intoxication is _____.

4. An emotional dependence, desire, or compulsion to continue to take a drug is _____.

5. Define tolerance.

Match the following:

6. Amphetamines
7. Opioids
8. Cannabis
9. Deleriants
10. Barbiturates

a. Can be a stimulant or depressant; mild hallucinogen
b. Fumes or vapors producing mild intoxication
c. Relaxes CNS and slows down the body processes
d. Narcotic drugs to relieve pain or induce sleep
e. Stimulates the CNS

11. Explain the purpose of a "test dose" or pentobarbital during detoxification.

12. Differentiate between "cold turkey" and methadone substitution.

13. State the more common medical problems of substance abuse.

14. List supportive care available to persons who abuse drugs.

15. Discuss short-term goals during drug withdrawal.

16. State the client-care goals during recovery from drug dependence.

REFERENCES

Altrocchi J: Abnormal Behavior. New York, Harcourt Brace Jovanovich, 1980

Burgess A: Psychiatric Nursing in the Hospital and the Community, 3rd ed. Englewood Cliffs, Prentice–Hall, 1981

Daniel WA Jr: Adolescents in Health and Disease. St. Louis, CV Mosby, 1977

Donlon PT, Rockwell DA: Psychiatric Disorders: Diagnosis and Treatment. Bowie, Robert J. Brady, 1982

Drug Abuse: The Chemical Cop-Out. National Association of Blue Shield Plans, 1973

Haber J, et al: Comprehensive Psychiatric Nursing, 2nd ed. New York, McGraw–Hill, 1982

Kelly M: For Kids Only: What You Should Know About Marijuana. Alcohol, Drug Abuse and Mental Health Administration, Rockville, MD, U.S. Department of Health and Human Services, 1980

Lancaster J: Adult Psychiatric Nursing. Garden City, NJ, Medical Examination Publishing, 1980

Lego S: The American Handbook of Psychiatric Nursing. Philadelphia, JB Lippincott, 1984

Liska K: Drugs and the Human Body. New York, MacMillan, 1981

Marder L: Drug Dependency—Techniques in Recognition and Treatment. San Francisco, American Medical Association, 1972

Marijuana Update: Pleasantville, NY, Reader's Digest Association, 1979

McLeod A et al: Questions and Answers (booklet). Rockville, MD, Biospherics, Inc. (in cooperation with Special Action Office for Drug Abuse Prevention and National Institute on Drug Abuse) 1973

Murray R, Heulskoetter M: Psychiatric Mental Health Nursing. Englewood Cliffs, Prentice–Hall, 1983

Parents, Peers and Pot: Alcohol, Drug Abuse and Mental Health Administration. Rockville, MD, U.S. Department of Health and Human Services, 1980

A Reason for Tears. Lexington, KY, H.E.L.P. Publishers, 1982

The parents' guide to drug abuse. Listen, Journal of Better Living. Narcotics Education, Inc. Washington, DC, 1978

Schultz J, Dark S: Manual of Psychiatric Nursing Care Plans. Boston, Little, Brown & Co, 1982

Stuart G, Sundeen S: Principles and Practice of Psychiatric Nursing, 2nd ed. St. Louis, CV Mosby, 1983

Vourakis C, Bennett G: Angel dust: Not heaven sent. Am J Nurs: Apr, 1979

Walker JI: Everybody's Guide to Emotional Well-Being. San Francisco, Harbor Publishing, 1982

Wilson H, Kneisl C: Psychiatric Nursing, 2nd ed. Menlo Park: Addison Wesley Publishing, 1983

Yowell S, Brose C: Working with drug abuse patients in the ER. Backer et al (eds): Psychiatric Mental Health Nursing: Contemporary Readings. New York, D. Van Nostrand, 1978

21

DISORDERS OF INFANCY,

CHILDHOOD, AND

ADOLESCENCE

CHILDREN LEARN WHAT THEY LIVE

If children live with criticism,
They learn to condemn.

If children live with hostility,
They learn to fight.

If children live with ridicule,
They learn to be shy.

If children live with shame,
They learn to feel guilty.

If children live with tolerance,
They learn to be patient.

If children live with encouragement,
They learn confidence.

If children live with praise,
They learn to appreciate.

If children live with fairness,
They learn justice.

If children live with security,
They learn to have faith.

If children live with approval,
They learn to like themselves

If children live with acceptance and friendship,
They learn to find love in the world.

Dorothy Law Nolte

LEARNING OBJECTIVES

1. Discuss the following causative factors pertaining to disorders of infancy, childhood, or adolescence:
    Constitutional factors
    Effects of physical disease or injury
    Temperamental factors
    Environmental factors
2. Differentiate the four types of mental retardation.
3. List the clinical symptoms of a hyperactive child with an attention deficit disorder.
4. State the characteristics of an anorectic personality.
5. Differentiate bulimia from anorexia nervosa.
6. Explain the following diagnoses:
    Transient tic disorder
    Functional encopresis
    Functional enuresis
7. State the diagnostic criteria for infantile autism.
8. Plan nursing interventions for the following persons:
    A depressed 12-year-old boy with suicidal ideation
    A manipulative 19-year-old anorectic girl who refuses to eat
    A 7-year-old hyperactive boy
    A 4-year-old autistic boy who is mute

ISORDERS of infancy, childhood, or adolescence generally occur as a result of complex reactions during one's early developmental stages. The child's age, stage of personality development, motor and physical development, and ability to communicate, are a few of the factors influencing such reactions. Barker (1983) groups these factors into four main groups: constitutional factors, effects of physical disease or injury, temperamental factors, and environmental factors.

Constitutional factors are a result of genetic inheritance and the condition of the intrauterine environment during pregnancy. Genetic effects cause few psychiatric disorders in childhood; however, they can cause mental impairment or retardation, such as Down's syndrome (formerly called mongolism) and phenylketonuria. A decreased supply of oxygen and the presence of a disease such as syphilis create an adverse intrauterine environment that can affect the central nervous system (CNS) of the fetus. Fetal alcohol syndrome, which occurs in the pregnant woman who abuses alcohol, premature birth, and birth trauma are also causes of abnormal development, including mental impairment. Genetic counseling, good prenatal care, well-equipped and competently staffed labor and delivery units, and the presence of neonatal intensive care units all help to decrease the onset of abnormal development, which may be accompanied by emotional disturbance or mental impairment.

Severe malnutrition, physical disease (*e.g.,* diabetes, rheumatoid arthritis, or congenital heart defect), brain damage due to infection or trauma, and injuries such as severe burns or traumatic amputation all may lead to the development of a psychiatric disorder.

A temperamental factor is described by Webster as a "mode of emotional response," "disposition," or "excessive sensitiveness" exhibited by a person. Adverse or negative temperamental factors include withdrawal, slow or impaired adaptation to environmental change, unstable mood states, and exaggerated, intense reactions to an environmental stimulus. Heredity, interpersonal relationships, and the environment all influence one's temperament. Children with a positive temperament display a happy, contented mood, the ability to adapt readily, a positive approach to new situations, and a low-key or mild reaction to environmental stimuli. They are less apt to develop a behavior disorder than are children who exhibit adverse temperamental factors.

Environmental factors are considered to be the main cause of behavior disorders in children during early and middle childhood. One's family, school, and neighborhood are considered functioning systems of the environment shaping the child's development. The family provides a protective training ground for the child as he learns to adapt, to live as a member of society, and to become independent. Any negative or maladaptive responses learned within one of the functioning systems can be extended to the other systems. For example, a child who uses the maladaptive behavior of a temper tantrum at home to get his way will probably attempt to use such behavior at school until limits are set.

"Scapegoating" is a term used to describe the role of a person within a family who is the recipient of angry, hostile, frustrated, or ambivalent emotions experienced by various family members. Such a person is singled out as family members project their feelings onto him. As a result, the child may use acting-out behavior in an attempt to cope, to decrease anxiety, to receive love and attention, or to preserve his self-esteem.

Placing too much responsibility on a child, making him a "little adult," is an abnormal family role that can cause a behavior disorder. Such a child might be expected to baby-sit siblings, to help with adult tasks, or even to fulfill the role of an absent adult. The child does not have the opportunity to progress through the normal stages of growth and development.

A child whose mother is depressed or is experiencing severe emotional trauma is at risk because of the influence of a negative environment. Mental or physical abuse may occur in such a setting. The child generally receives little love and attention, if any, and lacks a close interpersonal relationship as he attempts to relate to others, develop trust, and gain independence.

Barker (1983) lists the characteristics of a school environment that influence the development of normal, positive behavior in children. A study of secondary school children was done in London by Rutter (1981). The characteristics are summarized as follows:

1. An integration of the intellectually able and less able children provides for a well-balanced classroom, encouraging normal growth and development.

2. Acknowledgement and praise by teachers promotes the development of a positive self-concept.

3. Encouragement of participation in running of the school fosters responsibility.

4. Placing moderate emphasis on academic achievement permits the child to participate in a variety of activities and to develop a well-rounded personality.

5. Good role modeling by teachers promotes positive behavior in children.

6. A comfortable, pleasant, and attractive environment is conducive to the development of mentally healthy persons.

Neighborhoods also can influence the development of behavior disorders. Poor socioeconomic conditions in crowded inner cities produce higher rates of psychiatric disorders in children than are seen in suburban areas. Delinquency, substance abuse, childhood depression, and antisocial personalities are just a few examples of disorders prevalent in such neighborhoods.

CLASSIFICATION OF CLINICAL DISORDERS

Disorders of infancy, childhood, or adolescence are separated into five major groups by the DSM-III. They include intellectual, behavioral, emotional, physical, and developmental disorders. Each of these groups is subdivided as follows:

1. Intellectual disorders

    Mental retardation

2. Behavioral disorders (overt)

    Attention deficit disorder

    Conduct disorder

3. Emotional disorders

    Anxiety disorders of childhood or adolescence

    Other disorders of infancy, childhood, or adolescence

4. Physical disorders

    Eating disorders

    Stereotyped movement disorders

    Other disorders with physical manifestation

5. Developmental disorders

    Pervasive developmental disorders

    Specific developmental disorders

Other categories discussed in this text are also appropriate for children or adolescents, and age-specific features are included in each chapter. They include diagnoses such as affective disorders, personality disorders, psychosexual disorders, organic mental disorders, substance use disorders, and adjustment disorder.

Many texts present an excellent summary of psychological development, focusing on the developmental stage, motor and physical development, language or communication, cognitive behavior, interpersonal behavior, developmental crisis, and the most frequent disturbing behaviors in each developmental stage. The reader is referred to such texts on growth and development for additional information as it is important in the assessment and treatment of disorders affecting infants, children and adolescents.

INTELLECTUAL DISORDER: MENTAL RETARDATION

Mental retardation is described by the DSM-III as the presence of a subaverage general intellectual functioning associated with or resulting in impairments in adaptive behavior. The onset occurs before age 18. Altrocchi (1980) describes persons with mental impairment as unable to think abstractly, adapt to new situations, learn new information, solve problems, or profit from experience. Causative factors are numerous. They include defective genes, an abnormal number of chromosomes, malnutrition, radiation exposure, maternal infections, Rh incompatibility, syphilis, anoxia, birth injury, brain tumor, head trauma, early infant infections (*e.g.,* meningitis), and deprivation of normal growth and development experience (seen in a low socioeconomic status).

Mental retardation is classified by intelligence quotient (IQ) scores and deficits in adaptation. The following chart illustrates the categories of mild, moderate, severe, and profound mental retardation.

Subtype	IQ Level	Deficits	Comments
Mild	50–70	None in early childhood Difficulty adapting to school Achieve to 6th grade level by late teens May need assistance when experiencing social or economic stress	80% of all MR groups Can achieve social and vocational skills "Educable"
Moderate	35–49	Poor awareness of needs of others Need moderate supvervision due to self-care deficit Generally does not progress beyond 2nd grade level Require supervision and guidance under mild social or economic stress	12% of all MR groups May profit from vocational training Can function in sheltered workshops as unskilled or semiskilled persons "Trainable"
Severe	20–34	Poor motor development and minimal speech noted Unable to learn academic skills but may learn to talk and be trained in elementary hygiene skills or activities of daily living	7% of all MR groups Require complete supervision in a controlled environment May learn to perform simple work tasks
Profound	Below 20	Requires total nursing care and a highly structured environment with supervision due to a self-care deficit Possesses a minimal capacity for sensorimotor functioning	Less than 1% of all MR groups May learn some productive skills "Custodial"

Please note that there may be quite a variability in the relationship of categories. For example, a severely retarded person living with a very loving and supportive family may function as well, if not better, than a moderately retarded individual living in less advantageous circumstances.

Various associated features of mental retardation include irritability, aggressiveness, temper tantrums, stereotyped repetitive movements, nail-biting, and stuttering. Mental retardation is twice as common in males as in females.

Mental Retardation, Severe Level: Clinical Example

MW, 21 years old, was born by a normal spontaneous vaginal delivery without any complications. Two months after birth MW developed a temperature of 105°F and had a grand mal seizure. He was admitted to the neonatal intensive care unit with the diagnosis of fever of undetermined origin (FUO). Diagnostic tests revealed the presence of encephalitis. MW recovered but his parents were cautioned about the possibility of CNS damage because of the severity of his illness. During early childhood, ages 1 to 5, MW was able to communicate with his parents to some extent but exhibited poor motor development. His need for complete supervision in a controlled environment became evident because he also was unable to learn basic skills such as reading, writing, and arithmetic. IQ testing revealed MW's IQ to be that of a severely retarded or mentally impaired person. At age 21 he continues to live at home with very supportive parents who have been able to teach him some self-care activities. He relates well to a pet cat, helps his mother with simple household chores and helps his father with gardening and lawn care.

ATTENTION DEFICIT DISORDER WITH HYPERACTIVITY (BEHAVIORAL DISORDER)

Characteristics of an attention deficit disorder include a short attention span, impulsivity, and distractibility with or without hyperactivity. More familiar terms include hyperkinetic syndrome, hyperactive child, and minimal brain dysfunction.

Causative factors of hyperactivity may include an inherited temperament, in which the child displays symptoms since birth, cardiac abnormality, electrophysiologic abnormality of the cortex, stressful interpersonal family relationships, or an organic brain disorder.

Clinical symptoms may include stubbornness, negativism, temper tantrums, obstinacy, inability to tolerate frustration, deficit in judgment, poor self-image and aggressiveness. Symptoms may occur around age 3 but generally are not diagnosed until the child enters school, at which time academic and social functioning may be impaired. Boys are affected approximately ten times more often than girls. Of all elementary school children, 5% to 10% are affected by this disorder.

The DSM-III diagnostic criteria describe the child who has an attention deficit disorder with hyperactivity as follows:

1. Inattention resulting in failure to complete a task, failure to pay attention or listen, distractibility, inability to concentrate, and difficulty participating in play activity over a period of time.

2. Impulsivity, since the child often acts before thinking, shifts frequently from one activity to another owing to a short attention span and inner "drivenness," is unable to organize work, requires much supervision, disrupts class or groups by frequently speaking out of turn, and is unable to sit still and await his turn.

3. Hyperactivity, demonstrated by fidgeting, the inability to sit still, running or climbing on things, moving about in one's sleep, and appearing to be in high gear all the time. The child's "motor" or inner drivenness never "idles" or "stalls."

4. Onset before age 7 and lasting at least 6 months. The behavior is not caused by disorders such as schizophrenia, affective disorder, or severe or profound retardation.

Attention deficit disorder without hyperactivity contains all the features described with the exception of no symptoms of hyperactivity.

Attention Deficit Disorder With Hyperactivity: Clinical Example

BS, aged 6, diagnosed as having an attention deficit disorder with hyperactivity, was interviewed by a clinical psychologist in the presence of several student nurses. When BS first entered the room he jumped up and down several times, giggled nervously, and then said "I'm sorry." The psychologist asked BS to sit still as he attempted to time his ability to remain immobile for a period of time. One minute seemed an eternity to BS, who insisted time was up in fifteen seconds. When asked to draw a picture of the psychologist, BS was unable to sit still long enough to complete the drawing. He ran about the room investigating electrical outlets and various pieces of equipment in the room. After he knocked over a table lamp, BS repeatedly stated that he was sorry. As the psychologist asked him to participate in a ring-toss game, he stated "You go first, I always go last." He was unable to stand still as he awaited his turn.

The student nurses who observed BS's behavior stated they were exhausted after 30 minutes. "How do his parents keep up with him 24 hours a day?", "Does he ever unwind?", "Does he always break things?", and "Why does he say that he is sorry so often?" are just a few of the comments by the students. One student questioned how his behavior would affect other children when he played with them. Another student wanted to know how long BS would remain hyperactive. Postclinical conference discussion focused on assessment of BS's behavior and the development of a nursing care plan.

CONDUCT DISORDER (BEHAVIORAL DISORDER)

Conduct disorders generally occur just before, during, or immediately after puberty. Causes of such behavior may include

1. A poor parent–child interpersonal relationship

2. Lack of a father figure

3. Parental rejection

4. Lack of a secure, permanent family group as experienced by orphans or foster children during institutional living

5. Failure to bond during infancy

6. Incompatibility of the child's and parents' temperaments

7. Inconsistency in setting limits and disciplining a child by parents or authority figures

8. Large family size

9. Association with lower socioeconomic class children, including exposure to "delinquent groups"

Conduct disorders, as stated earlier, generally are seen during the developmental stages before, during, or just after the onset of puberty. Interpersonal behavior at this time consists of developing peer relationships, participating in activities outside the family, lessening family ties, and exhibiting independence. If the child does not successfully complete these developmental stages of industry versus inferiority (ages 6 to puberty) and identity versus role confusion (puberty and adolescence) as described by Erikson (1963), he may develop a sense of inferiority, may experience difficulty learning and working, and may fail to develop a sense of identity.

Symptoms may develop first within the family unit when the child attempts to cope with anxiety or resolve an inner conflict. Involvement in adolescent gangs also may precipitate the onset of antisocial behavior. In either case, there are usually unstable or poor interpersonal relationships within the family.

Generally, such a disorder is seen more frequently in boys, is more common in children whose parents display antisocial behavior or alcohol dependence, and may occur in varying degrees of impairment from a mild to a severe form.

Conduct disorder is classified into four subgroups: Undersocialized, aggressive; undersocialized, nonaggressive; socialized, aggressive; and socialized, nonaggressive. Following is a brief description of each type:

TYPE	CHARACTERISTICS AND BEHAVIOR
Undersocialized, aggressive	Displays persistent, aggressive behavior directed toward people or property
	Violates basic rights of others
	Inability to show affection, empathy, or develop a positive interpersonal relationship with others
	Examples of aggressive behavior: Rape, vandalism, assault and battery, or armed robbery involving confrontation with others
Undersocialized, nonaggressive	Although unable to show affection, empathy, or develop a positive interpersonal relationship, this person does not direct physical violence against others.

TYPE	CHARACTERISTICS AND BEHAVIOR
	Examples of nonaggressive behavior: Violation of important rules, disobedience in general, disapproved sexual behavior, truancy, solitary stealing without confronting a person, substance abuse, persistently telling lies, or running away from home
Socialized, aggressive	Displays a genuine concern for the welfare of others Able to form social attachment to others Avoids blaming others Able to experience guilt Although able to socialize, this person will exhibit aggressive behavior and violate the rights of others. Examples of aggressive behavior were cited earlier.
Socialized, nonaggressive	Ability to socialize as described above; however, displays nonaggressive behavior avoiding confrontation with people such as disobedience and telling lies

The DSM-III states that the pattern of conduct must exist for at least six months and not meet the criteria for antisocial personality if the person is 18 or older. Various complications are listed as the result of conduct disorder. They include suspension from school, difficulty with the law, and physical injury from accidents, fights, or other physical encounters.

ANXIETY DISORDERS (EMOTIONAL DISORDERS)

The DSM-III lists three categories of anxiety disorders: separation anxiety disorder, avoidant disorder, and overanxious disorder.

SEPARATION ANXIETY

Separation anxiety disorder may occur as early as 6 to 12 months of age as the child experiences the developmental crisis of trust versus mistrust. It is characterized by excessive anxiety, which is severe and persistent when the child is separated from a parent (usually the mother), significant other, home, or familiar surroundings. As the child grows older he may refuse to travel independently from home, or to spend the night at a friend's house, attend camp, or go to school (school-phobia). Psychophysiologic symptoms, such as headache, nausea, vomiting, and stomachache, are seen frequently when the child anticipates separation or when it actually occurs. He may show a reluctance or refusal to go to sleep at night or to stay alone in the home and withdraw socially. The child may become housebound or incapacitated in the severe form of separation anxiety disorder owing to the presence of morbid fears of illness, injury, danger, or death. Duration of such a disturbance must be at least 2 weeks before a diagnosis is made.

Separation Anxiety Disorder: Clinical Example

CW, 5 years old, began to complain of a stomach ache each morning as her mother prepared to go to work. The complaint persisted for approximately a week when CW began to wander into her parents' bedroom each night after she had gone to bed. During the day the babysitter noticed that CW would follow her from room to room and refuse to play outside. The baby-sitter brought CW's behavior to the attention of her parents who decided to consult the pediatrician. A diagnosis of separation anxiety disorder was made. Fortunately CW's behavior was identified early in its development, and she responded well to the pediatrician's suggestions for managing her anxiety.

AVOIDANT DISORDER

Avoidant disorder may manifest itself as early as 2½ years of age. Stranger anxiety generally occurs at the age of 6 months to 1 year and usually is resolved before the second year when the child learns to trust people and establish faith and hope about the environment and future. If such fears are unresolved, the child may begin to avoid contact with strangers and display an undue desire for affection and acceptance with members of his family. Clinging, tearful, unassertive, or mute behavior may occur, interfering with peer relationships. Symptoms must persist for at least 6 months for a diagnosis to be made.

OVERANXIOUS DISORDER

Overanxious disorder is characterized by excessive concern about future events, minor procedures, personal competency, and social acceptance; excessive need for reassurance; self-consciousness; somatic complaints; and feelings of tension. Typical somatic complaints include headache, dizziness, shortness of breath, or a "lump-in-the-throat" feeling when the person complains of feeling nervous. The comment "Worry is the price you pay for something that may never happen" applies to such a person who may be referred to as a worrywart. No specific age is listed in the DSM-III regarding onset of this disorder.

OTHER DISORDERS (EMOTIONAL DISORDERS)

Five disorders are included in this category. They are briefly summarized as follows:

DISORDER	CHARACTERISTICS
Reactive attachment disorder of infancy	Failure to thrive or develop physically Failure to respond to the caretaker's voice Does not reach for mother Apathy Hypomobility Excessive sleep Poor appetite, resulting in weight loss or failure to gain weight Onset before the age of 8 months owing to lack of adequate care, emotional deprivation, strict parents, malnutrition, or lack of a stimulating environment Occurs during developmental crisis of human interactive and relational capacities versus a deficit to these capacities (initial 6 mo) or during basic trust and affiliation versus mistrust (6–12 mo)
Schizoid disorder	Inability to form social relationships Little desire for social involvement Sensitive to criticism Occasional aggressive behavior Onset as early as age 5 More common in boys Occurs during the developmental crisis if initiative and assertion versus fear and guilt
Elective mutism	Continuous refusal to talk Able to comprehend language Able to speak when electing to Extremely shy Withdrawn More common in girls Considered a rare disorder Usually occurs before age 5
Oppositional disorder	Negative, oppositional behavior or nonconformity, generally directed toward parents, teachers, or other authority figures Generally occurs after age 3 during the developmental crisis of independence and autonomy versus shame and doubt
Identity disorder	Inability to establish an identity during the developmental crisis of identity versus role confusion (puberty and adolescence) The individual may be uncertain about a career, life goals, religious affiliation, moral values, sexual orientation, etc. Considered to be more prevalent than in the past due to conflicts of adolescent and parental values and life-styles

EATING DISORDERS (PHYSICAL DISORDERS)

Five eating disorders are classified by the DSM-III. They include anorexia nervosa, bulimia, pica, rumination disorder of infancy, and atypical eating disorder.

ANOREXIA NERVOSA

Anorexia nervosa, a condition that is seen mainly in young women, has become increasingly prevalent. Characterized by an aversion to food, it may result in death owing to serious malnutrition. The age of onset is usually late adolescence; however, diagnosis has been in young girls, 8 to 11 years of age, as well as women over age 30. Statistics reveal that:

1. Of all anorectics, 92% to 95% are female
2. Of diagnosed anorectics, 15% to 21% die
3. Anorexia occurs mainly in upper middle class families; however, victims may be from any socioeconomic group
4. Usually the youngest daughter of several children is afflicted

   Some factors that may contribute to the development of this disease include disturbed self-image, parent–child conflicts, past and present experiences resulting in feelings of dependency and helplessness, the adolescent's desire to return to the alleged comfort and safety of childhood, a stressful life situation, psychotic depression, or early manifestation of schizophrenia. Starvation is an attention-getting device that permits the anorectic patient full control of her body, allows her to remain in or revert to a prepubital state, and is considered manipulative behavior.

   The DSM-III states that the anorectic has an intense fear of becoming obese although weight loss occurs. The person insists that she is fat even when emaciated, displaying a disturbance of body image. A weight loss of at least 25% of the original body weight is seen, as well as the refusal to maintain at least minimal body weight for age and height. No known physical illness or disease is responsible for the weight loss.

   Various methods are used to lose weight. They include induced vomiting, laxatives, enemas, diuretics, diet pills, excessive exercise, binging and purging, stimulants, or refusal to eat. Deceitful behavior may prevail as the anorectic patient disposes of food she is supposed to eat. The following symptoms occur as the disorder progresses. Not all persons who are anorectic exhibit all the symptoms listed.

1. Dry skin
2. Brittle hair and nails, hair beginning to fall out
3. Amenorrhea
4. Constipation

5. Hypothermia

6. Decreased pulse, blood pressure, and basal metabolic rate

7. Skeletal-like appearance

8. Presence of lanugo (downy-soft body hair seen in newborn infants)

9. Intense fear of becoming obese

10. Distorted body image as patient continues to see self as fat

11. Loss of appetite

12. Dehydration, malnutrition, and electrolyte imbalance, which can result in death

13. A total lack of concern about her symptoms

The preanorectic person is generally considered to be a "model child and student" who is meek, compliant, perfectionistic, and an over-achiever. She is usually overly sensitive, fears independence and sexual relationships, has a low self-concept, and is resistant to growing up and maturing.

As the eating disorder progresses, the anorectic person presents behaviors such as manipulation, stubbornness, hostility, and deceitful-ness. Defense mechanisms used are denial, displacement, projection, rationalization, regression, isolation, and intellectualization. Fadiman's article, "The Skeleton at the Feast" (*Life,* February 1982), is an excellent presentation of a 16-year-old's struggle with anorexia, focusing on behav-ior, symptoms, family dynamics, and treatment. *The Best Little Girl in the World* (Levenkron, 1978) is also a highly recommended book about anorexia nervosa.

Warning signs that should alert parents, teachers, or others to the pos-sibility of anorexia include

1. Drastic weight loss in the presence of unusual eating habits, such as fasting, binging, or refusal to eat excepting tiny portions

2. Obsession with neatness or personal appearance, including frequent mirror gazing. The person constantly checks her appearance, fearing unattractiveness and obesity.

3. Hostility and the desire to control others

4. Calorie counting, dieting, and excessive exercise

5. Weighing oneself several times daily

6. Depressed mood

7. Amenorrhea or irregular menses

8. Wearing loose-fitting clothing to hide her physical appearance as it changes

9. Denying hunger

Living in an environment that is overprotective, rigid, or lacks conflict resolution, the anorectic achieves secondary gains such as love and undue attention because she is considered to be a special or unique person.

Anorexia Nervosa: Clinical Example

MJ, 19 years old, was a sophomore in college when her psychology professor noted a change in classroom behavior as well as a sudden weight loss. When questioned about her behavior, MJ told the professor that she was losing weight to compete for a position on the track team, although she was unable to give him a specific goal regarding her desired weight. She began to wear clothing that was loose fitting and would refer to herself as overweight although others commented about her thinness. MJ's meek, compliant behavior changed to that of a deceitful, hostile, and manipulative person. She isolated herself at mealtime and engaged in various exercises after eating. At times she would eat large amounts of food and then induce vomiting. A close friend observed MJ taking large amounts of over-the-counter diet pills as well as laxatives. In an effort to continue her weight loss, MJ would set her alarm so that she could exercise during the night and also awaken for early morning jogging. She became obsessed with exercising. Her physical appearance deteriorated as her hair began to fall out, her skin became quite dry, and acne developed. MJ also complained of being chilly all the time and wore layered clothing. During track practice, MJ became light-headed, felt irregular heart beats, perspired profusely, and experienced severe fatigue. The track coach took her to the college health clinic to be examined by the physician. Physical examination revealed poor skin turgor, as well as other symptoms of dehydration. The physician also suspected a potassium and protein deficit, although MJ denied any eating problems. Her weight was approximately 15 pounds under the desired weight for her height and body build. She had lost 25 pounds in a four-month period and experienced amenorrhea for two months. The college physician recommended that MJ see the school counselor regarding her concern about weight loss.

During clinical rotation at a psychiatric hospital, several students had the opportunity to observe and communicate with an anorectic 20-year-old woman. They were amazed at her willpower during breakfast, lunch, and midmorning snack time as she limited her caloric intake. For breakfast she consumed black coffee and a piece of dry toast. For a midmorning snack, she drank ice water, and for lunch she had lettuce salad without dressing. The students were startled by her physical appearance because her cheek bones, clavicles, and iliac crests were quite prominent. One student commented that she looked like "death warmed over" and another noted that she looked much older than her age. As the students communicated with the woman, they noted that she continually referred to herself as being fat and her conversation focused on her weight. The students were unable to understand why a person would go to such extremes to lose weight and still be unsatisfied with the results.

BULIMIA

Episodic binge eating with a rapid consumption of a large amount of food in under 2 hours is classified as bulimia. The person is aware that the behavior is abnormal, fears the inability to stop eating voluntarily, is self-critical, and may experience depression after each episode.

According to the DSM-III criteria, the bulimic person consumes high-calorie, easily ingested food, eats inconspicuously, and terminates binging or gorging by self-induced vomiting, going to sleep, or engaging in social activities. The person may stop eating because of abdominal pain. Repeated attempts are made to lose weight by fasting or dieting, abusing laxatives, enemas, or diuretics; by self-induced vomiting; or by abusing over-the-counter weight control medications. Weight fluctuation is seen owing to alternating dieting or fasting and binging. Onset of bulimia occurs in adolescence or early adult life. It may become chronic and occur intermittently over several years.

The psychiatric implications are significant because approximately 30% of those patients with bulimia also experience depression and require antidepressant medication.

Serious medical complications that may occur because of alternating binging and purging include

1. Chronic inflammation of the lining of the esophagus

2. Rupture of the esophagus

3. Dilatation of the stomach

4. Rupture of the stomach

5. Electrolyte imbalance or abnormalities, leading to arrhythmias of the heart and metabolic alkalosis

6. Heart problems, irreversible congestive heart failure, and death due to abuse of ipecac syrup

7. Chronic enlargement of the parotid gland

8. Dehydration

9. Irritable bowel syndrome or abnormal dilatation of the colon

10. Rectal prolapse or abscess

11. Rupture of the diaphragm, with entrance of the abdominal contents into the chest cavity

12. Dental erosion

13. Chronic edema

14. Fungal infections of the vagina or rectum

Bulimia: Clinical Example

LR, a 21-year-old secretary, was seen in the emergency room of a local community hospital with complaints of weakness, rapid pulse, dizziness, and difficulty swallowing. A physical assessment disclosed symptoms of dehydration, with a possible electrolyte imbalance. On being questioned further, LR confided to the physician that she was concerned about her weight and had tried various measures to control her appetite. She found herself craving sweets and other high-calorie food. When such feelings occurred she would devour "everything in sight" that was easily ingested, eating for 1 to 2 hours at times. Her grocery bills were quite high, over $100.00 per week, because of such cravings. After such binging episodes, LR would induce vomiting to avoid weight gain. She stated that she felt "out of control" and anxious when she binged. Her main fear was that of becoming fat, and when she vomited she was able to relieve herself of guilt feelings due to overeating. Recent publicity about anorexia and bulimia had caused her to seek help for physical symptoms that had been present for several weeks. LR agreed to a complete physical examination and referral to a counselor who had experience working with bulimic persons.

PICA

Persistent eating of non-nutritive substances such as clay, paint, plaster, ice, starch, or the compulsive eating of one food is referred to by the DSM-III as pica. Such behavior may occur between 1 and 2 years of age and may persist into adolescence or through adulthood. Although considered to be a rare disorder, possibly caused by mental retardation, neglect, poor supervision, or a mineral deficiency (*e.g.,* zinc or iron), pica can present serious health consequences. Behavior must occur for at least 1 month to be diagnosed as pica.

ATYPICAL EATING DISORDER

This catchall category is used for those eating disorders that cannot be classified in the previous categories.

STEREOTYPED MOVEMENT DISORDERS (PHYSICAL DISORDER)

Subclassifications of stereotyped movement disorders include transient tic disorder, chronic motor tic disorder, and tourette's disorder.

Tics, or habit spasms, are described as sudden repetitive, purposeless movements of muscles or groups of muscles that are not under voluntary control. Examples include repetitive rapid eye-blinking, facial contortions, head jerking, or involuntary production of noises or words.

Although the etiology of tics is unknown, possible causes include stress, tension, brain damage, or a decreased production of the neurotransmittors serotonin and dopamine.

Transient tic disorders generally begin during childhood or early adolescence, are recurrent, and can be suppressed voluntarily for a few minutes or hours. They disappear during sleep and lessen in intensity during absorbing activities. Tics generally last from at least 1 month to no more than a year.

Chronic tic disorder is described by the DSM-III as recurrent, involuntary, rapid, repetitive, and purposeless movements that involve no more than three muscle groups at a time, do not vary in intensity, and can be suppressed voluntarily for minutes or hours. The duration is at least 1 year. They may occur in childhood or after age 40.

Tourette's disorder or Gilles de la Tourette's syndrome is described as a combination of motor tics including involuntary vocal and verbal utterances that often are obscene. Corprolalia is an irresistible urge to utter obscenities and is present in approximately 60% of the disorders. Grunting, barking, sniffing, coughing, or yelping are various sounds heard. Onset occurs between ages 2 and 15; movements can be suppressed voluntarily for minutes or hours. Intensity of symptoms varies and the disorder lasts over 1 year. It can persist for a lifetime.

The classification of an atypical stereotyped movement disorder includes behavior such as head banging, rocking, and repetitive voluntary nonspasmodic movements of the fingers or arms. Persons with this disorder are not distressed by their symptoms and actually may enjoy such activities.

OTHER DISORDERS WITH PHYSICAL MANIFESTATIONS

Stuttering, functional enuresis (urination), functional encopresis (defecation), sleepwalking disorder, and sleep terror disorder are the categories described by the DSM-III.

STUTTERING

Stuttering is the presence of repetitious or prolonged sounds, syllables, or words. Characterized by frequent, unusual hesitations and pauses interrupting the flow of speech, it usually starts before the age of 12 and is present in approximately 1% of all children. It occurs four times as frequently in men as in women and becomes more severe in the presence of pressure to communicate. Stuttering may lessen or be absent when one is involved in singing or talking in a nonpressure situation (*e.g.*, to pets).

FUNCTIONAL ENURESIS

Functional enuresis is repeated involuntary urination day or night that is not due to a physical disorder. It is considered to be primary if urinary continence or complete bladder training has not been present for at least a year and secondary if it is preceded by complete bladder training for at least 1 year. Nocturnal enuresis or bedwetting occurs during sleep only; diurnal enuresis occurs during waking hours. Primary functional enuresis generally begins by age 5, whereas secondary functional enuresis occurs between the ages of 5 and 8.

Causative factors vary from case to case. These may be a small bladder capacity, urinary tract infection, structural abnormality, physical disease (*e.g.,* diabetes), regression, neurosis, adjustment reaction, or psychosis. A secondary emotional disorder may result owing to social ostracism by peers or familial attitude toward the child's behavior, such as anger, rejection, or punishment.

FUNCTIONAL ENCOPRESIS

Fecal soiling, or functional encopresis, is incontinence in one's clothing during the day or at night. It may occur voluntarily or involuntarily and is not due to a physical disorder. Primary encopresis occurs after age 4 and is not preceded by a period of complete bowel training, whereas secondary encopresis is preceded by fecal continence for at least 1 year and generally occurs between the ages of 4 and 8.

In the absence of a physical disorder, the main causative factor is said to be a disturbed relationship between the child and parents, usually the mother. Two types of soiling may occur: retentive soiling or nonretentive soiling. In retentive soiling, the child exhibits negativistic behavior by retaining fecal matter rather than releasing it when encouraged to do so. This is generally done in response to rigid or coercive toilet training, or may be a way of expressing anger and hostility. It also can be a form of regression in response to a real or perceived feeling of being unwanted or unloved. Such a child is generally immature and dependent on the mother. As feces is retained, leakage of liquid feces occurs. In nonretentive fecal soiling, lack of proper toilet training is usually the causative factor. Such a child may be poorly cared for, under stress, experiencing increased anxiety, immature, regressed, or mentally retarded.

Secondary Encopresis: Clinical Example

WJ, age 4½, was completely toilet trained by age 3. Her mother gave birth to a baby girl when WJ was 4 years old. Shortly after the birth of her sister, WJ began to have difficulty with retentive soiling. She refused to use the toilet when encouraged, only to be found later hiding behind a couch or drapes with soiled underwear. On one occasion, she disappeared from the living room while company was present and was later found in her bedroom closet grunting as though having a bowel movement. This behavior, which was quite frustrating to WJ's parents, continued for 3 months. At that time WJ's mother consulted with the pediatrician. With his help, Mrs. J was able to tolerate her daughter's behavior. She continued to reassure WJ that she was loved and wanted by her parents. WJ's behavior eventually subsided as she was allowed to help care for her baby sister.

SLEEPWALKING AND SLEEP TERROR DISORDERS (PHYSICAL DISORDERS)

Somnambulism, or sleepwalking, is a transient phase of development that generally begins between the ages of 6 through 12 and is seen more commonly in males than in females.

According to the DSM-III, the onset of sleepwalking occurs between 30 minutes and 3½ hours after one falls asleep. During this episode the person has a blank, staring face, appears nonresponsive to others, and is awakened with great difficulty. When awakened, the person is amnesic, recalling nothing of what happened. Although the person may be confused or disoriented for a brief period, no mental or behavioral impairment is noted.

Causative factors include normal stress and anxieties of childhood, undue fatigue, or medication (*e.g.,* a sedative or hypnotic).

Sleep terror, or night terror, is a disorder characterized by the child awakening in a frightened or terrified state with nonresponsivness to the environment. The child may appear to be talking to people who are not really present. For example, SA, 5 years old, awoke from sleep after 30 minutes, screaming as he sat up in bed. Although his mother responded to his panicky scream, SA was unaware of her presence. He appeared frightened, was perspiring profusely, and breathing rapidly as he muttered incoherently. After about 10 minutes, SA awakened momentarily to gaze at his mother, and then immediately fell back to sleep.

Behavior such as SA's generally occurs between the ages of 4 and 12 or may begin between the ages of 20 and 30. It is seen more frequently in males and occurs in approximately 1% to 4% of all children.

PERVASIVE DEVELOPMENTAL DISORDERS

The subtypes included in this category are infantile autism, childhood onset pervasive developmental disorder, and atypical pervasive developmental disorder, or disorders that affect basic psychological development during childhood. The terms symbiotic psychosis, childhood schizophrenia, and atypical children previously used as diagnoses are no longer part of the DSM-III classification.

INFANTILE AUTISM (DEVELOPMENTAL DISORDER)

Referred to formerly as infantile or autistic psychosis, infantile autism generally begins before 30 months of age and occurs three times more often in boys. Although causative factors are speculative they include genetic, environmental, and physical factors. Inherited cognitive defects, parental attributes, brain damage, or a metabolic disturbance are a few causes cited.

Symptoms include the inability to establish a meaningful relationship owing to the lack of responsiveness to others; gross deficits in language development, including mutism, echolalia, and the inability to name objects; withdrawal, which may be mistaken for deafness; obsessive ritualistic behavior, such as rocking and spinning; obsessional attachments to particular objects; and an anxiety or fear around harmless objects. Approximately 50% of autistic children have an IQ below 50.

Autistic children do not display an interest or need for cuddling, touching, or hugging. They ignore people as if they were inanimate objects or not present in the environment. Their interest may focus on mechanical objects as they participate in ritualistic behavior at a basic sensorimotor level.

Language skills may consist of pronominal reversal or the use of the pronoun *you* when *I* should be used, and immature grammer as well as echolalia and the inability to name objects. An obsessive desire for sameness is usually present. The child becomes resistant to change and is severely distressed if environmental change occurs.

Overactivity, distractibility, poor concentration, sudden unprovoked anger or fear, or aggressive outbursts also may occur. Autistic children do not experience delusions, hallucinations, incoherence, or looseness of association.

Intellectual functioning varies since children who are autistic may function at a normal, high, or retarded level. Memory may be exceptional, as observed in the behavior of an autistic child who played several pieces of complicated classical music on the piano.

Kaufman (1975) presents a vivid description of autistic behavior as he describes the diagnosis and treatment of his son, Raun Kahlil, and the impact of Raun's disorder on the family.

Infantile Autism: Clinical Example

TJ, age 16, was diagnosed as being autistic at age 2. Although he lives at home with his parents, TJ attends a school for developmentally disabled children. His ability to communicate verbally is minimally restricted to his making gutteral sounds at times. TJ requires constant supervision owing to masochistic behavior such as head banging and biting himself. Custodial care is also necessary to feed and toilet TJ. He has occasional outbursts in which he hits others and attempts to bite them. TJ responds to music, which seems to have a soothing affect on him, and he will stand on the basketball court for hours shooting baskets. Although he appears to be in his own world, TJ will unexpectedly respond to the voice of his classroom teacher by looking directly at her and nodding his head or making gutteral sounds. His parents report that his behavior at home fluctuates from manageable to hostile–aggressive outbursts, at which time he needs to be sedated.

CHILDHOOD-ONSET PERVASIVE DEVELOPMENTAL DISORDER

The term *pervasive* is used to describe the extent of a developmental disorder; that is, one in which many basic areas of psychological development are severely affected. A profound disturbance in social relationships is noted as well as various maladjusted behaviors. The DSM-III lists seven "oddities of behavior" used as diagnostic criteria. Summarized, these are:

1. A sudden onset of excessive anxiety, such as unexplained panic attacks
2. Inappropriate affect
3. Inability to tolerate change
4. Peculiar or odd motor behavior
5. Speech abnormalities
6. Hypersensitivity or hyposensitivity to sensory stimuli
7. Masochistic behavior

The onset of this disorder generally occurs after 30 months of age and before 12 years of age. It is seen most frequently in boys and children with low IQs, although it is considered to be a rare disorder. The person with this chronic disorder is unable to function independently, requiring supervision and financial support. As with infantile autism, this disorder does not exhibit clinical symptoms of delusions, hallucinations, incoherence, or marked loosening of associations.

The DSM-III states that the diagnoses of childhood type schizophrenia, atypical children, childhood psychosis and symbiotic psychosis have been replaced by infantile autism and childhood-onset pervasive developmental disorder. A child or adolescent who demonstrates the same symptoms as an *adult* schizophrenic is diagnoised as such, however. Schizophrenic children may not grow up into adult schizophrenics, although emotional problems may continue into adulthood to some extent. (Symptoms of schizophrenia are discussed in Chap. 25.)

SPECIFIC DEVELOPMENTAL DISORDERS

Within the classification of specific developmental disorders are developmental reading disorder, developmental arithmetic disorder, developmental language disorder, developmental articulation disorder, and mixed and atypical specific developmental disorders. The area of development is related to biologic maturation, and there may be no signs of psychopathology. Diagnoses and treatment usually occur within the educational system. Complications generally seen are academic failure, truancy, and antisocial behavior.

CHILDHOOD DEPRESSION

Although affective disorders were discussed in a separate chapter, childhood depression or the "killer blues" should be addressed at this time. Research has revealed that severe childhood depression is more common than is realized. It can interfere with a child's development and may result in suicide. Children are capable of experiencing deep pervasive, persistent unhappiness. Approximately 400,000 cases of childhood depression were diagnosed in 1983 (Lake, 1983). The following is a list of clinical symptoms generally present during childhood depression:

1. A pervasive sadness that is constantly present
2. Withdrawal
3. Irritable, negative behavior demonstrating the inability to have fun; destructive behavior
4. A poor or low self-esteem
5. Excessive guilt feelings, especially over minor incidents or situations that are not one's fault
6. Disturbance in sleep (*e.g.,* insomnia, night terrors, or excessive napping)
7. Running-away behavior
8. A change in appetite (either decrease or lack of appetite, or overeating)
9. Somatic or physical complaints (*e.g.,* headaches, stomachaches, and earaches)
10. Difficulty in school (*i.e.,* inattention, school anxiety, or sudden change in performance, resulting in poor grades)
11. Preoccupation with death such as undue concern about the health of a parent, death of a pet, or suicidal thoughts.

Causes of childhood depression are not cited specifically. Possible factors include poor or stressful environmental conditions, biochemical malfunction of the brain, genetic overload, or unusual sensitivity. Various theories also are discussed in the chapter on affective disorders, including precipitating events such as illness, trauma, or death of a loved one.

The following warning signs of depression are cited by Dr. Puig-Antich (Lake, 1983):

1. The child appears to be sad for at least 1 week.

2. He refers to himself as being unhappy.

3. He discusses suicide.

4. The child refuses to attend school.

If one or more of these warning signs is present, professional help should be sought.

Childhood Depression: Clinical Example

JK, a 13-year-old male athlete who was an excellent student, began doing poorly in class, skipping basketball practice, and staying out later than usual. His behavior resulted in arguments at home with his parents, especially his father, who attempted to discipline him. On one occasion, JK was caught smoking marihuana on the school grounds. JK's basketball coach, who had a good relationship with JK, asked him to stop by his office about 2 weeks after he began skipping practice. JK revealed to the coach that his parents were both very involved in their jobs and seemed to be too busy to enjoy family life. Everyone was going his separate way. JK was referred to the school counselor, who recognized the symptoms of depression.

TREATMENT

The following is a list of various methods used to treat infant, childhood, and adolescent disorders that require psychiatric help. Such disorders include anorexia nervosa, depression, conduct disorders, and pervasive developmental disorders.

Individual psychotherapy

Family therapy or systems therapy

Group therapy

Play therapy

Behavioral therapy

Art therapy

Music therapy

Drug therapy

Hospitalization

Day hospitals

Alternative families

A brief summary of each therapy is given below. (For more in-depth discussion, see Chap. 5.)

Individual Psychotherapy

Individual psychotherapy, according to Barker (1983), should include the following principles. These principles may serve as guidelines for a therapeutic nurse–patient relationship.

1. Accept the child but not necessarily the behavior. Remember that all behavior has meaning. The child may be acting out to receive attention or love. Limit setting may be necessary to protect the patient or therapist.

2. Do not criticize the child.

3. Avoid discussing symptoms with the child unless the child refers to them.

4. Attempt to understand the child's feelings and point of view.

Individual psychotherapy may focus on specific problems, such as poor self-concept, feelings of depression, extreme dependency, or the inability to communicate.

Family Therapy (Systems therapy)

The family is viewed as a biosocial subsystem that may be functional or dysfunctional (faultily integrated). Dysfunctional families may display poor interpersonal relationships, power struggles, extreme interdependency or disintegration. Disturbed behavior often is seen in children, who become the focus of such family problems. Family therapists attempt to provide help for disturbed children and families as a whole. This may include altering the family situation rather than treating the child individually.

Group Therapy

Children and adolescents may be treated in groups. Peer relationships play an important part in group therapy because peers often help each other by exchanging information, identifying with the group, expressing feelings openly, and suggesting solutions to problems. Group therapy is used in the treatment of disorders such as substance abuse, oppositional disorders, depression, and anorexia nervosa.

Play Therapy

Play therapy generally is used with children between the ages of 3 and 12. The child is given the opportunity to act out feelings such as anger, hostility, frustration, and fear. Various toys, puppets, or materials such as crayons and fingerpaints may be used. A doll house and dolls can be used to simulate family, sibling, or peer relationships. For example, a young girl may play with a doll and punish it or refer to it as a "bad girl," treating the doll the way she is treated by her parents. Watching a child at play allows the care-giver the opportunity to learn about a child's real and imaginary emotional life.

BEHAVIORAL THERAPY

Behavioral therapy attempts to alter a person's behavior and modify or remove symptoms such as temper tantrums or bedwetting. It often is used with hyperactive children to reduce the activity and to organize play. This is done by altering the circumstances before or after a particular behavior by using learning theory.

Operant conditioning, or behavior modification, is a second type of behavioral therapy used to modify behavior through manipulation. The person is reinforced or given a reward for desired behavior, whereas undesired behavior receives negative reinforcement. This type of therapy is used in the treatment of anorexia nervosa, delinquent behavior, enuresis, mental retardation, and several other disorders or problems.

Art and Music Therapy

Therapies involving art or music allow the child to express himself in these disciplines and can be effective with those who have difficulty communicating with others. For example, a 7-year-old depressed child was able to draw a picture of his fear of death after separation from his father, who was hospitalized for treatment of Hodgkin's disease. He had overheard family conversation regarding the seriousness of his father's condition and feared that his father would never return home.

Drug Therapy

Drugs are used to control hyperactivity or attention deficit disorder, depression, anxiety, and epilepsy.

Hyperactivity may be treated with a central nervous system stimulant such as methyl phenidate hydrochloride (Ritalin) or dextroamphetamine sulfate (Dexedrine) to prevent flooding of the cerebral cortex by a stream of impulses. Other medications include chlorpromazine hydrochloride (Thorazine) or haloperidol (Haldol), tranquilizers or anticonvulsants if epilepsy is present.

Antianxiety agents (*e.g.,* Valium and Librium), tricyclic antidepressants (*e.g.,* Elavil and Tofranil), and lithium all are used to treat children with anxiety or depression. Antipsychotic drugs, specifically phenothiazines (including Thorazine, Mellaril, Prolixin, and Trilafon), are used to treat children with psychotic symptoms. Haloperidol (Haldol), a butryophenone, also may be used to treat psychosis.

Sedative–hypnotics are prescribed for anxiety and sleep disturbances (*e.g.,* drugs such as Noctec and Triclos). These agents are used as an adjunctive, symptomatic treatment to alleviate distress.

Hospitalization

Hospitalization of children or adolescents serves various purposes, for example, removal of the child from a dysfunctional environment; treating severely disturbed behavior (*e.g.,* psychosis) in a controlled setting; providing protective care for suicidal, destructive, aggressive or hyperactive behavior; or treating severe anxiety disorders.

Day Hospitals

Treatment in a day hospital setting provides a therapeutic milieu for children. It serves as an extended outpatient clinic during the day, yet allows them to return home to their families evenings, nights, and weekends. It is quite useful in the care of emotionally disturbed children providing observation, treatment and care.

Alternative Families

Runaways, delinquents, and disturbed children often benefit from placement in the homes of alternative families. Children's services, group homes, and foster homes may provide much-needed physical and emotional care.

NURSING INTERVENTIONS

The nurse may participate in several of the therapies just described as well as provide nursing interventions in a hospital setting. Dreyer and colleagues (1979) list "ground rules" for establishing a therapeutic relationship with a child. They can be expanded to apply to adolescents as well as children and are summarized as follows:

1. Accept a child or adolescent as an equal when able, keeping in mind the person's age.

2. Do not use baby talk, substandard English, or talk down while communicating with the child or adolescent. Listen to the emotions expressed while talking, and encourage verbalization of feelings.

3. Do not force yourself on the patient or push him to confide in you.

4. Accept the person but discuss any undesirable behavior. Ignoring behavior such as tics also may be acceptable. Each behavior needs to be evaluated to decide the appropriate approach.

5. Be a good role model.

Another suggestion is to watch one's body language or nonverbal communication. Children and adolescents are quite observant of what adults say and how they can communicate feelings. They should know that adults have good and bad days that can affect their interpersonal relationships, especially the area of communication.

Walker (1982) lists rules for parents to live by that were published by Ann Landers several years ago. They were written by boys in a reform school for delinquent behavior. Briefly summarized, they state

1. Don't lose control in stressful situations because children are great imitators of parental behavior.

2. Don't use alcohol or pills as a crutch. Your behavior tells children it's okay to do the same.

3. Be a strict and consistent disciplinarian. Call a bluff. Don't compromise. Such an attitude denotes love and provides security. Children don't always want what they ask for; they just test parents.

4. Set a good spiritual example. Children need to know that a supreme being exists.

5. Don't try to imitate your children by dressing, talking, or acting younger. Children need good role models, not parents who try to be peers.

6. Be honest and give a few compliments if they are deserved.

Such suggestions are "a word to the wise" for nurses who work with children and adolescents in the psychiatric setting.

Other aspects of nursing interventions include helping the child to master developmental tasks to overcome regressive, slow, or impaired developmental behavior; establishing a method of communication with persons who have difficulty communicating, such as the withdrawn, disoriented, mute, hostile, preoccupied, or autistic child; identifying stimuli that might foster abusive, destructive, or otherwise negative behavior; and allowing time for the person to respond to therapeutic interventions.

The nurse should be aware of her own reaction to patients' behaviors. If unable to handle feelings or behaviors, she should seek assistance from peers or supervisory personnel. She also should respect the child's spatial territory and not invade his privacy. Therapeutic touch is used only after exploring the person's feelings about being touched (*i.e.,* a battered or abused child would probably withdraw and resist touch).

Nursing personnel may plan activities appropriate for the child's developmental level and age. They should consider his energy level and need to calm down after an activity.

Specific nursing interventions are discussed here for the following disorders of infancy, childhood and adolescence: mental retardation, attention deficit disorder, conduct disorder, anorexia nervosa, infantile autism, and childhood or adolescent depression. Examples of nursing diagnoses and nursing interventions are included at the end of the chapter.

Mental Retardation

As stated previously, mentally retarded persons may be educable, trainable, or require custodial care. Such persons may have dual diagnoses of mental retardation and mental illness, as well as a physical disability or limitation.

The nurse working in an institutional setting is challenged to provide environmental stimulation as well as to meet the needs of the child emotionally and physically because mentally retarded persons do not always communicate physical symptoms. Helping the child to master the activities of daily living may be a slow process involving behavioral therapy. Protective care may be necessary if the person is epileptic, prone, to acting-out behavior, disoriented, or masochistic (head banging or biting self). The administration of anticonvulsant and psychotropic drugs is also the responsibility of the nurse.

Education of the family is an important factor not to be overlooked because often the person attends an institution during the week but goes home for weekend or holiday visits. He also may attend a day hospital, special school, or sheltered workshop, and may return home at night as well as weekends. The nurse is the patient's advocate, both in the institutional setting and when relating to the family. Identifying the family's ability to cope and continue with the therapy at home is important to promote progress as well as to minimize the stress that can occur when changing environments.

Attention Deficit Disorder With Hyperactivity

The main treatment for an attention deficit disorder compounded with hyperactivity is to change the environment so that the child is able to alter or improve his reaction to the environment. Environmental stimuli are kept at a minimum while the child is medicated with CNS stimulants (*e.g.,* Ritalin, Dexedrine, or Benzedrine) that prevent flowing of the cerebral cortex by impulses (this in effect slows the child down). The role of the nurse is to identify, reduce, or eliminate such stimuli as well as to administer the medication. She may also work with the family or teachers to plan a firm, consistent, predictable environment. Limits and standards must be set while employing behavior therapy. The symptoms generally subside at puberty.

Conduct Disorder

The suggestions by delinquents listed earlier serve as a basic list of approaches when dealing with conduct disorders. Stated positively, they are included in the following list of interventions:

1. Establish trust by being honest.
2. Maintain control by setting limits for manipulative, acting-out behavior.
3. Be consistent with limit setting.
4. Respect the person's age and maintain an adult–child or adult–adult relationship, whichever is appropriate.
5. Establish realistic expectations. Discuss such expectations with the person and encourage verbalization of feelings.

Anorexia Nervosa

The chance of successful treatment is better if the patient maintains a body weight greater than 90 pounds. The weight appears to be a critical turning point in the anorectic patients response to therapy.

Various treatment approaches are used with anorexia nervosa. If the patient is in no physical distress, outpatient therapy may be employed. If an underlying depression exists, protective care may be necessary. In either case, the nurse plays an important role in the care of the anorectic person. She needs to adjust readily to mood swings and changes of behavior. This is done effectively by

Being matter-of-fact, friendly and casual if the patient is withdrawn or sullen

Setting limits to avoid manipulative behavior

Remaining uninvolved when the patient is indecisive or ambivalent

Avoiding confrontation when the patient exhibits hostility or anger

Stating that eating three nutritional meals a day is necessary to maintain a healthy body

Avoiding long discussions or explanation about food or the body

Approaching the person with positive expectations in spite of negative behavior

Allowing the patient to maintain some control, for example, in decision making

The nurse also plays an important role in a behavior modification program to help the person to alter inappropriate eating habits and gain weight. Privileges are earned if weight is gained or lost if there is a weight loss. The anorectic patient can be quite manipulative as she attempts to divert attention from her eating habits, which may include eating slowly, hiding food, or giving food to other persons. She needs to be supervised on a one-to-one basis to discourage such manipulative ploys.

Other nursing interventions may include monitoring intake and output, weighing the patient weekly, setting activity limits, insertion of a nasogastric tube and intravenous therapy if the physical condition warrants such care.

Medications that may be given include antidepressants (*e.g.,* Elavil, Sinequan and Tofranil), antianxiety agents (Valium), insulin therapy to stimulate the appetite, and hormones to correct amenorrhea or irregular menses.

If the anorectic is treated at home, the approach generally used is to ignore eating habits as well as the self-induced vomiting. Parents are instructed not to engage in conversation about eating, exercising, or weight.

Infantile Autism

Infantile autism is very difficult to treat because it is considered the most irreversible illness. The nurse is challenged as she assesses the child and

Helps the child establish a meaningful interpersonal relationship

Develops an effective way to communicate

Provides a safe, consistent environment to prevent self-destructive behavior

Allows time for the patient to develop tolerance for physical closeness

Encourages the child to participate in self-care

Administers medication for symptomatic relief (*e.g.,* Haldol)

Helps the child's family to handle difficult behavior effectively by employing behavioral therapy

As stated earlier, Kaufman's (1975) article on autism describes a long-term, deeply committed, two-phase program for his son, Raun. The first phase was to motivate Raun to explore the world outside him. The second phase focused on a program of instruction to master developmental tasks.

In 3 months, he accomplished 14 months of development. Not all autistic children make such progress, but Raun's story is encouraging.

Childhood and Adolescent Depression

Childhood and adolescent depression can go unrecognized or untreated, resulting in a chronic or severe form of depression, possibly leading to suicide. The nurse needs to be aware of the differences between childhood or adolescent depression and adult depression if effective nursing intervention is to be provided.

A comparison of the depressions follows.

CHILDHOOD/ADOLESCENT DEPRESSION	ADULT DEPRESSION
Constant depression, involving every aspect of one's world	Depression usually improves during the day Worse in the early morning hours
It can paralyze emotional growth and social development.	
Anger or hostility leads to aggressive behavior.	Not normally aggressive
Reality testing reinforces feelings of depression.	Reality testing allows the adult an opportunity to examine feelings and events regarding depression objectively.
Higher percentage of suicidal ideation than adults	
Does not recognize need for help	Generally recognizes need and seeks help

The nurse's role is to assist the depressed child or adolescent in:

Verbalizing feelings, including exploration of suicidal thoughts

Developing a positive self-image

Developing independence

Taking prescribed psychotropic drugs, such as antidepressants or antianxiety drugs

The nurse also encourages participation in therapies such as individual, family, or peer group counseling. (Other nursing interventions are discussed in Chap. 23.)

Following are nursing diagnoses and nursing interventions relating to both children and adolescents who exhibit emotional problems:

NURSING DIAGNOSES	NURSING INTERVENTIONS
Disturbance in self-concept, resulting in suicidal thoughts	Establish rapport and trust. Explore the child's or adolescent's thoughts about death, including future plans. (Refer to chapter on self-destructive behavior.) Identify strengths and positive coping mechanisms.

(continued)

NURSING DIAGNOSES	NURSING INTERVENTIONS
	Assist the child in finding alternative ways to handle his feelings.
	Use play, art, or music therapy to encourage expression of feelings. Adolescent may respond to psychodrama.
	Encourage participation in individual, group, or family therapy to share feelings, discuss problems, make decisions, and test reality.
Sleep pattern disturbance: Insomnia	Establish a bedtime routine after exploring personal habits.
	Provide for quiet, relaxing activities before the hour of sleep. Children need time to relax.
	Assign a staff person to stay with the child before bedtime to discuss reasons for insomnia, such as fear of the dark or homesickness.
	Administer sedative–hypnotics if necessary, as prescribed.
Noncompliance: Manipulative behavior	Limit setting should be done with consistency by all shifts.
	One staff member on each shift should be responsible for decision making.
	Be nonpunitive in attitude when confronting the patient about behavior.
Alteration in nutrition: Less than body requirements owing to self-induced vomiting after eating	Insert a nasogastric tube or begin IV therapy if the patient's condition warrants such interventions.
	Monitor intake, vomitus, and elimination.
	Structure meals and snack times.
	Use limit-setting regarding the use of the bathroom immediately after eating to prevent vomiting or disposal of concealed food.
	Monitor weight at least once a week.
	Monitor electrolytes, as well as hemoglobin, hematocrit, and blood sugar level if ordered.
	Monitor vital signs and blood pressure.
Ineffective individual coping: Poor impulse control	Anticipate anger or loss of control.
	Set limits, stating that the person will be held accountable for his or her actions.
	Encourage verbalization of feelings.
	Reinforce good behavior with positive feedback.
Social isolation because of withdrawal	Seek out the person daily and spend time with him or her.
	Establish rapport and trust.
	Meet the person at his present level of functioning.
	Explore his feelings regarding withdrawal.
	Slowly encourage contacts with other people.

SUMMARY

This chapter focused on the disorders of infancy, childhood, and adolescence, classified according to intellectual, behavioral, emotional, physical, and developmental symptoms. Factors influencing the onset of such disorders were discussed. These include constitutional, temperamental, and environmental factors, as well as the effects of physical disease or injury. Diagnostic criteria, etiology, treatment, and nursing interventions were described for each of the following subclassifications: mental retardation; attention deficit disorder with or without hyperactivity; conduct disorders; anxiety disorders; emotional disorders, such as reactive attachment; eating disorders, such as anorexia nervosa; stereotyped movement disorders such as tics; disorders with physical manifestations, such as enuresis and encopresis; pervasive developmental disorders, such as infantile autism; and childhood depression. Clincial examples of severe mental retardation, attention deficit disorder with hyperactivity, anorexia nervosa, bulimia, secondary encopresis, infantile autism, and childhood depression were given. A brief summary of treatment regimes discussed individual psychotherapy, as well as family, group, play, behavioral, art, music, and drug therapy. Hospitalization, day hospitals, and alternative families were also presented. Nursing interventions focused on the basics for establishing a therapeutic relationship with a child or adolescent, suggested rules for parents to live by, and therapeutic approaches for specific behaviors. Examples of nursing diagnoses and nursing interventions were given, including disturbance in self-concept, sleep pattern disturbance, noncompliance (manipulative behavior), alteration in nutrition less than body requirements because of self-induced vomiting, ineffective individual coping (poor impulse control), and social isolation because of withdrawal.

LEARNING ACTIVITIES

I. Clinical activities
   A. Care for a patient exhibiting a disorder of infancy, childhood, or adolescence.
   B. Identify the developmental level of the patient. State the tasks appropriate for the developmental level and identify those tasks uncompleted. State nursing interventions to facilitate meeting such tasks.
   C. Assess the patient's ability to relate to others. Consider peers, family, and members of the health team. In what manner does the patient communicate?
   D. Review the patient's treatment plan. Is it appropriate? If not, what changes or additions would you make?

    II. Case study: Anorexia nervosa

Read Anne Fademan's article "A Case Study of Anorexia Nervosa: The Skeleton at the Feast" (*Life:* Feb., 1982) and discuss the following questions:

    A. What clinical symptoms did Jane Daly present?

    B. Describe her interpersonal relationship with her family.

    C. State the reactions of Jane's family to her illness.

    D. Summarize the treatment Jane received. Was it effective?

    III. Independent activity

    A. Identify facilities in your community that provide care for infants, children, or adolescents with psychiatric disorders. Consider hospitals, foster homes, children's services, and rehabilitative services.

    B. Investigate the role of the school psychologist in the diagnosis and care of a child with a behavioral disorder.

    C. Contact a local law enforcement agency and obtain information regarding the various types of disturbed or disturbing children or adolescents who are brought to their attention. What options are available when handling such people?

SELF-TEST

1. List three causes of disorders in childhood.

2. State four behaviors that could be warning signs of depression.

3. List two nursing interventions for a child experiencing insomnia.

4. Discuss the purpose of play therapy and when it would be an appropriate nursing intervention.

5. Describe infantile autism.

6. List two nursing interventions to help a child relate to an adult.

7. Differentiate between adolescent and adult depression.

8. State three nursing interventions for adolescent depression.

9. List three ways in which a family may promote a positive interpersonal relationship with a disturbed adolescent.

10. State four nursing interventions appropriate to increasing an adolescent's self-esteem.

11. Define anorexia nervosa.

12. State five clinical symptoms of anorexia nervosa.

13. List a nursing intervention for each of the symptoms listed in the previous question.

14. Discuss the rationale for using behavior modification when caring for an anorectic patient.

15. Define the following terms:
Tics
Elective mutism
Functional encopresis
Functional enuresis
Pervasive developmental disorder

16. List five symptoms of attention deficit disorder with hyperactivity.

17. State nursing interventions for each of the symptoms listed in the previous questions.

18. Differentiate the levels of mental retardation.

19. List five causes of conduct disorder.

20. List two examples of undersocialized aggressive behavior.

21. Describe separation anxiety disorder.

22. List five characteristics of reactive attachment disorder of infancy.

23. Give a brief explanation of the following therapies as they apply to children and adolescents:
Individual psychotherapy
Group psychotherapy
Art therapy
Music therapy
Drug therapy

24. Discuss the rationale for the following environmental changes for children and adolescents:
Hospitalization
Day hospital
Alternative families.

REFERENCES

Agee V: Treatment of the Violent Incorrigible Adolescent. Lexington Ky, Heath & Co, 1979

Altrocchi J: Abnormal Behavior. New York, Harcourt Brace Jovanovich, 1980

Barker P: Basic Child Psychiatry, 4th ed. Baltimore, University Park Press, 1983

Bruch H: Eating Disorders: Obesity, Anorexia Nervosa and the Person Within. New York, Basic Books, Inc., 1973.

Buchanan D, Rogers A: A comprehensive adolescent treatment program: An inpatient, interdisciplinary approach. J Psych Nurs:July, 1980

Burgess A: Psychiatric Nursing in the Hospital and the Community, 3rd ed, New Jersey, Prentice–Hall, 1981

Crowl M: Art therapy with patients suffering from anorexia nervosa. The Arts in Psychotherapy, Vol 7, 1980

Dreyer S et al: Guide to Nursing Management of Psychiatric Patients, 2nd ed. St. Louis, CV Mosby, 1979

Erikson E: Childhood and Society, 2nd ed. New York, WW Norton & Co, 1960

Fademan A: A Case Study of Anorexia Nervosa: The Skeleton at the Feast. Life Magazine, February, 1982.

Fox K: Adolescent ambivalence: A therapeutic issue. J Psych Nurs: Sept. 1980

Freedman, Kaplan, Sadock: Comprehensive Textbook of Psychiatry. Baltimore, Williams & Wilkins, 1975

Frisch A: Depression. In Josephson M, Proter R (eds): Handbook of Childhood Psychopathology. New York, Janson Aronson, 1979

Haber J et al: Comprehensive Psychiatric Nursing. New York, McGraw–Hill Book, 1982

Hafen B, Peterson B: Preventing adolescent suicide, Nurs 83: Oct, 1983

Harlin V: The hyperkinetic child: His management in the school environment. School Health Review: March-April, 1973

Harris F, Wilson L: Mental Health Problems in Children. In Snider J (ed): McGraw-Hill Handbook of Clinical Nursing. New York, McGraw–Hill, 1979

Harris M: Understanding the autistic child. Am J Nurs: Oct, 1978

Hart N, Keidel G: The suicidal adolescent. Jan, 1979

Kaufman B: Researching the "unreachable" child. New York Magazine: Feb, 1975

Kaye E: On starving oneself to death. Family Health: Sept, 1979

Kolb L: Modern Clinical Psychiatry. Philadelphia, WB Saunders, 1977

LaVigna GW: The behavioral treatment of autism. Psychiatr Clin North Am: Aug, 1978

Marholin D, Luisille JK: Children's problems. Psychiatr Clin North Am: Aug, 1978

McNelly P, Hickey P: Anorexia nervosa: A challenge to the nurse. Nurs Mirror: Sept, 1978

Mellencamp A: Adolescent depression: A review of the literature, with implications for nursing care. J Psych Nurs: Sept, 1981

Melton JH: A boy with anorexia nervosa. Am J Nurs, Sept, 1974

Minuchin SB, et al: Psychosomatic Families. Cambridge, Harvard University Press, 1978

Moore JA, Coulman MU: Anorexia nervosa: The patient, her family and key family therapy interventions. J Psych Nurs: May, 1981

Moss GR, Mann RA: A behavioral approach to the hospital treatment of adolescents. Psychiatr Clin North Am: Aug, 1978

Murray R, Zentner J: Nursing Assessment and Health Promotion Through the Life Span. Englewood Cliffs, Prentice–Hall, 1979

Nolen W: Anorexia nervosa: The dieting disease. McCalls: June, 1977

O'Neill CB: A different kind of weight problem. Guideposts: Sept, 1981

Ritvo E: Autism—Diagnosis—Current Research. New York, Haisted Press, 1976

Roberts S: Behavioral Concepts and Nursing Throughout the Life Span. Englewood Cliffs, New Jersey: Prentice-Hall, 1978.

Ryan BA: We played a game with Jill . . . and Jill won. Nurs 80: Dec, 1980

Schlemmer J, Barnett P: Management of manipulative behavior of anorexia nervosa patients. J Psych Nurs: Nov, 1977

Schulterbrandt J, Raskin A (eds): Depression in Childhood: Diagnosis, Treatment, and Conceptual Models. New York, Raven Press, 1977

Schultz J, Dark S: Manual of Psychiatric Nursing Care Plans. Boston, Little, Brown & Co, 1982

Stunkard A, Surwit R: Behavioral treatment of the eating disorders. In Leitenburg

H (ed): Handbook of Behavior Modification and Behavior Therapy. Englewood Cliffs, Prentice–Hall, 1976

Trubo R: Eating Disorders: The price of society's desire to be thin. Medical World News, July 12, 1984

Walker P, Brook B: Community homes as hospital alternatives for youth in crisis. J Psych Nurs: Mar, 1981

Wilson H, Kneisl C: Psychiatric Nursing. Menlo Park, Addison–Wesley, 1983

22

IMPAIRED THOUGHT

PROCESSES RESULTING IN

PARANOID BEHAVIOR

LEARNING OBJECTIVES

1. Define the term *paranoid*.

2. Describe the clinical features of paranoid persons.

3. Differentiate among the following:
   Acute paranoid disorder
   Shared paranoid disorder
   Paranoia

4. Discuss the psychiatric management of paranoid disorders.

5. State nursing interventions for the following nursing diagnoses related to paranoid behavior:
   Alterations in thought processes because of inaccurate interpretation of environmental stimuli, resulting in feelings of suspicion and fear
   Potential for violence owing to unpredictable, hostile, aggressive behavior related to delusions
   Noncompliance by refusal to eat or take medications because of delusional thoughts
   Disturbance in self-concept because of low self-esteem
   Ineffective individual coping exhibited by repeated somatic complaints

PARANOIA is a lay a term commonly used to describe a person who exhibits overly suspicious behavior. The technical use of the term is used to describe a wide range of behaviors that range from aloof, suspicious, and nonpsychotic to well-systematized and psychotic symptoms. Paranoid disorders are not due to any other mental disorder such as schizophrenia, affective, or organic mental disorders. They do not involve periodic mood shifts and are not associated with hallucinations, cognitive disorganization, or emotional deterioration. The DSM-III classifies paranoid disorders as acute paranoid disorder (a disorder with a duration of under 6 mo), shared paranoid disorder (a chronic disorder), and paranoia.

ETIOLOGY

Several predisposing factors have been identified in the development of paranoid disorders. They include relocation due to immigation or emigration; sensory handicaps, such as deafness or blindness; severe stress; low socioeconomic status, in which the person may experience feelings of discrimination, powerlessness, or low self-esteem; trust–fear conflicts; or altered perceptual states from the abuse of drugs or alcohol. The age of onset is generally middle-aged to late in life.

CLINICAL FEATURES

The paranoid person generally exhibits extreme suspiciousness, jealousy, and distrust, as well as being convinced that others intend to do him harm.

He may exhibit persecutory delusions, in which he feels he is being conspired against, spied upon, poisoned or drugged, cheated, harassed, maliciously maligned, or obstructed in some way. Conjugal paranoia or delusional jealousy, in which the person is convinced without due cause that his mate is unfaithful, may exist. He refuses to acknowledge negative feelings, thoughts, motives, or behaviors in himself, and projects such feelings onto another person by blaming that person for his problems. Paranoid persons spend much time confirming suspicions and defending themselves against imagined persecution. Such self-centered thoughts, in which everything is taken personally, are called ideas of reference.

Paranoid persons often exhibit resentment, anger, grandiose ideas, social isolation, seclusiveness, or eccentric behavior. Such people may resort to complaining about various injustices and instigate legal actions frequently. They rarely seek treatment and are brought to the attention of mental health professionals by friends, relatives, or associates who are concerned about their behavior. Social and marital functioning often are impaired, although the person preserves daily, intellectual, and occupational functioning.

DSM-III CRITERIA OF PARANOID DISORDERS

Paranoid disorders or psychotic states are characterized by moderately impaired reality testing, affect, and sociability. Some of the milder features of paranoid schizophrenia may be present but do not include hallucinations, bizarre delusions, incoherence, or loosening of association. Delusions may be persecutory, grandiose, erotic, or jealous in thought content. The person's emotion and behavior are appropriate to the content of the delusional system. The duration of the illness is at least 1 week.

Acute paranoid disorder meets the criteria for paranoid disorder but lasts less than 6 months. It is seen most frequently in persons who experience drastic changes in their environment such as prisoners of war, people leaving home for the first time, and refugees. This disorder develops suddenly and rarely becomes chronic.

Shared paranoid disorder develops as the result of a close relationship with a person who already experiences persecutory delusions. The sharing of such delusions by two closely related persons usually in the same family is referred to as *folie à deux*.

Paranoia is a rare condition characterized by a delusional system that develops gradually, becomes fixed, and is based on the misinterpretation of an actual event. The thought process appears clear and orderly, reality testing is intact, affect remains appropriate, sociability is maintained, and delusions are persecutory or grandiose in content. The paranoid person generally considers himself to be endowed with unique, superior ability. Such a chronic, stable delusional system lasts at least 6 months. This rare psychotic state generally is diagnosed between ages 25 and 40, in persons who possess a superior intellectual ability and find rationalization and projection to be satisfactory mechanisms of defense.

Shared Paranoid Disorder: Clinical Example

In October or November of 1982, two friends disappeared from California only to be found several weeks later on a snow-covered mountain top near a snowbound auto. The woman died of hypothermia but the man was able to crawl several miles for help. She had convinced her male companion that she was receiving signals from aliens who gave her special instructions to wait for them on a mountain top. Believing in her special powers, he accompanied her on the trip. Reality set in when the man recognized the fact that the woman was dying.

Rowe (1978) states that separation is unendurable in this disorder, which could account for the man's not leaving her until he realized that his own life was at stake. His thought disorder may clear up without formal treatment due to separation from the woman, the primary psychotic partner in *folie à deux*.

Acute Paranoid Disorder: Clinical Example

A 45-year-old Cuban man who recently moved to Florida with his family suddenly becomes suspicious that Fidel Castro is "out to get him." He barricades the windows and doors of his home, has his telephone number unlisted, and warns his family to be careful whenever they leave the house. Although he displays this delusion of persecution and exhibits hypervigilance, he is able to function with minimal impairment. When questioned, his wife states that he has felt guilty about leaving his parents behind in Cuba.

Working with such a patient would be extremely difficult because his delusional system may have an element of truth in it. People who have emigrated from Cuba to the United States have related stories of persecution for crimes they did not commit, whereas others have fled to avoid persecution for crimes committed. Living in such an environment could predispose someone to the development of a highly suspicious thought process.

TREATMENT

Donlon and Rockwell (1982) state that the treatment of paranoid disorders is difficult because of the denial by the patient, the presence of suspicion, and resistance to therapy because of the paranoid delusions. The person is highly threatened by any personal contact required during treatment.

Treatment depends on the severity of the disorder and the ability of the person to function outside the hospital setting. It may occur in private practice by a psychiatrist or in a mental health clinic, where symptoms are alleviated to the degree that is essential for continued employment and community living. If feelings of persecution persist, and the tendency toward impulsive, destructive behavior presents a problem to the family and community, hospitalization may be required.

"The initial treatment plan is threefold: evaluate safety, provide symptom remission, and establish rapport" (Donlon and Rockwell, 1982, p. 73). If the person is extremely belligerent, injectable neuroleptics are very effective in controlling distressing feelings. Once such feelings are alleviated and psychotherapeutic intervention begins, the therapist must be honest and straightforward while focusing on the patient's emotional response to the environment. He also must convey to the patient that although he does not agree with any delusions, he is interested in the patient's welfare. Confronting delusions directly may increase agitation and usually is not beneficial to the patient. Long-term management generally consists of low-dosage antipsychotic or neuroleptic drugs and individual psychotherapy.

NURSING INTERVENTIONS

Nursing care of paranoid patents focuses on establishing rapport; enhancing self-esteem; decreasing fears and suspicion; handling hostility, aggression, delusions, and ideas of reference; observing for suicidal ideation; and assisting the patient in the activities of daily living (ADL). Long-term goals generally focus on assisting the patient in developing alternative ways to cope with stress and loss, develop feelings of trust toward family or close associates, and comply with a medication regime.

Paranoid persons may make the nurse feel as if she were being attacked, assaulted, and belittled. She may see herself as stupid because the paranoid person blames her or others for his or her difficulties (Murray and Huelskoetter, 1983). The nurse should be aware that delusions protect patients from recognizing or coping with feelings that are often the opposite of those represented by the delusion, result from overwhelming anxiety, represent an exaggerated picture of what the person believes, and often result in the use of the defenses such as projection or intellectualization. Barile (Lego, 1984) lists five nonproductive reactions to delusional patients. These responses include becoming anxious and avoiding the patient; reinforcing delusions by actually believing the patient; attempting to prove that the patient is mistaken by presenting a logical argument; setting unrealistic goals that lead to disappointment, frustration, or anger; and being inconsistent with nursing interventions.

The following are examples of nursing diagnoses and interventions for paranoid persons:

NURSING DIAGNOSES	NURSING INTERVENTIONS
Alterations in thought processes because of inaccurate interpretation of environmental stimuli, resulting in feelings of suspicion and fear	Establish rapport and a trusting relationship by listening, showing acceptance of the patient, and being consistently reliable. Be genuine and honest. Provide a nonthreatening environment. Respect the patient's desire for privacy. Allow the patient physical distance to increase comfort. Present detailed information when talking with the patient. Explore feelings of fear or distrust.
Potential for violence owing to unpredictable hostile aggressive behavior, related to delusions	Speak clearly and concisely. Do not whisper or act secretive in the presence of the patient (avoid creating suspicion). Observe closely for clues to unpredictable behavior. Offer concern and protective intervention to prevent injury to self and others. Avoid physical contact, unless acceptable by the patient or it is necessary to restrain the patient. Accept rebuffs and abusive language as symptoms. Be honest, Do not argue or disagree. Attempt to modify nursing care to reduce outbursts or aggression toward staff or other patients. Limit social participation. Avoid competitive, aggressive activities or close physical contact.
Noncompliance by refusal to eat or take medications due to delusional thoughts	Attempt to understand what the patient is trying to say. Allow patient to choose food. Provide food not handled by others (*i.e.,* boxed cereal, unopened milk container). Do not mix medicine with food. Obtain order for IM administration if patient refuses oral preparation. Observe patient closely while administering medication.
Disturbance in self-concept because of low self-esteem	Attempt to reinforce self-esteem by showing recognition and offering praise when appropriate. Encourage decision making.

(continued)

NURSING DIAGNOSES	NURSING INTERVENTIONS
	Do not retaliate to anger or suspicious behavior.
	Provide opportunities for the patient to accomplish the task.
Ineffective individual coping exhibited by repeated somatic compliants.	Try to direct the patient's interest to other persons or things.
	Do not show undue concern about complaints.
	Report complaints to attending physician.

SUMMARY

This chapter focused on the classification of paranoid disorders, including those disorders not due to any other mental diseases such as schizophrenia, and affective or organic mental disorders: acute paranoid disorder, shared paranoid disorder, and paranoia. The etiology or predisposing factors were stated and clinical features discussed. The DSM-III criteria of each disorder also was listed. Examples of shared paranoid disorder and acute paranoid disorder were given. The treatment approaches were discussed, focusing on the administration of neuroleptic medication and individual psychotherapy to control distressing feelings. Nursing interventions, including nonproductive reactions to delusional patients, were presented. Examples of nursing diagnoses and nursing interventions discussed included alterations in thought processes; potential for violence owing to unpredictable, hostile, aggressive behavior related to delusions, noncompliance by refusal to eat or take medications due to delusional thoughts, disturbance in self-concept due to low self-esteem, and ineffective individual coping, exhibited by repeated somatic complaints.

LEARNING ACTIVITIES

I. Clinical objectives
   A. Focus on at least one patient who is demonstrating suspicious behavior.
   B. Identify the use of projection as you interact with the patient.
   C. Identify delusional thinking and the purpose it serves (*i.e.,* grandiose thinking to enhance one's self-esteem).
   D. Observe how the patient's behavior affects the staff.
   E. List specific activities aimed at establishing rapport and enhancing self-esteem.
   F. Does the patient express fear verbally or nonverbally, and in what situations?

    G. If possible, discuss with the patient ways to alter or cope with one situation that produces fear.

    H. Attempt to identify a person in the community who may become a support person and to whom this patient might relate on a continuing basis.

II. Independent activity

    A. Complete the programmed instruction "Understanding Hostility" (Am J Nurs: Oct, 1967).

    B. Review "The Client Who Is Delusional" by Linda Barile (Lego, 1984) and complete the following:

        1. Define paranoid, grandiose, sexual, religious, somatic, and inferiority delusions.

        2. Discuss the five examples of nonproductive reactions to delusional persons.

SELF-TEST

1. What is the overused defense mechanism in paranoid disorders?

2. *Folie à deux* is a term used to identify _____.

3. A rare psychotic state in which judgment is impaired only in relation to a delusion but the rest of the personality is intact is known as _____.

4. Define acute paranoid disorder.

5. State the reason a therapist is challenged when working with a paranoid patient.

6. Explain the rationale for administering neuroleptic drugs to a paranoid patient.

7. State the reason the behavior of a paranoid patient may be unpredictable.

8. List nursing actions for unpredictable, hostile, aggressive behavior.

9. List several nursing interventions appropriate for a patient who refuses to eat or take medication because he fears he is being poisoned.

10. State nursing actions for disturbance in self-concept due to low self-esteem.

REFERENCES

Altrocchi J: Abnormal Behavior. New York, Harcourt Brace Jovanovich, 1980

American Psychiatric Association: A Psychiatric Glossary, 5th ed. Washington, American Psychiatric Press, Inc., 1980

Bailey D, Dreyer S: Care of The Mentally Ill. Philadelphia, FA Davis, 1977

Burgess A: Psychiatric Nursing in the Hospital and the Community, 3rd ed. New Jersey, Prentice–Hall, 1981

Carpenito LJ: Nursing Diagnosis: Application to Clinical Practice. Philadelphia, JB Lippincott, 1983

Donlon P, Rockwell D: Psychiatric Disorders Diagnosis and Treatment. Bowie, Robert Brady Co, 1982

Freedman, Kaplan, Sadock: Comprehensive Textbook of Psychiatry. Baltimore, Wilkins & Wilkins, 1975

Kolb L: Modern Clinical Psychiatry. Philadelphia, WB Saunders, 1977

Kyes J, Hofling CK: Basic Psychiatric Concepts in Nursing. Philadelphia, JB Lippincott, 1980

Lancaster J: Adult Psychiatric Nursing. Garden City, NY, Medical Examination Publishing, 1980

Lego S: The American Handbook of Psychiatric Nursing. Philadelphia, JB Lippincott, 1984

Murray R, Huelskoetter M: Psychiatric Mental Health Nursing: Giving Emotional Care. Englewood Cliffs, Prentice–Hall, 1983

Rowe CJ: An Outline of Psychiatry. Dubuque, William Brown, 1980

Schultz J, Dark S: Manual of Psychiatric Nursing Care Plans. Boston, Little, Brown & Co, 1982

Stuart GW, Sundeen SJ: Principles and Practice of Psychiatric Nursing. St. Louis, CV Mosby, 1983

Wilson H, Kneisl C: Psychiatric Nursing, 2nd ed. Menlo Park, Addison–Wesley Publishing, 1983

23

DISTURBANCES IN MOOD

DUE TO AFFECTIVE

DISORDERS

LEARNING OBJECTIVES

1. Define affective disorder.
2. Describe how the following theories relate to the development of an affective disorder:
   Genetic predisposition theory
   Biochemical theory
   Environmental theory
3. List those persons more prone to the development of depression because of the stress of environmental factors.
4. Differentiate first-level, middle-level, and severe-level depression.
5. List the somatic and psychological symptoms of dysthymic disorder (depressive neurosis or exogenous depression).
6. Define cyclothymic disorder (cyclothymic personality).
7. List symptoms of hypomanic behavior.
8. Differentiate dysthymic disorder from major depressive disorder (endogenous depression).
9. Define the following terms:
   Melancholia
   Physiologic signs of depression
   Bipolar disorder
   Manic episode or disorder
10. Differentiate the three subclassifications of bipolar disorder: mixed, manic, and depressed.
11. Compare the three phases of manic behavior.
12. Discuss the rationale for the following modes of treatment in affective disorders: psychotherapy, chemotherapy, occupational or recreational therapy, and electroshock therapy.
13. Describe therapeutic nursing interventions when planning care for patients with affective disorders.

EPRESSION is a natural emotion that most people experience sometime during their lives. It can manifest itself as the "blues" or sadness; grief; mourning; nonpathologic or neurotic depression; pathologic or psychotic depression; or in the form of hyperactivity and manic behavior.

Statistics provided by the National Institute of Health in 1980 state that approximately 20 million Americans between the ages of 18 and 74 suffer from serious depressive disorders yearly. Of these 20 million people, about 25% seek help. Over one fourth of the population will exhibit signs of a *severe* depressive episode during a lifetime.

Depression can occur at any age. Infants may exhibit signs of anaclitic depression or failure to thrive when separated from their mothers. School-aged children may experience depression along with anxiety and exhibit signs of hyperactivity. (Approximately 400,000 children yearly suffer from depression.) Teenage depression and suicide rates have risen dramatically within the past few years because of feelings of loneliness, low self-concepts, and drug abuse. Neurotic or nonpathologic depression occurs most frequently between ages 20 and 40 and affects twice as many women as men. Psychotic or pathologic depression generally occurs later in life, and appears equally in both sexes.

Affective disorder is a DSM-III classification that refers to a mental disorder exhibiting prominent and persistent mood changes of elation or depression accompanied by associated symptoms such as fatigue and insomnia. An abnormality of affect, activity, or thought process is noted. The mood changes appear to be disproportionate to any cause and may continue over an extended period. Specific diagnostic criteria and presenting symptoms will be discussed within each subclassification of affective disorders.

ETIOLOGY

Causative factors have been classified as genetic, biochemical, and environmental. A summary of each of these theories follows.

Genetic Predisposition Theory

According to the National Institute of Health, various studies of adoptees have found higher correlations of depression between depressed adoptees and biologic parents than with adoptive parents. Studies of twins also have shown that if an identical twin develops an affective disorder, the other twin has a 70% chance of also developing the disorder. The risk decreases to about 15% with siblings, parents, or children of the afflicted person. Grandparents, aunts, or uncles have about a 7% chance of developing an affective disorder.

Theorists also state that a dominant gene may influence or predispose a person to react more readily to experiences of loss or grief, thus manifesting symptoms of depression.

Biochemical Theory

Biogenic amines, or chemical compounds known as norepinephrine and serotonin, have been shown to regulate one's mood and to control drives such as hunger, sex, and thirst. Increased amounts of these neurotransmitters at receptor sites in the brain cause an elevation in mood; decreased amounts can lead to depression. This explanation is termed the *biogenic amine hypothesis*.

High levels of the hormone cortisol have also been observed in depressed persons. Normally cortisol levels peak in the early morning, level off during the day, and reach the lowest point in the evening. Cortisol peaks earlier in depressed persons and remains high all day.

ENVIRONMENTAL THEORY

Financial problems, any type of loss, physical illness, perceived or real failure, or midlife crises are all examples of environmental factors contributing to the development of a depressive disorder. Examples of persons at risk or more prone to depression from environmental factors include:

1. Separated, divorced, or widowed persons who lack companionship and generally suffer from loneliness

2. Young, poor mothers who are single heads of households. This group generally is faced with raising children and maintaining a household without emotional or financial support and are particularly prone to depression.

3. Persons who abuse alcohol or drugs. Alcohol is a depressant; many drugs also depress the central nervous system (CNS) when they are abused. Depression may occur secondary to psychological dependency.

4. Young women who have been taught to be helpless. They are unable to assert themselves to face realities, solve problems, or make decisions.

5. Parents experiencing the "empty-nest syndrome." When children leave home, parents who have devoted their lives to raising them no longer feel needed and experience feelings of uselessness or loneliness.

6. Patients with a chronic, debilitating, or terminal illness (*e.g.,* multiple sclerosis or cancer). These people may experience feelings of loneliness, helplessness, and hopelessness, with a low self-concept and loss of independence.

7. Children who experience a real or perceived loss of a valued object. The dynamics of depression during childhood begin as the child develops a low self-esteem followed by a real or imagined loss such as parental love or attention. The child experiences ambivalent feelings toward the loss and develops guilt feelings as he experiences the negative or "hate" half of the ambivalence. Repression occurs as the child buries or hides such negative feelings. Any time negative feelings toward the valued object occur, the child becomes angry and experiences feelings of hostility and aggression turned inward.

8. People who think negatively. Norman Vincent Peale, author of *The Power of Positive Thinking,* and Aaron Beck, a noted psychiatrist, have both stated that a person's mood can be influenced by the way

he thinks. If a person is negative about himself, the world, and the future, negative memories occur at the expense of positive experiences. Behaviorists and cognitive therapists propose that people become depressed because of having learned negative ways of acting and thinking. They believe that such persons need to reinterpret negative or distorted thoughts and actions more realistically and positively.

9. Persons who are taking prescribed drugs such as phenothiazines, steroids, and reserpine. Drug-induced depression can occur in persons who take such medication over an extended period.

Depression has been categorized in many ways. One method is by placing depressive behaviors on a continuum from first-level, or transitory depression to severe-level depression. First-level depression is exhibited by affective symptoms of sadness or "the blues"—an appropriate response to stress. The person who experiences such depression may be less responsive to the environment and may complain of physical discomfort; however, he usually recovers within a short period. For example, a person may become disappointed when told that he was not chosen as a representative to a conference that he hoped to attend. During this time he may be unable to concentrate, may communicate less with co-workers, may appear less productive than normal, and may isolate himself at work and at home.

Middle-level depression is the depressive state that includes the DSM-III subclassifications of dysthymic and cyclothymic disorders. Other terms that refer to dysthymic disorder are depressive neurosis, neurotic depression, exogenous depression and reactive depression.

Severe-level depression is a category for persons with the DSM-III subclassifications of major depressive disorder, bipolar disorder, and manic disorder. Persons with severe depressive disorders can exhibit psychotic symptoms such as delusions and hallucinations. Major depressive disorders also are referred to as endogenous depression, a depression that appears to develop from within a person with no apparent cause or external precipitating factor. Depression caused by biochemical imbalance is such an example.

DYSTHYMIC DISORDER (DEPRESSIVE NEUROSIS)

Symptoms of dysthymic disorder are similar to those of a major depressive disorder or severe-level depression; however, they are not as severe and do not include psychotic symptoms such as delusions, hallucinations, and impaired communication or incoherence. Clinical symptoms generally persist for 2 years or more and may be present all the time or may occur intermittently with normal mood swings present for a few days or weeks.

Persons who develop dysthymic disorders are generally overly sensitive, often have intense guilt feelings, and may experience chronic anxiety.

Clinical symptoms of middle-level and severe-level depression can be classified as somatic, or physical, and as psychological. Somatic symptoms are as follows:

1. *Chronic fatigue:* Approximately 80% of those persons complaining of fatigue, lethargy, the inability to perform normal tasks, or lack of energy, suffer from depression.

2. *Psychomotor retardation or pronounced reduced mental and physical activity:* The person may lack motivation, be indecisive, exhibit a slumped posture and awkward body movements, and appear lethargic. The person generally complains of an inability to concentrate and may exhibit slowed or muffled speech when communicating.

3. *Psychomotor agitation or pronounced agitated mental and physical activity:* These symptoms may occur as a result of increased anxiety experienced by the depressed person. Restlessness, pacing, or constant walking, purposeless movements, or an inability to concentrate may occur.

4. *Chronic generalized or local pain:* The person is assessed to be an apparently healthy person, but complains of persistent headaches, back pain, or some other chronic pain.

5. *Sleep disturbances:* Depressed persons complain either of insomnia or of fatigue and lethargy that result in excessive sleeping. Sleep patterns may consist of difficulty falling asleep, difficulty staying asleep, difficulty sleeping soundly, or early morning awakening.

6. *Disturbances in appetite:* Persons who are depressed may experience symptoms of anorexia or loss of appetite, or they may be compulsive overeaters.

7. *Gastrointestinal complaints:* Nausea, diarrhea, and constipation are complaints frequently voiced by depressed persons.

8. *Impaired libido:* Depressed interest in sex or decreased responsiveness to sexual stimuli may be a concern of the depressed person.

9. *Anhedonia:* The inability to experience pleasure when participating in acts that normally produce pleasure.

10. *Lack of interest in self-care:* The person loses interest in personal appearance and neglects washing, grooming, and changing clothes.

Psychological symptoms of depression are as follows:

1. *Deep sense or feeling of sadness:* Characterized by crying, gloom, and a sad facial expression.

2. *Anxiety:* Depressed persons may experience internal feelings of anxiety or psychomotor agitation that interfere with daily functioning.

3. *Unconscious anger or hostility directed inward:* Described in the dynamics of childhood depression. Such persons are irritable, restless, or easily annoyed.

4. *Guilt feelings:* Pertaining to real or imagined failures.

5. *Indecisiveness:* Doubt about life and the future.

6. *Lack of self-confidence:* A poor self-concept; this may result in feelings of self-destruction.

Depression: Clinical Example

JW, a 30-year-old air traffic controller, is married and has three children. He is an overly sensitive person who experiences much stress in his occupation. Approximately 2 weeks ago JW began having work-related problems that caused him to consider resigning his position. He told his wife that he was having difficulty concentrating while at work, felt nervous, was unable to sleep, and had lost his appetite. His wife encouraged him to see his family doctor because he was experiencing recurrent episodes on a daily basis. During the intake interview, JW related to the doctor that he no longer felt happy nor was he able to experience pleasure when he went out to dinner with his wife or on picnics with the family. He expressed concern over his loss of interest in sex, his inability to concentrate, insomnia, restlessness, and occasional thoughts of suicide.

Dysthymic Disorder: Clinical Example

KD, an elderly widow, was admitted to a nursing home with the diagnosis of depression. KD's husband had died 4 years earlier when she was 72 years old. At that time, she had moved into a senior citizen's apartment complex but was unable to care for herself because of crippling arthritis. She was transferred to a nursing home, at which the staff noted that KD would become extremely agitated at times, complain of shortness of breath, and refuse to leave her room. Although the staff attempted to communicate with KD, she would tell them to leave the room. One of KD's nurses found her to be extremely apprehensive, crying, and complaining about nursing care. She confided in the nurse that she prayed every night that she would die. KD refused to participate in her care and dismissed the nurse from her room. The second day the same nurse noticed a change in KD's behavior as the patient apologized for her irritability and rudeness. She confided that various problems had been upsetting her. Later she agreed to take a walk with the nurse but was unable to tolerate the noise and activity in the hall and asked to return to her room.

The student nurse shared in a multidisciplinary team conference that KD had been diagnosed as neurotic or dysthymic depression 3 years before her admission. KD appeared to be depressed "most of the time," and frequently talked about death. The nurse shared her "innermost" feelings when she stated "I felt so helpless when she became upset and questioned why God didn't let her die." The next day the nurse was able to bring a volunteer's dog to KD's room and noticed that she responded with a smile while she petted the dog and talked to it. The staff commented that the only time KD appeared happy was when the dog visited twice a week. The conference focused on underlying emotions and psychological symptoms of depression that KD exhibited.

CYCLOTHYMIC DISORDER (CYCLOTHYMIC PERSONALITY)

The DSM-III subclassification of a cyclothymic disorder is also a middle-level depression involving periods of depression and hypomania or a mood somewhere between euphoria and excessive elation. Rapid or accelerated speech, increased activity, and a decreased need for sleep are symptoms of hypomania. Depressive and hypomanic moods may occur alternately, may be intermixed, or may be separated by intervals of normal mood level lasting for several months.

Other symptoms of hypomania include

1. Increased energy level and productivity
2. Egotistical behavior since the person gives the impression that he thinks a lot of himself
3. Increased ability to think creatively
4. Uninhibited gregariousness or seeking the company of others
5. Increased sexuality with no regard for consequences
6. Increased pleasurable activities, for example, shopping sprees and chance business investments
7. Restlessness or excessive motor activity
8. Pressure of speech or rapid, accelerated talking
9. Inappropriate laughter or telling of jokes
10. Bragging about or exaggeration of past accomplishments

Cyclothymic disorder is a chronic condition that usually occurs in early adulthood, is more common in women, and can interfere with social and occupational functioning.

Cyclothymic Disorder: Clinical Example

WB, a 35-year-old plumber, was repairing a water heater when he began to talk rapidly and tell one joke after another to the homeowner. He laughed inappropriately and began to brag about his ability to "outwork" other employees. When WB returned to the company warehouse, his supervisor told him that the homeowner had called to inform him about WB's job performance and behavior. The supervisor expressed concern about WB's actions; the past several months he had noted that WB appeared to be either very happy or depressed. He described WB's mood as similar to the tracks of a roller coaster with several ups and downs. WB was advised to see his family physician before he would be permitted to continue to work.

It may be easy to become caught up in such a person's jovial mood when he appears to be the center of attention as he jokes and teases the nursing personnel. The patient's endless energy keeps the staff busy as he attempts to involve everyone in various activities. It may be difficult to tolerate such loud, boistrous behavior 24 hours a day. Symptoms of depression are usually a part of the history before the patient's admission to the hospital.

MAJOR DEPRESSIVE DISORDER (ENDOGENOUS DEPRESSION)

(Somatic and psychological symptoms of depression were discussed earlier). DSM-III diagnostic criteria state that persons with a major depressive disorder *do not* experience momentary shifts from one dysphoric or unpleasant mood to another, as is seen in dysthymic and cyclothymic disorders. Depressive symptoms such as insomnia, poor or increased appetite, loss of interest in activities, decreased communication, psychomotor agitation or retardation, and suicidal thoughts must be present almost every day for at least 2 weeks. Persons also may experience loss of contact with reality, delusions, and hallucinations. Such a disorder then is categorized as a psychotic depressive disorder and may be seen in persons with the diagnosis of schizophrenia or substance abuse, or in geriatric patients.

Melancholia is another DSM-III subclassification used to describe a severe form of depression that includes anorexia or weight loss, inappropriate or excessive guilt feelings, increased psychomotor retardation or agitation, awakening at least 2 hours earlier than usual in the morning, early morning depression, inability to react to pleasurable stimuli, and loss of pleasure in all or almost all activities. Such persons may be unable to engage in the activities of daily living (ADL), have difficulty with verbal communication, withdraw, and display poor body posture.

The terminology physiologic signs of depression should be noted at this time. Physiologic signs are considered to be classic symptoms of depression and are used as a quick reference when diagnosing depressive behavior. They include

Anorexia and weight loss	Insomnia
Constipation	Fatigue
Lack of interest	

The depressed person displays little interest in self-care. Posture, communication, and clothing reflect the mood, in addition to poor personal hygiene. Patients who are profoundly depressed are unable to plan and carry out a suicide attempt. The time of greatest danger for self-destruction may occur when the patient begins to feel better but still has periods of hopelessness (see Chap. 24).

Major depressive disorders may occur as a single episode or may be recurrent in nature and occur at any age.

BIPOLAR DISORDER (DEPRESSION AND MANIA)

Bipolar disorder is to the severe-level depression what a cyclothymic disorder is to a middle-level depression. It also is referred to as manic-depressive disorder because it involves two cycles, depression and mania.

The sudden onset of a bipolar disorder usually occurs with the manic phase before age 30, can last from a few days to months, and ends abruptly. The depressive phase may occur suddenly or may develop over time. A normal phase may occur between the depressive and manic phases, lasting a short period or for several years. DSM-III classifies these cycles as

1. *Bipolar disorder, mixed:* The person experiences both manic and major depressive phases cyclically or alternating every few days.

2. *Bipolar disorder, manic:* The person is currently experiencing, or has just recently experienced, a manic episode.

3. *Bipolar disorder, depressed:* The person is currently experiencing, or has just recently experienced, a major depressive episode. One or more manic episodes have been previously experienced.

When the person is in the depressive phase of the cycle, he may exhibit any of the symptoms seen in a major depressive disorder.

Clinical symptoms of the manic phase may include the following behaviors:

1. Psychomotor overactivity or excitement. The person may become involved in numerous activities owing to an excessive amount of energy. He may believe he is capable of doing anything and everything.

2. Insomnia without fatigue. The manic person is unable to sit still or sleep for any length of time.

3. Euphoria or an elated mood. The person may exhibit different states of elated behavior: Hypomania, acute mania, or delirious mania. Hypomania can be difficult to detect because the person experiences increased happiness or optimism, a heightened emotional tone, and becomes frustrated easily. Hypomanic persons are oriented in all three spheres and are not delusional. Remission can be spontaneous and

occur without treatment. The acute state is manifested by excessive elation, agitation, accelerated thinking and speaking, hyperactivity, and pressure of speech. Normally, such persons are seen for treatment as inpatients. The delirious state is characterized by extreme excitement, disorientation, agitation, delusions, and hallucinations. Exhaustion, injury, and death may occur if this stage occurs. With the advent of lithium and major tranquilizers, delirious mania rarely is seen.

4. Distractibility. The person is easily distracted owing to a short attention span and increased energy levels.

5. Pressured speech. The person talks rapidly and loudly.

6. Flight of ideas. This thought disorder, defined as jumping from one idea to another with no apparent connection, may occur along with pressured speech. Impaired communication occurs when this thought process is present.

7. Manipulative or demanding behavior. Such behavior may occur as a result of impatience or feelings of self-importance.

8. Destructive or combative behavior. Manic persons may experience paranoid ideation or hallucinations, which can cause destructive or combative behavior.

9. Delusions of grandeur. This thought disorder is characterized by an inflated self-esteem. The person may believe that he has a special relationship with well-known individuals such as political figures or entertainers.

10. Impaired judgment. Psychomotor excitability, distractibility, delusions, hallucinations and other thought disorders may impair one's judgment.

During the manic phase, the individual may dress in a bizarre manner such as wearing bright-colored clothing, several hats, excessive jewelry, and the like. He may telephone various people such as the mayor, governor or congressman regardless of the time of day; go on shopping sprees; believe he is an important person with a special mission; or exhibit incoherent speech.

Manic Bipolar Disorder: Clinical Example

MS, a 45-year-old housewife, was admitted to the psychiatric unit with the diagnosis of bipolar disorder, manic type. The student nurse who assisted with the admission procedure noted that MS was wearing excessive rouge, eye shadow, and lipstick. Her purple dress was adorned with several necklaces, two neck scarves, and two belts. MS's fingernails and toenails were covered with purple nail polish. Every time the student attempted to question her, she would respond in a rapid, loud voice. The student noted that MS was easily distracted and appeared to jump from one idea to another while talking. She also described herself as an "indispensible" member of her church's governing board and stated "I need to get home so that I can help the pastor make some important decisions." During the next several days, the student noted that MS was unable to sleep at night. Although she participated in numerous activities during the day, MS was not able to complete any projects successfully owing to a short attention span and distractibility. She would approach various patients and share intimate personal secrets with them.

During the postclinical conference, students who had attempted to relate to MS made various comments such as, "I can't believe someone really dresses like that," "Does she really believe she is needed by the pastor to make decisions?" and "How can I communicate with someone who talks so fast? I have difficulty understanding her."

MANIC EPISODE OR DISORDER

DSM-III reserves this subclassification for persons who exhibit persistent manic behavior as a prominent part of an illness. The elevated or irritable mood may alternate with, or exist concurrently with, a depressive mood.

Such symptoms must persist for 1 week or more with at least three behavioral symptoms described under bipolar disorder, manic phase.

TREATMENT OF DEPRESSION AND MANIA

Hospitalization is recommended for those persons who are severely depressed, displaying suicidal ideation, or requiring medical care secondary to depression. Persons displaying symptoms of acute manic behavior require hospitalization as well.

Antidepressant drugs generally are started immediately, when it is necessary, because symptomatic relief usually is not achieved for approximately 2 to 4 weeks after therapy has been initiated. Tricyclic antidepressants (*e.g.,* Elavil, Norpramin, Sinequan, and Vivactil) may be prescribed for persons with symptoms such as a decreased appetite, weight loss, decreased energy, or poor sleep. Monoamine oxidase (MAO) inhibitors (*e.g.,* Marplan, Nardil, and Parnate) are usually prescribed for patients who fail to respond to trycyclic antidepressants, experience several physical complaints, or experience anxiety or phobic attacks while depressed. Amoxapine (Asendin) and Trazodone hydrochloride (Desyrel) also are prescribed for depression.

Lithium also is started immediately to treat bipolar disorder since it is quite effective in controlling mania. It is considered a potentially dangerous drug because the therapeutic level is slightly less than the toxic level. Serum levels must be monitored for toxic level, and the patient should be observed for side-effects. Patients usually respond to levels of 0.8 mEq/

liter to 1.5 mEq/liter. Toxic levels occur above 1.5 mEq/liter or 2.0 mEq/liter. Since lithium takes approximately 2 weeks to effect change in the patient's symptoms, a major tranquilizer also is prescribed until the lithium is effective.

Individual, family, group, or behavioral psychotherapy may be prescribed to treat depression. Manic persons should show some response to medication before therapy sessions, such as decreased agitation and restlessness, and an increased attention span.

In addition, occupational or recreational therapy is used to channel the activity level of persons exhibiting manic behavior or psychomotor agitation and to increase the self-esteem of depressed persons.

Antianxiety agents (*e.g.,* Equanil, Tranxene, Ativan, and Serax) may be prescribed for persons who manifest symptoms of anxiety. Sedative–hypnotics, such as barbiturates, may be ordered to treat underlying anxiety and sleep disturbances.

Psychotropic drugs (*e.g.,* Haldol, Mellaril, or Thorazine) may be prescribed to treat acute psychotic symptoms, such as hallucinations and delusions, as well as symptoms of agitation, overactivity, and combativeness.

Electroconvulsive (electroshock) therapy is effective in the treatment of depression, especially for persons who are nonresponsive to chemotherapy or who require a rapid remission of symptoms. (Electroconvulsive therapy is generally effective within a few days).

Some types of depression are considered treatable by a family physician; however, the following behaviors should be referred to a mental health care specialist: failure to respond to drug therapy, suicidal ideation, recurrent manic episodes, and irrational thinking.

The assessment, treatment, and nursing intervention for persons who express feelings of hopelessness, helplessness, worthlessness, and suicidal thoughts are discussed in the chapter on self-destructive behavior.

NURSING INTERVENTIONS FOR DEPRESSION AND MANIA

Persons who are depressed may be difficult to communicate with or approach. Isolation, withdrawal, ambivalence, hostility, guilt, or impaired thought processes are but a few symptoms that can interfere with the development of a therapeutic relationship. The manic patient's hyperactivity, pressured speech, and manipulation also interfere with attempts at communication.

The nurse must be aware of personal vulnerability to depressive behavior. Working with such persons may cause one to react to the depressed atmosphere and in turn experience symptoms of depression. The following is a list of attitudes that the nurse should display toward depressed and manic persons:

1. *Acceptance.* The nurse should spend time with the patient and accept him for what he is. Depressed persons are not always able to express feelings and may exhibit peculiar behavior. Because depressed persons exhibit a low self-esteem, the care-giver should avoid acting in any manner that could be interpreted as rejection or criticism. The manic patient's manipulative, demanding behavior may elicit feelings of disgust and nonacceptance. The nurse should make the manic person aware that she will accept him but not his behavior. Limit setting is one way of displaying acceptance.

2. *Honesty.* The nurse should be truthful, not making promises that she is unable to keep, nor should she provide false reassurance. The depressed person is less able to tolerate disappointment.

3. *Empathy.* Any attempts to cheer up a depressed person will be viewed as an inability to understand his feelings or problems. Such an approach may cause further withdrawal, isolation, and depression. The care-giver should provide the person with an opportunity to express negative, painful feelings and respond in such a way as to convey the message that one recognizes and empathizes with the emotions, thoughts, or feelings of another.

4. *Patience.* Depressed persons may be unable to make decisions as simple as what to eat for breakfast or what items of clothing to wear. The nurse should be aware of the impact of psychomotor retardation on decision making. Psychomotor agitation also requires patience. Underlying anxiety in the depressed person may cause hyperactivity, anger, and hostile behavior. The nurse also must demonstrate patience while setting limits with the demanding, manipulative, manic patient. Such persons can try one's patience, resulting in feelings of frustration, irritation, and anger on the part of the care-giver.

Assessment focuses on mood, affect, behavior, and appearance. Body language replaces communication skills because the person is unable to convey feelings of anger, hostility, and ambivalence.

Questions the nurse can ask the patient to assess the level of depression, while observing facial expressions, body posture, tone of voice, and overall appearance, include:

1. Do you have difficulty falling asleep at night?
2. Do you experience middle-of-the-night awakening?
3. If so, are you able to return to sleep?
4. Do you awaken earlier than usual in the morning?
5. Are you alert or depressed when you get up in the morning?
6. Do you sleep excessively?
7. Have you been experiencing feelings of worthlessness, self-reproach, or inappropriate guilt?

8. Do you have difficulty concentrating or making decisions?

9. Can you watch an entire movie or television show?

10. Does your mood change or fluctuate during the day?

11. Has your sex drive lessened?

12. Are you frequently constipated?

13. Has your energy level decreased?

14. Have you lose interest in life?

15. Has there been a change in your appetite?

16. Do you feel alienated from those around you?

17. Have you every considered or attempted suicide? (If so, ask the patient when and whether he has a plan at present.)

Nursing intervention includes assisting the person in meeting basic human needs. The more severe the depression, the more important becomes physical care since the person loses interest in self-care. Patients who exhibit manic behavior also may neglect personal hygiene. The caregiver may need to assist the person with bathing and grooming, as well as with personal hygiene. Because appearance is neglected, the patient may need help with selecting the appropriate attire to wear, as well as with washing and pressing clothing.

Dietary needs should be monitored. The depressed person may be too uninterested to eat, whereas the manic person may be too hyperactive to eat. Intake and output (I & O) should be monitored until the patient is able to take the responsibility of meeting nutritional needs.

Periods of rest and activity need to be evaluated because depressed patients may sleep continuously in an attempt to avoid the problems and anxieties of reality. Neurotic or dysthymic depression is characterized by increased feelings of depression as the day progresses. Such persons generally "feel better in the morning." Persons with major depressive disorders or psychotic depression fall asleep easily, awaken early, and feel better as the day progresses.

Simple activities are most effective for a person with a short attention span or an inability to concentrate. Completion of such tasks enhances one's self-concept because the person feels more worthwhile after the job is done. One also must consider the person's energy level; the more energy the task requires, the less energy he will have to engage in hostile, aggressive behavior.

Protective care may be necessary for the manic as well as for the depressed person. Persons who exhibit manic behavior may injure themselves owing to excessive motor activity, inability to concentrate, distractibility, and poor judgment. Their destructive tendencies may include self-inflicting behavior and accidental injury. They also may provoke self-defensive actions unintentionally from others who fear injury.

Depressed persons may attempt self-inflicted harm or suffer injury owing to severe depression, lack of interest, psychomotor retardation, the inability to concentrate, or the inability to defend themselves against aggressive persons. The nurse should be aware of the potential for self-destructive behavior. Such an action may occur as the person's psychomotor retardation lessens, the ability to concentrate returns, and the person is able to formulate a plan of action.

Assisting with electroconvulsive or electroshock therapy is another nursing intervention while caring for depressed patients. Such persons are given a complete physical examination before treatment. The nurse's role before treatment is to withhold breakfast and to administer an anticholinergic medication to decrease or dry up body secretions to lessen chances of aspiration during treatment. The nurse must be available to answer any questions the patient may have, to provide supportive care, and to assist with the treatment and monitor the person's responses during a recovery period that usually lasts from a half hour to 1 hour. Care of the patient undergoing electroconvulsive therapy is described in detail in Chapter 3.

Observing for side-effects of psychotropic drugs is another responsibility of the nurse. Tricyclic antidepressants may cause dry mouth, blurred vision, drowsiness, difficulty with urination, and constipation. Antipsychotic drugs may produce extrapyramidal side-effects. (Refer to chapter on psychotropic drugs for additional information.)

MAO inhibitors require strict dietary adherence. Foods to be avoided include yogurt, cheese, wine, beer, pickled herring, chopped liver, sour cream, yeast extracts, and chocolate. Hypertensive crisis may occur after the administration of such drugs if the person combines the drug with food containing tryamine.

Lithium blood levels must be monitored frequently during an acute phase of bipolar depression and on a routine basis during the maintenance phase because toxicity may occur in response to excessive doses of the drug or in the presence of a decreased serum sodium level. The therapeutic level is usually between 0.8 to 1.5 mEq/liter. Diuretics, profuse diaphoresis, a low-salt diet, or diarrhea may result in lowered serum sodium levels and higher lithium levels. Symptoms of lithium toxicity include vomiting, diarrhea, weight loss, excessive thirst, abnormal muscle movement, muscle twitching, slurred speech, blurred vision, dizziness, stupor, and an irregular heart beat.

Patient education is another nursing intervention for depressed and manic persons. Such persons should be informed about the importance of outpatient treatment as well as the continuation of prescribed drugs. They may be placed on long-term maintenance levels of medication and could suffer a relapse if they discontinued the drugs. They should be taught to recognize the onset of side-effects, as well as the recurrence of symptoms, to avoid rehospitalization. A person diagnosed as having bipolar depression, mixed type, was able to describe the changes in affect and behavior in the initial phases of his illness. He related to the student nurse that "I could feel the changes coming on." He had been instructed to notify his attending physician or psychiatrist whenever he experienced such changes so that his outpatient treatment could be reevaluated in an effort to prevent the development of severe symptoms.

Manic patients should be cautioned not to take on too many responsibilities or to overextend themselves. Depressed persons should be instructed to contact a support person if feelings of depression return or increase in intensity.

Another aspect of nursing care is that of being supportive during psychotherapy sessions. The person may have difficulty expressing feelings of hostility, ambivalence, and guilt. Feelings of anxiety may occur or increase as the person begins therapy sessions. Such sessions may be directed at exploring feelings about self and relationship with the environment in an attempt to improve the person's self-esteem and decrease feelings of helplessness, hopelessness, and powerlessness. The nurse can be supportive simply by making herself available to the patient and by recognizing symptoms such as anxiety.

The following are examples of nursing diagnoses and nursing interventions for depressed and manic patients:

NURSING DIAGNOSES	NURSING INTERVENTIONS
Potential for injury: Suicidal ideation	Suicide precautions Suicide rating scale (See Chap. 24 for protective care of the suicidal patient.)
Social isolation	Establish trust. Assign the same staff members to work with the person whenever possible. Accept the patient as he is. When approaching the person, avoid being overly cheerful, sympathetic, or superficial. Display empathy. Use therapeutic communication skills such as silence and active listening. Encourage ventilation of feelings.
Dysrhythmia of sleep–rest activity	Observe for signs of fatigue. Provide opportunities for rest. Set limits regarding time to arise in morning and the amount of time spent in bed during the day. Decrease external stimuli before hour of retiring.

NURSING DIAGNOSES	NURSING INTERVENTIONS
	Offer warm milk and backrub at bedtime. Administer prescribed medication for insomnia.
Alterations in nutrition: Less than body requirements	Monitor I & O. Provide a high-protein, high-calorie diet as needed. Attempt to include the patient's favorite foods. Provide frequent, nutritional snacks in the form of "finger foods." Encourage adequate fluid intake. Offer high-calorie drinks. Weigh the patient weekly or as ordered.
Alteration in bowel elimination: Constipation	Monitor I & O. Encourage fluids. Encourage exercise. Provide bulk and fiber in diet. Administer laxatives as needed.
Alteration in self-concept	Involve in activities directed toward raising self-esteem. Display a sincere interest and offer praise or recognition for accomplishments.
Activity intolerance because of hyperactivity and distractibility	Decrease or limit environmental stimuli. Provide adequate room for hyperactivity. May need a private room to reduce external stimuli. Limit social interactions initially to prevent intrusive behavior. Select activities that provide an outlet for excessive energy yet do not trigger loss of control. Administer drugs as ordered to decrease hyperactivity.
Manipulation	Give simple explanations regarding hospital routine and nursing care. Contact the patient frequently but briefly to reassure him. Set limits and be consistent. Avoid arguing with the patient.

SUMMARY

Depression, a natural emotion that most people experience at one time or another, can manifest itself along a continuum from feelings of sadness to psychotic depression. Symptoms of depression can occur at any age, including infancy. Depression also may manifest itself in the form of hyperactivity and manic behavior. Such persons are thought to be using manic behavior as an effort to deny or repress feelings of depression unconsciously. Theories pertaining to the causative factors of depressive and manic behavior were discussed. They include the genetic predisposition theory, the biochemical theory, and the environmental theory. The following subclassifications of affective disorders were discussed: dysthymic disorder (depressive neurosis and exogenous depression), cyclothymic disorder (cyclothymic personality), major depressive disorder (endogenous depression and psychotic depression), bipolar disorders, and manic episode. Treatment of depression was discussed focusing on the use of psychotropic drugs to achieve symptomatic relief as soon as possible. Side-effects of tricyclic antidepressants and MAO inhibitors were discussed as well as lithium toxicity. Other treatments listed include psychotherapy, occupational therapy, recreational therapy, electroconvulsive or electroshock therapy, and referral, in the event that the person does not respond to traditional treatment. Nursing intervention focused on nursing attitudes toward depressed and manic persons, assessment, implementation of care to meet physiologic and psychological needs, observation for side-effects of prescribed drugs, and patient education. (The reader is directed to Chap. 24 for detailed information pertaining to protective care of suicidal patients and to Chap. 3 for information pertaining to electroconvulsive therapy.) Examples of nursing diagnoses and nursing interventions focused on social isolation, dysrhythmia of sleep–rest activity, alterations in nutrition, alteration in bowel elimination, alteration in self-concept, activity intolerance, and manipulation.

LEARNING ACTIVITIES

  I. Clinical activities
    A. Begin a relationship with a person experiencing symptoms of an affective disorder.
      1. Identify the person's level of depression or manic behavior.
      2. List physiologic and psychological symptoms.
      3. Describe the person's appearance, behavior, and ability to communicate.
      4. Does the person exhibit any signs of suicidal intent?
      5. List any psychotropic drugs ordered, evaluate their action, and observe for any side-effects. State what nursing management and health teaching should be done for each drug taken.
      6. List therapies being used and discuss value or effectiveness of each.
    B. Familiarize yourself with the agency's precautions for suicidal patients, as well as seclusion and restraint procedures.
    C. Chart your observations and interactions.
    D. Develop a nursing care plan for this person.

II. Affective disorder situation

KJ, a 39-year-old widow, is seen in the emergency room with the complaints of difficulty sleeping at night, headache, fatigue, and an uneasy feeling that she is unable to explain. These symptoms have persisted over the past several months and have become increasingly worse. She has lost approximately 8 lbs owing to anorexia and is having difficulty with constipation. KJ is diagnosed as having a dysthymic disorder.

Develop a brief but specific nursing care plan for this patient.

III. Independent activity

A. Complete the Programmed Instruction "Helping Depressed Patients in General Nursing Practice" (Am J Nurs: June, 1977).

B. List at least three situations in which you have observed persons who appeared to be depressed. Was the cause of the mood change identifiable? Was the mood change appropriate to the cause? What coping mechanisms or support systems did the person use?

C. Assess your own mood states for 1 week by plotting a daily graph. Using a scale of 1 to 10, indicate feelings of sadness at the lower level of the scale and feelings of well-being or elation at the higher level with 5 as the normal level. List those situations influencing any changes in your mood directly under the number and day of the week indicated on the scale.

Example:

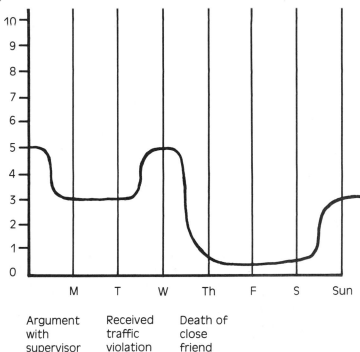

SELF-TEST

1. State three theories pertaining to the development of an affective disorder.
2. List five examples of persons who are more at risk to develop depression.
3. Describe symptoms of first-level depression.
4. List two DSM-III classifications that are considered to be middle-level depressive disorders.
5. Clinical symptoms of middle-level depression can be classified as _____ and _____.
6. Anxiety, unconscious anger, guilt feelings, indecisiveness, and self-doubt are psychological symptoms of which disorder (also called depressive neurosis)?
7. Cyclothymic disorder is a _____-level depression with clinical symptoms of hypomania as well as depression.
8. List five symptoms of hypomania.
9. Define anhedonia.
10. State the DSM-III criteria for the diagnosis of a major depressive disorder or endogenous depression.
11. State the five physiologic signs of depression.
12. Differentiate the three cycles of bipolar disorder.
13. Describe the three states or levels of mania.
14. List at least five clinical symptoms of manic behavior.
15. List various treatment modes of affective disorders.
16. State the therapeutic blood or serum level of lithium.
17. State the rationale for doing serum lithium levels.
18. List nursing interventions for dysrhythmia of sleep–rest activity.
19. Describe nursing interventions for alterations in nutrition: less than body requirements.
20. State nursing interventions for activity intolerance.
21. List psychotropic drugs used to treat depression.

REFERENCES

Altrocchi J: Abnormal Behavior. New York, Harcourt Brace Jovanovich, 1980
Authier J, Authier K, Lutey B: Clinical management of the tearfully depressed patient: Communication skills for the nurse practitioner. J Psych Nurs: Feb, 1979
Beck C: The occurrence of depression in women and the effect of the women's movement. J Psych Nurs: Nov, 1979
Benfer BA: Mood swings. Nurs 72: Aug, 1972

Ciba Pharmaceutical Co: Depression (pamphlet), Chap. 2. Summit, Ciba–Geigy Corporation, 1981

Clifford RH, Thompson ML: Depression suicide attempt/chronic. In Case Studies of Nursing Intervention. New York, McGraw–Hill, 1974

Dixson DL: Manic depression: An overview. J Psych Nurs: May, 1981

Donlon P, Rockwell D: Psychiatric Disorders: Diagnosis and Treatment. Bowie, Robert Brady, 1982

Freedman et al: Comprehensive Textbook of Psychiatry. Baltimore, Wilkins & Wilkins, 1975

Haber J et al: Comprehensive Psychiatric Nursing, 2nd ed. New York, McGraw–Hill, 1982

Harris E: The dexamethasone suppression test. Am J Nurs: May, 1982

Knowles RD: Dealing with feelings: Coping with lethargy. Am J Nurs: Aug, 1981

Knowles RD: Dealing with feelings: Handling depression by identifying anger. Am J Nurs: May, 1981

Knowles RD: Handling depression through activity. Am J Nurs: June, 1981

Kolb L: Modern Clinical Psychiatry. Philadelphia, WB Saunders, 1977

Lancaster J: Adult Psychiatric Nursing. New York, Medical Examination Publishing, 1980

Mellencamp A: Adolescent depression: A review of the literature, with implications for nursing care. J Psych Care: Sept, 1981

Programmed instruction: Helping depressed patients in general nursing practice. Am J Nurs: June, 1977

Robinson L: Psychological Aspects of the Care of Hospitalized Patients. Philadelphia, FA Davis, 1984

Rosenbaum M: Depression: What to do, what to say. Nurs 80: Aug, 1980

Rowe CJ: An Outline of Psychiatry. Dubuque, William Brown, 1980

Schneider JS: Hopelessness and helplessness. J Psych Nurs: Mar, 1980

Schultz J, Dark S: Manual of Psychiatric Nursing Care Plans. Boston, Little, Brown & Co, 1982

Sills G, Wise D: The depressed client. New York, American Journal of Nursing

Smith M: Depression. Nurs 78: Sept, 1978

Swanson AR: Communicating with depressed persons. In Backer B, Dubbert P, Eisenman E (eds.): Psychiatric/Mental Health Nursing: Contemporary Readings. New York, D. Van Nostrand, 1978

Treating the Emotions: Part III: Depression. Life Magazine: Apr, 1982

Valente S: Stalking patient depression. Nursing 84: Aug, 1984

Walker JI: Everybody's Guide to Emotional Well-Being. San Francisco, Harbor Publishing, 1982

White CL: Nurse counseling with a depressed patient. Am J Nurs: Mar, 1978

24

SELF-DESTRUCTIVE

BEHAVIOR: SUICIDE

She put on her new blue nightgown
And combed her hair.
Painted her eyes and mouth.
Used some of the Christmas cologne
And then she swallowed the pills.

When they brought her to us,
Her gown was soiled and twisted around her body.
Her hair was damp and knotted.
The cosmetics grotesquely smeared on the tear-wet face.
She could still talk.
She took few enough pills for that:
"Let me alone, let me sleep."

We didn't have time to sympathize.
There was a man on the pacemaker in the next room.
A child had died an hour ago.
It was a Sunday, too, and naturally
We were short of help.
She was, frankly, a nuisance.

The resident passed the slender plastic tube
While she wept and fought, and we held her down.
The new nurse said, "Poor thing. . ."
I said, "Poor thing, nothing. If they're going to do it,
I wish they'd do it right and save us all this bother."
I didn't know she heard me. Maybe I didn't care.

That must have been a month ago.
Tonight she came in again,
D.O.A.
This time she'd hanged herself. The way I knew her
Was the same blue nightgown- her face was changed.
The police had found a note.
All it said was, "This time I'll do it right."

Only a couple of hours till midnight.
I'll be glad to finish up and go home.
I'm tired, as usual and though it's warm in here
I'm cold and not as unshaken as they think.
I know why I'm cold.
Death touched me again tonight.

Don't worry, I'm not going to brood about it.
It couldn't help her and I know it wouldn't help me.
You can't go back. You can't take back the words,
But I would if I could,
If I only could
This once.

Author Unknown

LEARNING OBJECTIVES

1. Describe the relationship between depression and suicide.
2. State several causative factors or motives for self-destructive behavior.
3. List those persons considered to be at risk or prone to self-destructive behavior.
4. State examples of verbal and behavioral suicidal clues.
5. Differentiate among primary, secondary, and tertiary prevention in relation to nursing care.
6. Explain the importance of self-assessment when working with suicidal pateints.
7. Explain the term *postvention.*
8. Discuss the medical treatment of suicidal persons.
9. Discuss the therapeutic milieu for a patient on suicidal precautions.
10. List therapeutic nursing interventions when caring for a person exhibiting self-destructive behavior.

SUICIDE is considered to be one of the ten leading causes of death among adults in the United States. The need to be loved and accepted, along with a desperate wish to communicate feelings of loneliness, alienation, worthlessness, helplessness, and hopelessness, often result in intense feelings of anxiety, depression, and anger or hostility directed toward the self. If no one is available to talk to or listen to such feelings of insecurity or inadequacy, a suicide attempt may occur In an effort to seek help or end an emotional conflict.

Approximately 25,000 people commit suicide each year. The following statistics have been made available by various sources such as the National Institute of Health, the Harvard School of Public Health, the *American Journal of Epidemiology,* the Center for Disease Control, and researchers such as Resnick and Farberow.

1. Suicide is the third leading cause of death among American teenagers and young adults in their early twenties. It is the second leading cause of death among college students. Approximately 18 American adolescents commit suicide daily.

2. One person out of every one hundred threatens suicide. There are approximately 250,000 attempts yearly.

3. One out of every ten persons entertains recurrent or persistent thoughts of suicide (suicidal ideation).

4. Approximately 1% of the annual deaths in the United States are reported as suicide. A more realistic figure is 2% to 3%; however, such attempts generally are reported as accidents to spare families the stigmatizing impact of suicide and to facilitate insurance coverage that otherwise would not occur in the event of suicide.

5. Approximately 75% of those persons contemplating suicide consult their family physician about some other matter before such an attempt. Such a visit may be a cry for help because of feelings of ambivalence about suicide or part of a well-planned scheme to obtain lethal material (*e.g.,* sleeping pills).

6. Approximately 25% of all suicides are persons 65 years of age and over.

7. Approximately 80% of those persons attempting suicide give clues. Such clues are categorized as verbal or behavioral. Verbal clues include talking about death, making comments that significant others would be "better off without" the person, and asking questions about lethal dosages of drugs. Behavioral clues include writing forlorn love notes, writing angry messages directed at a significant other who has rejected the person, giving away personal items, or taking out a large life insurance policy. A third category, situational clues, is used to describe those events or situations that present themselves when something happens either around or within the person, such as the unexpected death of a loved one, divorce, job failure, or diagnosis of a malignant tumor. Such situational clues may place the person at risk for potential suicide.

8. Approximately 2 million Americans survive suicide attempts yearly.

9. Men accomplish suicide more often than women; however, women attempt suicide three times as often.

10. Suicide represents a loss of over 16 billion dollars each year considering productivity, medical care, and welfare payments to survivors.

11. 65% to 75% of those persons who successfully commit suicide have made previous attempts.

12. In 1979 approximately 151 suicides occurred among children aged 10 to 14. Documented cases reveal self-destructive characteristics of children as young as 4 years of age. Examples of suicidal acts include attempts to strangle oneself, to set fire to clothing, and to jump out of windows. Statistics reveal that five youngsters between the ages of 5 to 9 killed themselves in 1976.

ETIOLOGY

Suicide is defined by Webster as the act of direct self-destructive behavior by purposely killing oneself. Why does a person contemplate such an act? Causative factors, or motives for attempting suicide, include

1. A progressive failure to adapt. The person no longer is able to cope in a world of stressors that are overwhelming.

2. Feelings of alienation or isolation, especially in teenagers. The isolation may occur gradually, resulting in a loss of all meaningful social contacts and relationships. Isolation can be self-imposed or can occur

as a result of the inability to be assertive, express feelings, cope posi-tively, or develop meaningful relationships with others.

3. Feelings of anger or hostility. A person may harbor feelings of intense hostility toward a significant other and intend to get revenge or manipulate the person. For example, a woman deserted by her hus-band may feel that her suicidal act will cause him to suffer guilt feel-ings and loss of self-esteem among friends and relatives or that per-haps the attempt will force him to return home. Feelings of hostility may also be directed inward owing to self-hatred. The suicide then is a form of self-punishment. For example, an army officer broods over the orders he gave to his company that resulted in killing several young children. Suicide would be a form of self-punishment and atonement for a sin or crime he feels that he committed.

4. A reunion wish or fantasy. A newspaper article recently described the death of an elderly man whose wife had just died. He left a note to his children stating that he did not want to live without his wife, and because of his belief in life after death, he planned to join his wife.

5. A way to end one's feelings of hopelessness and helplessness. Hope is a sense of the possible; it gives promise for the future and an expec-tation of fulfillment. Persons who experience hopelessness feel inse-cure and believe that there are no solutions to various problems. They experience a sense of the impossible. Helplessness is a feeling that everything that can be done has been done; there is nothing left to sustain hope.

6. A cry for help. Some people attempt suicide hoping to draw attention to themselves to receive help. For example, a 49-year-old woman in financial distress attempted suicide by taking a moderate overdose of sleeping pills, hoping that her boyfriend, who never displayed an interest in her business, would come to her rescue financially as well as emotionally.

7. A deliberate gamble with death from feelings of frustration, self-hatred, or ambivalence. Persons who are ambivalent harbor feelings of self-preservation and self-destruction. Such persons may threaten or attempt suicide and then seek help. Stuntmen, daredevil drivers, and persons who play such games like Russian roulette are deliber-ately gambling with death and often harbor feelings of ambivalence, or self-hatred. Such persons appear to be living on "borrowed time" because they live with the risk of death frequently.

8. An attempt to "save-face" or seek a release to a better life. Persons who were involved in the stock market crash of 1929 during the depression jumped from windows in suicide attempts caused by feel-ings of failure. These people had viewed themselves as competent, successful, and respected prior to the crash. The suicides were an effort to save face, relieving them of the responsibility of dealing with business failures.

9. Terminal or chronic illness. People with a terminal or chronic illness may attempt suicide as a last chance to maintain control of their lives or a wish to be released from pain. Noncompliance, or refusal to follow the prescribed medical care, is a passive or indirect form of suicide seen among the chronic or terminally ill. For example, a patient with advanced emphysema refused to follow the doctor's advice to quit smoking although he was maintained on oxygen per nasal cannula. The patient died as a result of noncompliance.

10. Impaired thought processes (*e.g.,* delusions or hallucinations). Persons who hallucinate or entertain delusional thoughts may respond to persistent thoughts or "voices" that tell them to follow through with life-threatening acts.

The following is a list of those persons considered to be at risk or prone to self-destructive behavior:

1. Older single, divorced, or widowed men

2. The elderly

3. Unemployed persons

4. People in poor physical health

5. People living alone

6. Minority groups

These six groups of people may experience feelings of dependency, loneliness, and worthlessness as they attempt to care for themselves in a society that places much emphasis on youth, physical fitness, success, and independence. Other at-risk groups include:

7. Alcoholics and substance abusers: Persons who are alcoholics are considered suicidal because of the effect of high consumption of alcohol on the body over a period of time, as well as its depressing effect on the central nervous system. The mixing of drugs and alcohol increases the chance of drug-alcohol interaction that could result in death. Many drugs cause psychological or physiologic dependency, thus creating emotional conflict and depression as well as physiologic deterioration. Drug–drug interactions also increase the likelihood of death as a result of self-destructive impulses.

8. People such as air traffic controllers whose occupations require selfless public service and dedication, and who work under high pressure: The lives of physicians and policemen also are often stressful due to the long work hours and disruption of family and social life.

9. Adolescents: Causative factors that place adolescents at risk include the dependence–independence conflict, uncertainties about sexual role and sexual adequacy, peer group influences, and drug experimentation or abuse (see Chap. 21).

10. Chronic or terminally ill persons whose life-styles are disrupted by the illnesses: Persons with anorexia nervosa or bulimia are definitely at risk. They are committing a passive form of suicide that could become acute and is caused by feelings of frustration, guilt, anger, or loss of control.

11. Accident-prone individuals: Such persons, who experience repeated accidents in which their lives are in jeopardy, may be attempting suicide unconsciously.

12. Previous attempters: Persons who have not developed adequate coping mechanisms or who lack sufficient support systems are at risk each time they experience increased stress.

13. Persons who engage in autoerotic sexual acts: The use of chains, shackles, ropes or other devices to enhance autoerotic feelings often restrict or immobilize the person and create a level of semiconsciousness that could result in accidental death or suicide.

Hatton, Valente, and Rink (1977) have developed a method of assessment of a person's degree of suicidal risk (see table on p. 472).

MISCONCEPTIONS ABOUT SUICIDE

Several misconceptions exist regarding the dynamics of suicide. They are presented in an attempt to inform the reader of such fallacies.

1. *Suicidal individuals give no warning of their intent.* Eight out of ten persons give some type of verbal or behavioral clue prior to a suicide attempt.

2. *Suicidal persons want to die; therefore, once suicidal, always suicidal.* In reality the person is generally suicidal for a limited period termed the *suicidal crisis* period. During this crisis, the person is undecided about living and dying (ambivalent) and gambles with death. He leaves his destiny or fate in the hands of others. Those saved are usually quite grateful.

3. *Once a suicidal attempt has failed, the suicidal risk is over.* Persons who attempt suicide remain at risk during the period of improvement because they experience increased energy levels and are able to put morbid thoughts and feelings into action. Persons recovering from a severe depression are considered to be at high risk for approximately 9 to 15 months.

4. *Suicidal tendencies are inherited.* There is no evidence to support this misconception. Suicide is an individual pattern of behavior.

5. *Only "crazy" people commit suicide.* Approximately 10% of all suicides occur as a result of major psychological breakdowns. Farberow states that studies of genuine suicide notes show that the people were extremely unhappy but not mentally ill.

ASSESSING THE DEGREE OF SUICIDAL RISK

Behavior or Symptom	Intensity of Risk		
	Low	Moderate	High
Anxiety	Mild	Moderate	High, or panic state
Depression	Mild	Moderate	Severe
Isolation-withdrawal	Vague feelings of depression, no withdrawal	Some feelings of helplessness, hopelessness, and withdrawal	Hopeless, helpless, withdrawn and self-deprecating
Daily functioning	Fairly good in most activities	Moderately good in some activities	Not good in any activities
Resources	Several	Some	Few or more
Coping strategies and devices being used	Generally constructive	Some that are constructive	Predominately destructive
Significant others	Several who are available	Few or only one available	Only one, or none available
Psychiatric help in past	None, or positive attitude toward	Yes, and moderately satisfied with	Negative view of help received
Life-style	Stable	Moderately stable or unstable	Unstable
Alcohol and drug use	Infrequently to excess	Frequently to excess	Continual abuse
Previous suicide attempts	None, or of low lethality	None to one or more of moderate lethality	None to multiple attempts of high lethality
Disorientation and disorganization	None	Some	Marked
Hostility	Little or none	Some	Marked
Suicidal plan	Vague, fleeting thoughts but no plan	Frequent thoughts, occasional ideas about a plan	Frequent or constant thoughts with a specific plan

(Hatton D, Valente S, Rink A: Suicide Assessment and Intervention, p. 56. New York, Appleton–Century–Crofts, 1977)

6. *Suicide occurs more frequently among the very rich or very poor.* Suicide occurs among all levels of society, regardless of socioeconomic status.

ASSESSMENT

Suicide is considered more preventable than any other cause of death. This statement is based on the assumption that all suicidal persons are ambivalent about life and therefore are never 100% suicidal.

Assessment of the person who is self-destructive includes the application of close observational and listening skills to detect any suicide clues, the specificity of the plan, and its degree of lethality. As stated previously, 80% of all potential suicide victims give some type of clue. Clues that might lead one to suspect that a patient is in danger of making a suicide attempt include any person who

1. Has a history of suicidal attempts

2. Talks about death, suicide, wanting to be dead, and appears to be in deep thought

3. Asks suspicious questions such as "How often do the night personnel make rounds?", "How many of these pills would it take to kill a person?", "How high is this window from the ground?", "How long does it take to bleed to death?" and so forth

4. Fears being unable to sleep and fears the night

5. Is depressed and cries frequently

6. Keeps away from others owing to self-imposed isolation especially in secluded areas or behind locked doors

7. Is tense, worried, and has a hopeless, helpless attitude

8. Imagines he has some serious physical illness like cancer or tuberculosis. He may want to end his suffering or decrease the imagined burden to his family.

9. Feels very guilty about something real or imaginary or who feels worthless. He may feel he is not worthy to live.

10. Talks or thinks about punishment, torture, and being persecuted

11. Is listening to voices (The voices may tell him to try to take his life.)

12. Suddenly seems very happy, without any apparent reason, after being very depressed for some time. (He may be happy now that he has figured out a method of committing suicide.)

13. Collects and hoards strings, pieces of glass, a knife, or anything else sharp that he might use to hurt himself

14. Is very aggressive or very impulsive, acting suddenly and unexpectedly

15. Shows an unusual amount of interest in getting his affairs in order

16. Gives away personal belongings

During the assessment process, the nurse begins to establish a therapeutic relationship based on trust as she displays an attitude of acceptance, empathy, and support. Such a response is supportive to persons who experience feelings of worthlessness, helplessness, and hopelessness. The encouragement of verbalization of negative feelings is essential, as well as the direct questioning about suicidal intent.

1. Be alert to diagnose the potentially suicidal patient. Failure to recognize such patients is generally due to the lack of adequate assessment skills, inability to recognize suicidal behavior, or presence of a value system in which suicide is taboo and is therefore not discussed.

2. Assess the person for any biologic or organic cause of depression. Various illnesses are accompanied or occupied by a depressive reaction. Such a depression is real and presents the various clinical symptoms as discussed in Chapter 23. Drugs and alcohol also may cause a biologic depression. Statistics show that 3% to 25% of those people on prescribed medications experience depression. A urine and blood drug screen as well as blood alcohol level should be performed if substance abuse is suspected.

3. Once a suicidal patient is identified, evaluate the person's intent on suicide. Does the individual have a plan? How lethal is it? How accessible are the weapons or equipment?

The most common methods of self-destruction include guns and poisoning (prescribed medication), which are generally readily accessible. The method of choice is usually an indication of the person's degree of intent to complete the attempt successfully. Other lethal methods include hanging, strangulation, jumping, cutting or piercing, and drowning. Men generally choose the more violent methods of firearms, explosives, hanging, and strangulation; whereas women generally elect to overdose on medication or cut their wrists. Removing lethal methods from the environment may prevent an impulsive attempt at self-destruction. Hospitalization may be necessary to protect the person from self-destructive behavior, particularly when he or she has no one living with him or no support system.

NURSING INTERVENTION

Nursing intervention focuses on prevention of self-destruction and is classified as primary, secondary, and tertiary prevention. Primary prevention focuses on the elimination of factors causing or contributing to the development of an illness or disorder. Secondary prevention is described as an attempt to identify and treat physical or emotional disorders in the early stages before they become disturbing to an individual. For example, a 24-year-old schoolteacher experiences feelings of increased anxiety and mild depression when told by her fiancée that he is breaking the engagement. Effective assessment or secondary prevention should alleviate such symptoms and prevent the onset of self-destructive behavior. Tertiary prevention is intervention aimed at reducing residual disability after an illness. A residential treatment center, halfway house, or rehabilitation center may be used to treat a recovering alcoholic patient who previously attempted suicide, is recovering from a severe depression, but needs the supervision and support of others as he handles his drinking problem.

Crisis intervention is performed in emergency situations in which a suicidal crisis exists. The nurse assesses the person and the problem, plans therapeutic interventions, intervenes, and assists the person in making realistic plans for the future while he uses successful coping mechanisms to reduce anxiety and tension (see Chap. 6).

Self assessment (autognosis) is imperative if the nurse expects to handle self-destructive persons effectively. Haber (1982) lists several questions the nurse can use as a self-assessment guide. In short, they refer to evaluating one's

Values and belief about life versus death

Positive and negative feelings about the suicidal person

Ability to be nonjudgmental

Energy level, mentally and physically, when working therapeutically with a suicidal person

Ability to let the person assume the responsibility for his actions

Suicide precautions vary according to the person's intent on self-destruction. Bailey and Dreyer (1977) discuss a suicidal intention rating scale (SIRS) that provides a guide in the management of hospitalized persons considered to be self-destructive. A person who displays no evidence of past or present suicidal ideation is given a rating of 0. Nursing intervention consists of the normal hospital care. A person who shows evidence of suicidal ideation, has not made an attempt at self-destruction, and has not threatened suicide is given a rating of 1+. The nurse observes and evaluates the person for evidence of recurrent suicidal thoughts. Actively thinking about suicide or evidence of a previous attempt is given a rating of 2+. Such a person should be protected from self-destructive impulses. Personal items are made available for use but must be returned to the staff and kept under lock and key if they are potentially dangerous. These items include glass containers, sharp objects, hard plastics, belts, ties, pins, and any liquid cosmetics or deodorants that could be drunk and result in poisoning. A person who makes a suicide threat, such as "Leave me alone or I'll kill myself," is assigned a rating of 3+. Such a person should be searched at the time of admission for the possession of lethal instruments. Any carry-in items such as luggage also should be checked. Potentially dangerous items (*e.g.,* a razor, mirror, or nail file) are to be used only under the direct supervision of a hospital employee. Protective care includes periodic checks at least every 30 minutes, limited visits by family members only, and no privileges to leave the unit unless otherwise specified by the physician. If the person does leave the unit, he is to be accompanied by a member of the staff. A 4+ rating is reserved for the person who actively attempted suicide or is hospitalized to prevent self-destructive impulses. Nursing intervention for a 4+ rating may include the following protective care. An explanation should be given to the patient so that he understands what is being done and why.

1. Confinement to a security room to observe the person's behavior more readily. The door is locked whenever the patient is left alone, and frequent, periodic checks are made at irregular intervals. The nurse can provide constant watchful care by staying with the person, and by listening and being supportive. The use of leather restraints, full or belt, is used as a last resort to immobilize agitated, self-destructive persons. Windows in the room should be locked, with screens covering the glass to prevent self-harm. Seclusion must be used judiciously because it can isolate a person further and enhance feelings of worthlessness, helplessness, and hopelessness.

2. Removal of objects that could prove to be dangerous to the person. This is done by searching the person's clothing, carry-in items, and body in a dignified or professional manner. The body search includes checking any part of the body in which harmful objects might be stored, such as body orifices and the hair. One female patient concealed Librium in a plastic bag in her vagina, with the intent of overdosing at some future time during hospitalization.

3. Removal of street clothes and placing the person in a hospital gown. Removal of bed linens. Suicide attempts have been made by a patient's attempting to hang himself with linen or clothing.

4. Feeding the patient in the seclusion room. Food is served on paper dishes if one of the staff is unable to stay with the patient during meals. Sharp utensils are removed from the tray to prevent an impulsive attempt at self-destruction.

5. Direct supervision of the person whenever he is removed from the security room to prevent impulsive self-destructive behavior.

6. Restricted visitation privileges. Such visitors require special permission by the attending physician. After visitors have departed, the patient should be checked for items that may have been left behind accidently or innocently given to him.

7. Securing a verbal stated promise not to attempt suicide. Instead the

patient will seek out a staff member if he experiences suicidal thoughts.

8. Giving a message of hope by being optimistic that life can be better and the patient will receive help in an attempt to solve his problem.

9. Medicating, if necessary. Injections usually are given to persons in security rooms to facilitate rapid absorption and to prevent noncompliance, such as refusal to take medication or hoarding of it.

If a patient is admitted to a general hospital following a suicide attempt, 24-hour supervision is required at the expense of the family because seclusion rooms are not usually available.

Once the person has inner control over self-destructive behavior, he is removed from seclusion or the security room. He should be encouraged to engage in an activity that is an outlet for tension and hostility. Participating in an active sport like volleyball, working with sandpaper, or pounding wood are examples of such an outlet. The room assignment should be near the nurses' station to provide close observation. Having another patient in the same room offers support to the person and lessens feelings of loneliness.

The patient should be monitored while he is taking any prescribed medication because patients have been known to save medication for future suicide attempts. As the depression lessens, the person acquires energy to follow through with another self-destructive attempt.

Participation in group, individual, or family psychotherapy is encouraged. As the patient recovers and discharge planning occurs, he is encouraged to identify agencies or support systems in the community that he can contact to alleviate recurrent suicidal feelings. The patient and family should be educated about signs and symptoms of depression, warning signs of suicidal thoughts, and effects of medication, including any special precautions.

It would be wrong to suggest that closely supervised patients do not succeed in suicide attempts. A clinical example of a person who did succeed in a suicide attempt during hospitalization follows.

SM, a 35-year-old engineer and father of three children, had been admitted to the neuropsychiatric unit of a state hospital with the diagnosis of depression. During the intake interview, SM exhibited symptoms of suicidal ideation because he made statements such as, "I'd be better off dead", "My family would be better off without me", and "Yes, I have thought about killing myself." SM was placed on strict suicide precautions and antidepressant medication, and began attending therapy sessions on the unit. Within 3 weeks the suicidal precautions were lifted, and SM was granted lawn privileges but was to be supervised by one of the hospital employees. SM appeared to be improving and was granted a day pass to visit his family 4 weeks after his admission. At approximately 3 o'clock the day after SM visited his family, he asked for lawn privileges to play tennis. Although SM was supervised by a hospital employee, he was able to run away and leave the hospital grounds. Later that evening SM's family notified the hospital that he had secured a handgun and committed suicide by firing the gun into his mouth.

The student nurse who had begun to develop a therapeutic relationship with SM was shocked by the news and immediately experienced guilt feelings. She stated, "Did I say something to upset him that much? Was it my fault he committed suicide?" She questioned whether there were some verbal clues that she should have noticed. The staff was quite helpful in explaining to the student that patients may commit suicide in spite of all the precautions taken during hospitalization. They further explained to her that in her capacity as a student, she was not with the patient 24 hours a day to observe him continuously as the three shifts did. She should therefore not blame herself for his actions.

Survivors of a successful suicide attempt are victims also. They initially experience feelings of confusion, shock, or disbelief. Once they recover from the psychological impact of a loved one's death, feelings of guilt, grief, and possible rejection emerge. Postvention, a therapeutic program for bereaved survivors of suicide, allows family members or other survivors to vent their feelings at a time of such trauma. This program provides immediate contact with the survivors (within 24 hours) to assist them in coping with their feelings of shock and grief. This is the first phase of postvention. During the second phase, survivors are given the opportunity to develop new coping methods in an effort to prevent the development of maladaptive or destructive behavior. The survivor learns to cope with feelings of lowered self-esteem, depression, and the fear of developing a close interpersonal relationship. The third phase focuses on helping the survivors view the grief experience as a growth-promoting experience and ends on the first anniversary of the suicide.

Special attention should be given to children who are survivors because they are quite vulnerable to the death of a parent. They may feel that they caused the death by "wishing mommy dead" or "telling mommy I hate her." As a result of such feelings, children may be unable to work through the grieving process, become preoccupied with the subject of suicide, develop self-destructive behavior, exhibit signs of depression, or have difficulty working through the developmental tasks of childhood.

Carr suggests that the following interventions are helpful as preventive and postventive measures with children who are survivors:

Allow the child to express feelings.

Assist the child in the development of a meaningful relationship with others.

Encourage the development of positive coping skills.

Teach the child assertiveness.

Allow the child to develop ideas and values.

Expose the child to courses on psychological principles and human behavior in the educational process.

Examples of nursing diagnoses and nursing interventions pertaining to the self-destructive person follow.

NURSING DIAGNOSES	NURSING INTERVENTIONS
Potential for injury: Self-destructive behavior due to the inability to cope with stress, feelings of guilt, and so forth	Determine the degree of suicidal intent or potential by noting any previous suicide attempts and asking the patient if he has a plan for suicide.
	Institute the appropriate suicide precautions by providing a safe environment, observing the patient's behavior, and maintaining close supervision.
	Explain suicide precautions to the patient
	Secure a suicide contract with the patient to seek out staff if thoughts of suicide occur.
	Provide for a one-to-one contact so that the patient is able to recognize, ventilate, and accept his feelings.
	Reinforce healthy coping mechanisms.
	Explore new coping mechanisms.
	Discuss alternatives to suicide.
Social isolation	Convey acceptance, interest, and a caring attitude.
	Provide opportunities for the patient to spend short periods with another person daily by assigning a staff member to seek out the patient for a one-to-one interaction.
	Assess the patient's response to a one-to-one relationship and gradually encourage him to participate in small-group activities.
	Explore support systems available to the patient.
	Mobilize social support systems.
Disturbance in self-concept: Feelings of worthlessness	Accept the patient for who he is.
	Convey a caring attitude.
	Encourage ventilation of feelings.
	Point out positive aspects about the patient (*e.g.*, his vocation, family, or accomplishments).
	Provide opportunity for the person to succeed in simple or minor tasks so that he will receive positive feedback and a sense of worth for his achievements.
	Avoid judgmental statements about self-destructive behavior.

SUMMARY

Suicide, one of the ten leading causes of death in the United States, often occurs as the result of intense feelings of anxiety, depression, anger, or hostility. Statistics pertaining to suicide were presented, as well as causative factors or motives for self-destructive behavior. Examples of persons considered to be at risk were cited such as persons living alone, adolescents, the elderly, the chronic or terminally ill, and psychotic persons. Hatton, Valente, and Rink's method of assessing a person's degree of suicidal risk was presented. Misconceptions about suicide were explored. Medical treatment of self-destructive behavior was discussed, focusing on identifying the potential suicide patient, assessing the patient for any biologic or organic cause of depression, evaluating the person's intent on suicide, maintaining an open communication system, prescribing antidepressant medication, consulting mental health care professionals, and hospitalizing the person for protective care if necessary. Nursing interventions described include primary, secondary, and tertiary prevention, as well as crisis intervention. The importance of self-assessment or autognosis was stressed. Behavioral clues pertaining to self-destructive behavior were cited. A discussion of the suicidal intention rating scale was included, focusing on nursing interventions appropriate for each rating. A detailed explanation of protective care for strict suicide precaution was given. Nursing measures, pertaining to the person removed from suicide precautions, were explained. Postvention, a therapeutic program for bereaved survivors of suicide, was described, with special attention given to children who are survivors. Examples of nursing interventions for the following nursing diagnoses were discussed: potential for injury due to self-destructive behavior, social isolation, and disturbance in self-concept due to feelings of worthlessness.

LEARNING ACTIVITIES

I. Clinical activities
  A. If possible, establish a therapeutic relationship with a suicidal patient.
  B. Rate the patient's suicidal ideation.
  C. Describe the type of protective care the patient is receiving.
  D. Using the nursing process, plan nursing care for the patient.
II. Independent activities
  A. Identify what makes you feel happy and sad.
  B. How do you cope with sad or depressed feelings?
  C. State what you do to cheer yourself up.
  D. List one or two situations in your life that caused you to be depressed. Why and for how long did you feel depressed?

E. Discuss the effect of weather and music on your mood.

F. Make a list of those things you like best about yourself and state why you like those things.

G. Identify agencies in your community that provide support for persons contemplating suicide.

SELF-TEST

1. State the classifications of clues to suicidal behavior and give examples of each.

2. List five causative factors that may lead to suicide.

3. State five categories of people considered to be at risk or prone to self-destructive behavior.

4. Discuss three misconceptions about suicide.

5. State the rationale for autognosis or self-assessment when working with suicidal patients.

6. State the purpose of the assessment process when admitting a self-destructive person to the hospital.

7. Explain the rationale for strict suicidal precautions.

8. List in detail those nursing interventions included in strict suicidal precautions.

9. Describe nursing care measures employed once a patient has gained control over self destructive behavior.

10. Describe the three phases of postvention for survivors or victims of a successful suicide attempt.

11. List nursing interventions for
Social isolation
Disturbance in self-concept

REFERENCES

Altrocchi J: Abnormal Behavior. New York, Harcourt Brace Jovanovich, 1980

Bailey D, Dreyer S: Care of the Mentally Ill. Philadelphia, FA Davis, 1977

Barry D: Psychosocial Nursing Assessment and Intervention. Philadelphia, JB Lippincott, 1984

Carmack B: Suspect a suicide? Don't be afraid to act. RN: Apr, 1983

Carr EG: The motivation of self-injurious behavior: A review of some hypotheses. Psychological Bulletin, 1977

Clifford RH, Thompson ML: Depression suicide attempt/chronic. Case Studies of Nursing Intervention. New York, McGraw–Hill, 1974

Colt G: Suicide in America. Reader's Digest: Febr, 1984

Diran O: You can prevent suicide. Nurs 76: Jan, 1976

DiVasto P et al: A framework for the emergency evaluation of the suicidal patient. J Psych Nurs: June, 1979

Donlon P, Rockwell D: Psychiatric Disorders: Diagnoses and Treatment. Englewood Cliffs, Prentice–Hall Publishing, 1982

Durkheim E: Suicide: A Study in Sociology. Glencoe, Gum Tree Press, 1951

Farberow N, Shneidman E: The Cry for Help. New York, McGraw–Hill, 1961

Grollman EA: Suicide: Prevention, Intervention and Postvention. Boston, Beacon Press, 1971

Haber J et al: Comprehensive Psychiatric Nursing. New York, McGraw–Hill, 1982

Hafen BQ, Peterson B: Preventing adolescent suicide. Nurs 83: Oct, 1983

Hart N, Keidel G: The suicidal adolescent. Am J Nurs: 1979

Hatton D et al: Suicide Assessment and Intervention. New York, Appleton–Century–Crofts, 1977

Hoff LA: People in Crises. Menlo Park, Addison–Wesley, 1978

Hoff LA, Resing M: Was this suicide preventable? Am J Nurs: July, 1982

Loughlin SN: Suicide: A case for investigation. J Psych Nurs: Febr, 1980

Mellencamp A: Adolescent depression: A review of the literature with the implications for nursing care. J Psych Nurs: Sept, 1981

O'Roark MA: The alarming rise in teenage suicide. McCall's Magazine: Jan, 1982

Reubin R: Spotting and stopping the suicide patient. Nurs 79: Apr, 1979

Rowe CJ: An Outline of Psychiatry. Dubuque, William Brown Co, 1980

Schneider JS: Hopelessness and helplessness. J Psych Nurs: Mar, 1980

Schneidman E: Voices of Death. New York, Harper & Row, 1980

Schultz J, Dark S: Manual of Psychiatric Nursing Care Plans. Boston, Little, Brown & Co, 1982

U.S. Department of Health and Human Services: Suicide Prevention: The Challenge for Nurses (pamphlet). Washington, DC, National Institute of Health Publication No. 82–2308, August, 1981

Wilson H, Kneisl C: Psychiatric Nursing, 2nd ed. Menlo Park, Addison–Wesley, 1983

25

IMPAIRED THOUGHT

PROCESSES:

SCHIZOPHRENIC

DISORDERS

LEARNING OBJECTIVES

1. List etiologic theories regarding the development of schizophrenic disorders.

2. Identify symptoms relevant to schizophrenia.

3. Differentiate between primary and secondary symptoms of schizophrenia.

4. Differentiate the five specific types of schizophrenic disorders by symptoms and developmental level of onset.

5. Differentiate between schizophrenic and schizophreniclike disorders.

6. Describe modes of treatment to aid the schizophrenic person with adaptation to stress.

7. State the rationale for the use of limit setting for overly aggressive behavior.

8. Describe therapeutic nursing intervention when planning care for patients with schizophrenia.

T HE following is an account of a hypothetical article that could have appeared in a local newspaper. The headline reads

LOCAL MAN GOES WILD IN SHOPPING CENTER

A local man was apprehended by police in Macy's Department Store Wednesday evening following an outburst of bizarre behavior.

According to a salesclerk, Robert Hayden, 25, was Christmas shopping when he suddenly began to accuse her of stealing his wallet and keys.

Before he was subdued by security, Hayden seized and opened several packages, examined them, and then threw the packages across the store, breaking several items. Hayden stated that he would get even with the people who were spying on him and trying to steal his personal property.

As he was led away by the police, the disheveled-looking Hayden stated that voices told him not to trust anyone. He has since been admitted to the local receiving hospital for psychiatric evaluation.

Actions similar to those described in the article may be indicative of psychotic behavior. Such a person has difficulty recognizing reality, and with communicating and relating to others. This behavior generally occurs because the person is no longer able to cope with or handle the demands of life.

One type of psychotic behavior is schizophrenia. Schizophrenic disorder, a more technically accurate term than schizophrenia, is considered to be a serious psychiatric disorder, which tends to be chronic and generally leads to severe disability. The main characteristics include impaired communication, with loss of contact with reality and deterioration from a previous level of functioning in work, social relations, or self-care. There is also a disturbance of language, thought process, perception, and affect or mood, lasting longer than 6 months. Onset of symptoms occurs before age 45.

Although schizophrenia occurs in approximately only 1% of the population, it continues to be a major health problem and occurs equally among men and women. According to Rowe (1980) approximately 2 million Americans suffered from schizophrenia in 1980. Freedman, Kaplan, and Sadock (1981) stated that in 1976 between 460,000 and 940,000 people required treatment yearly for schizophrenia. Approximately 150,000 new cases of schizophrenia occur yearly in the United States. One fourth of all hospital beds are occupied by schizophrenics.

THEORIES OF SCHIZOPHRENIA

Several theories have been proposed regarding the etiology or psychodynamics of schizophrenia although the exact cause has not been identified. A brief summary of the theories follows.

Psychological or Experiential Theory

Proponents of this most common theory state that schizophrenia develops early in life because of various stressors. Among these are poor mother–child relationships, deeply disturbed family interpersonal relationships, impaired sexual identity and body image, rigid concept of reality, and repeated exposure to double-bind situations. A double-bind situation is a "no-win" experience in which there is no correct choice. An example might be when a mother tells a child who is dressed in good clothes that he may go out and play but not get dirty. At the same time, the mother's body language conveys the message that she prefers that the child stay indoors. The child does not know which message to follow.

The following is an example of a home situation that could contribute to the development of schizophrenia if therapeutic intervention does not occur.

A 10-year-old boy lives with his parents, two siblings and an invalid grandmother. The mother works full-time and, because of physical disability, is unable to do the housework. The grandmother is unable to help with daily chores so the children are expected to help with various tasks such as sweeping, cleaning, ironing, and emptying the garbage. If the work is not done to the mother's satisfaction, the children are punished physically and are made to forfeit various privileges.

The mother does not communicate well with other family members. When she arrives home from work, she generally complains about work and the condition of the house. The children have learned to avoid her as much as possible.

The father is a traveling salesman and does not spend much time with the children. When the father is home, he and his wife argue about finances and disciplining the children. Because he is gone frequently, the

10-year-old boy has not had a father figure with whom he can identify. He has begun to show an interest in cooking and plays with dolls.

The mother and grandmother do not get along well. Both try to outdo each other with various somatic or physical complaints.

The boy has begun to withdraw to his room whenever his parents argue or his mother complains about the housework due to his fear of punishment. On occasion he has soiled his bed while sleeping and has resorted to babytalk.

Biologic Theory

Theorists have listed at least two subtitles under the biologic theory: these are genetic and biochemical predisposition to schizophrenic disorders.

The genetic (or hereditary) predisposition suggests that children of schizophrenic parents are more apt to develop schizophrenia than are other persons. Approximately 40% of children born to parents who are both schizophrenic will be affected. If only one parent is schizophrenic, approximately 10% of the children will be psychotic.

The biochemical or toxic psychosis theory lists possible contributive factors to the onset of schizophrenia. Substances similar to hallucinogens or mind-altering drugs, which accumulate excessively in the body and cause an elevated level of dopamine is a possible factor being considered. According to the theory, excessive dopamine allows nerve impulses to bombard the brain, resulting in schizophrenic symptoms. The administration of antipsychotic medication supposedly blocks the excessive release of dopamine. The cause of the release of high levels of dopamine has not yet been found.

Environmental or Sociocultural Theory

Theorists state that the person who develops schizophrenia has a faulty reaction to the environment and is unable to respond selectively to numerous social stimuli. Theorists also believe that persons who come from low socioeconomic areas or broken homes in deprived areas do not have the chance to experience achievement. An example of this theory can be seen in the following situation.

An 8-year-old girl lives in a two-room apartment infested with rats and roaches. Her mother, who is unwed, is on welfare and receives Aid for Dependent Children to support 6 children. The young girl is expected to babysit three younger children while her mother seeks employment and goes shopping for groceries. Consequently, she has missed much schooling and has been retained in the first grade for another year. Her occasional playmates consist of a 5-year-old boy and a 7-year-old girl, both of whom are also deprived children.

In response to this faulty environment, the young girl has learned to fantasize and to create her own playworld. She has created her own language so that others do not learn about her secret world. If this behavior continues without therapeutic intervention, the young girl could be presenting clinical symptoms suggestive of the development of schizophrenia.

Organic Theory

Those who suggest the organic theory offer hope that schizophrenia is a functional deficit, occurring in the brain and caused by such stressors as infection, poison, trauma, or abnormal substances. They also propose that schizophrenia may be a metabolic disorder.

Vitamin Deficiency Theory

The vitamin deficiency theory suggests that persons who are deficient in vitamin B, namely B_1, B_6, B_{12}, and vitamin C may become schizophrenic as a result of a severe deficiency.

Although this theory, as well as other theories, has not been confirmed, research continues in hope of isolating a chemical that might be responsible for the development of schizophrenia.

CLINICAL SYMPTOMS

DSM-III classification lists five classifications of schizophrenic disorder: disorganized, catatonic, paranoid, undifferentiated, and residual. Four other psychotic disorders classified as schizophreniclike disorders are schizophreniform disorder, brief reactive psychosis, schizoaffective disorder, and atypical psychosis. The five classifications of schizophrenic disorders will be discussed in this chapter as well as schizophreniclike disorders.

Although schizophrenia occurs between the ages of 15 and 45, some theorists feel the onset is diagnosed primarily between the ages of 17 and 27. Presenting clinical symptoms of schizophrenic disorder are listed as primary and secondary.

Bleuler developed the "4 As," which are considered primary symptoms. They include:

1. *Associative disturbance or looseness:* Associative disturbance is a thought disorder in which the person does not think logically. The ideas expressed have little, if any, connection. Ideas shift from one subject to another and cannot be followed by the listener. "Three ships are sailing. I like to swim. Look at the airplane" is an example of associative disturbance.

2. *Affective disturbance or inappropriate mood:* The person lacks the ability to show appropriate emotional response. Affect is described as inappropriate, flat, or blunt. An example of inappropriate affect occurs when a person laughs during a sad movie. A monotonous voice and expressionless face are examples of flat affect. Blunting refers to a reduction in the intensity of expression.

3. *Autism:* Autism is a thought process defined as a retreat from reality. The person feels unrelated to others or to the environment. Preoccupation with illogical ideas, fantasizing, and daydreaming are examples of autistic behavior. The person appears to be emotionally detached from others and lives in his own world.

4. *Ambivalence:* Ambivalence is described as experiencing contradictory or opposing emotions, attitudes, ideas, or desires for the same person, thing, or situation. The classic example is loving and hating someone at the same time.

Secondary symptoms were also identified by Bleuler. They include:

1. *Delusions:* A delusion is defined as a false or fixed belief that cannot be changed by logic. Delusions generally are classified according to thought content (*e.g.,* persecutory, grandiose, or religious). A person who believes she is the Queen of England is exhibiting a grandiose delusion. Someone with a religious delusion might believe that he is John the Baptist or that God has sent him on a specific journey to fulfill a prophecy. A persecutory delusion is experienced when a person believes that someone is spying on him or wants to harm him.

2. *Illusions:* An illusion occurs when a person falsely interprets or perceives a real environmental stimulus. It may involve any of the senses. An example of a visual illusion is looking at the moon on a clear night and seeing the "man-in-the-moon." Baking a cake and claiming that it smells like burning rubbish is an example of an olfactory illusion.

3. *Hallucinations:* Hallucinations are false perceptions without an external or environmental stimulus and can involve any of the senses. They occur while a person is awake but can occur in a delirious state. Substance abusers have experienced visual and tactile hallucinations while withdrawing from the influence of drugs. They have described seeing snakes coming out of the walls and feeling insects crawling over their bodies. Hearing voices telling one to seek revenge is an example of an auditory hallucination. A person who hallucinates is unable to discern that a hallucination is a created, not a real, perception. He does not view the world as it really is nor does he interact with it in normally acceptable behavior.

Other clinical symptoms may include

1. Loss of ego boundaries or the loss of one's identity. The individual is disturbed about his sense of self. He feels that he is unable to control his life.

2. Inadequate ability, interest, or drive to complete a task. The person may lose interest in his job, neglect personal hygiene, or be incapable of carrying out tasks as part of a daily routine. He may appear disheveled, dirty, or inappropriately dressed.

3. Impaired reaction to the environment resulting in withdrawal, or psychomotor behavior (*e.g.,* pacing, rocking, spinning, or repeated ritualistic behavior).

4. Mood swings, in which the person exhibits various emotions such as anger, anxiety, and depression, without any obvious reason for such behavior.

5. Unfounded somatic or bodily complaints (hypochondriacal)

6. Change in appetite. The person may lose interest in eating, display bizarre eating habits, or become overly concerned about food.

Three phases have been used to describe the development of schizophrenic disorders. The earliest phase of development is the *prodromal* phase, characterized by symptoms such as a deterioration in a previous level of functioning, bizarre or peculiar behavior, disturbed communication and social withdrawal. The *active* or second phase is characterized by the psychotic symptoms described by Bleuler. The *residual* or third phase is said to occur when the psychotic symptoms lessen in intensity.

Full recovery is possible; however, schizophrenic patients usually experience remissions (partial disappearance of clinical symptoms) and exacerbations (increase in seriousness or intensity of the clinical symptoms).

Symptoms of schizophrenia will be presented with the specific clinical types. Terminology related to psychosis is discussed at the end of this chapter under learning activities.

CLINICAL TYPES OF SCHIZOPHRENIA

Disorganized Type

The classification of disorganized type (previously called hebephrenic) is considered to be the most severe type of personality disorganization. Clinical symptoms occur because the person is unable to complete a transition from adolescence to maturity, thereby contributing to an early onset. Clinical symptoms include

1. Blunted, inappropriate, or silly emotions such as giggling or superficial sadness. An example would be to laugh when told someone had just been involved in a serious accident.

2. Incoherence or the inability to make sense or be understood when talking. The person appears to be mumbling words rather than speaking clearly.

3. Regression to an earlier developmental level even to the point of enuresis (bedwetting) or encopresis (fecal soiling).

4. Hypochondriasis, or being preoccupied with the condition of one's body. The person has an unrealistic interpretation of physical signs or symptoms, fearing that a disease is present.

5. Hallucinations and delusions that are not well organized

6. Absence of systematized or logically defined delusions

7. Extreme social withdrawal

The prognosis is poor, and a chronic condition is generally seen.

Disorganized Type: Clinical Example

MJ, a 19-year-old waitress, was seen in the admitting office of a psychiatric hospital. During the initial interview, she giggled inappropriately. Her long, uncombed hair fell over her face, concealing her facial expressions. She mumbled incoherently at times and displayed the behavior of a 13- or 14-year-old adolescent. She complained of numerous aches and pains and stated that voices told her she was being punished for not cleaning her room. MJ's mother stated that she remained in her room at home and did not socialize with friends. Her parents sought help when they noticed her behavior regressing during the past 2 months.

Because of the young age of most patients diagnosed as schizophrenic disorder, disorganized type, student reactions vary from shock to disbelief. They may identify with the patient who is close to their age or resembles someone that they know. This reaction could interfere with the development of a therapeutic relationship. Such feelings should be shared and explored with the clinical instructor.

Once the initial reaction has been examined and resolved, nursing care can be initiated based on the assessment of the patient. With a patient such as MJ, who mumbles and giggles inappropriately owing to feelings of discomfort or inadequacy, communication must be established. Reality should be stressed when the patient discusses the voices that talk to her (see nursing interventions for hallucinations at the end of the chapter).

A physical examination should be done within 24 hours to rule out any organic cause. Once the results are known, reality can be stressed if the patient continues to complain. Limit setting may be used to discourage complaints by refusing to discuss somatic concerns with the patient if there is no pathologic basis for the complaints. Regressive behavior occurs as the patient reverts to a more comfortable developmental stage to decrease feelings of anxiety. Social withdrawal occurs as the patient becomes preoccupied with thoughts and fantasies. (Nursing interventions for regression and withdrawal are discussed at the end of the chapter.)

Catatonic Type

Catatonic schizophrenia is differentiated from other types of schizophrenic disorders mainly by behavioral or psychomotor symptoms. Symptoms include

1. Abnormal or catatonic posturing, in which the person voluntarily assumes an unusual or bizarre position.

2. Catatonic stupor or withdrawal from the environment. Expressionless, the patient may stare into space. A decrease in spontaneous movements also may be noted, in which the person lies, sits, or stands still for long periods of time. Although the patient appears nonresponsive, he may still be in contact with the environment and aware of all that is happening. Catatonic patients have recalled detailed experiences after recovering from the stupor.

3. Catatonic rigidity. The patient will assume a position and will not move when efforts are made to change the position.

4. Catatonic negativism. The patient who is catatonic is resistant to all instructions or attempts to be moved.

5. Catatonic excitement. The person responds to stimuli from within and becomes extremely agitated. Movements may be purposeless or stereotyped. Such a person is to be considered potentially aggressive and capable of assault during this state.

6. Unexpected shifts from one behavioral state to another may occur.

7. Waxy flexibility. The person will maintain the position in which he has been placed.

8. Two mannerisms occasionally exhibited by the catatonic patient are *echolalia* (repeats all words or phrases heard) and *echopraxia* (mimics actions of others).

The sudden onset of catatonic behavior usually occurs between the ages of 15 and 25 and is short in duration. Statistics show that more females than males are diagnosed as catatonic schizophrenics. The prognosis is good for an acute state but many patients have recurrent episodes.

Catatonic Type: Clinical Example

CS, a 25-year-old engineer, was admitted to the hospital as a result of dehydration because of refusing to eat. During his hospitalization, CS was negativistic, refusing nursing care, food, and medication. He rarely spoke and assumed uncomfortable positions in bed for long periods. When placed in various positions by the nurse during the morning bath or shower, CS remained in the positions until they were changed by the nurse. He also exhibited purposeless movements of his hands and feet while sitting in the chair.

The student nurse's reactions to catatonic behavior generally consist of fear and frustration. Fear of unpredictable, abnormal behavior is a normal response that results in the exercise of caution when one is working with catatonic patients. Frustration is heightened when the patient exhibits negativistic behavior such as the refusal to eat or nonresponsiveness to the environment.

Basic human needs must be monitored to ensure adequate nutrition, elimination, activity, and rest. The patient may need to be protected during periods of unpredictable agitated behavior. (Nursing interventions for agitation are discussed at the end of this chapter.)

Paranoid Type

The main behavior identified in the paranoid schizophrenic is that of suspiciousness. Clinical symptoms include

1. Overuse of the defense mechanism projection. The person may blame others for failures in his life or his illness, or believe that people are talking about him because they do not like him. (Refer to *ideas of reference* in vocabulary list at the end of the chapter.)

2. Hostility and aggressiveness or violence. The person may display impulsive, hostile behavior to defend himself against suspected harm. Violence may be the result of auditory hallucinations (voices telling him to act in a certain way).

3. Argumentative behavior. Paranoid individuals are very defensive and prone to arguing owing to their suspicious nature.

4. Auditory hallucinations, which are persecutory or grandiose. The paranoid patient may state that voices are telling him he must die or that a specific person is going to harm him. While experiencing a grandiose auditory hallucination, the patient may state that the President of the United States has asked him to attend the Inaugural Ball, for example.

5. Delusions of grandeur, persecution, jealousy, or religion. Examples of delusions were cited earlier. The delusions of the paranoid schizophrenic are usually mystical and less organized than those seen in a patient with the paranoid disorder, paranoia.

6. Doubts about gender identity; that is, the patient may question his or her masculinity or femininity.

The onset of paranoid schizophrenia is usually seen in later adult life between the ages of 30 to 35 but can occur at any age.

Paranoid Type: Clinical Example

BW, a 35-year-old mechanic, was brought to the admissions office by his wife because he had exhibited strange behavior for several months. He accused his wife of poisoning his food, spending all his money, having an affair with his boss, and telling stories about him. He displayed no facial expressions during his initial interview and became quite argumentative when questioned about his job. At the end of the interview, BW confided in the interviewer that he had been receiving messages from Jesus Christ while watching television.

It is not unusual for the student nurse to react to the paranoid patient with feelings of fear because of his hostile, aggressive, argumentative, or unpredictable behavior. It is difficult to communicate with a patient who expresses a delusion or talks about hearing voices. Nursing interventions for the paranoid schizophrenic focus on behaviors such as suspiciousness, hostility, and aggression. These are discussed at the end of the chapter.

Residual Type

As stated earlier, the residual type can be described as the state of being in partial remission. The patient diagnosed as residual type has a history of one previous schizophrenic episode but no longer exhibits obvious or intense psychotic symptoms. He may exhibit clinical symptoms of social withdrawal, associative looseness, illogical thinking, or eccentric behavior. If the person is experiencing delusions or hallucinations, they are not readily discernible.

UNDIFFERENTIATED TYPE

This category is used for a person who exhibits a mixture of psychotic symptoms such as delusions, hallucinations, or grossly disorganized behavior, and cannot be classified in any of the other categories. The acute undifferentiated type is characterized by a sudden onset. Chronic undifferentiated type refers to symptoms of long standing.

The following is a clinical example of a patient diagnosed as schizophrenic disorder, acute undifferentiated type:

AB, a 52-year-old carpenter, was making a rocking chair in his workshop when he suddenly began to talk to the television set. When his wife stopped by to bring him supper she was shocked to find the rocking chair broken and the tools scattered on the floor. Her husband was huddled in the corner, curled up like a small child, talking to himself and singing Christmas carols. At times he mumbled incoherently. When Mrs. B attempted to talk to him, her husband did not recognize her or know where he was.

The more acute or sudden the onset of schizophrenic disorder, the more favorable is the prognosis. The earlier in life psychotic symptoms develop, the less favorable the prognosis.

SCHIZOPHRENICLIKE DISORDERS

The three subclassifications of schizophreniclike disorders are 1) schizoaffective disorders, 2) schizophreniform disorder, and 3) brief reactive psychosis.

The schizoaffective disorder is characterized by either depression or elation as well as the psychotic symptoms of schizophrenia and major affective disorders. Clinical symptoms of major affective disorders include behaviors auch as hyperactivity, euphoria, depression, pressure of speech, loss of interest, sleep disturbance, and loss of appetite (refer to Chap. 23 for a more detailed list of symptoms). The person presenting this diagnosis has a better prognosis than does the schizophrenic patient.

The diagnosis of schizophreniform disorder is used when the person exhibits features of schizophrenia for more than 1 week but less than 6 months.

Brief reactive psychosis may be seen when a person exhibits clinical symptoms of illogical thinking, incoherent speech, delusions, hallucinations, or disorganized behavior after psychological trauma (*e.g.,* the death of a loved one or an admission to an intensive care unit). Duration of symptoms is a few hours to 1 week. Shirley's article "ICU Psychosis: Helping Your Patient Return to Reality" in the January issue of *Nursing '82* is an excellent article depicting brief reactive psychosis.

TREATMENT

Four treatment modalities have been identified as being effective when treating the schizophrenic patient. The selection of the treatment modality depends upon the type of schizophrenic disorder and the severity of the psychotic behavior. All four modalities may be combined at one time. They are

1. *Psychotherapy:* Individual, group, behavioral, supportive, or family therapy may be used. Selection of the specific type of therapy depends on presenting clinical symptoms, the person's ability to communicate, and the relationship with the family. The therapist also will evaluate whether the patient will benefit more from an individual or a group approach.

2. *Milieu therapy:* A structured environment is used to minimize environmental and physical stress and to meet the individual needs of the patient until he is able to assume responsibility for himself.

3. *Chemotherapy:* Antipsychotic drugs or major tranquilizers (*e.g.,* Haldo, Stelazine, Mellaril, Prolixin, and Navane) may be prescribed. The choice of drug will depend on the presenting symptoms, patient's tolerance and response to the drug, and the expected outcome as a result of drug therapy. If the patient is acutely disturbed, he may

require an injectable form of fluphenazine (Prolixin). The cost of the drug also must be considered because the patient may discontinue taking the drug if he can not afford it. Most schizophrenic patients receive drugs over an extended period and usually continue them after discharge from the hospital.

Antiparkinsonian agents may be prescribed to prevent or decrease the extrapyramidal side-effects of psychotropic drugs. (Examples of such drugs are Cogentin, Artane, Akineton, and Symmetrel.) Refer to the Chapter 7 for more information.

4. *Somatic or electroconvulsive therapy.* These therapies may be used as a treatment for severe schizophrenic disorders if the patient is unresponsive to trials of psychiatric medication. The use of electroconvulsive therapy has declined owing to the introduction of psychotropic drugs during the late 1950s and early 1960s.

Statistics indicate that approximately one third of the schizophrenic patients receiving treatment will improve, one third will not respond to treatment, and one third will maintain an unchanged condition.

NURSING INTERVENTIONS

The nurse must establish a therapeutic relationship so that she can communicate effectively with the patient. Communication should be in simple or easy-to-understand terms and should be directed at the patient's present level of functioning. Schizophrenic patients may refuse to communicate or may communicate ineffectively as a result of

1. Self-contradictory or conflicting statements
2. Frequent changes in subject
3. Inconsistency in verbalization
4. Talking in incomplete or fragmented sentences
5. Presence of hallucinations and delusions

The nurse must remember that all behavior is meaningful to the patient, if not to anyone else.

Assessment of the schizophrenic patient includes identifying behavioral problems such as regression, disorientation, withdrawal, agitation, and acting out. Assessment of the patient's ability to perform activities of daily living (ADL) and meet basic human needs is imperative to maintain life. The patient's physical condition also should be assessed to plan appropriate nursing interventions. Schizophrenic patients may be unable to feed themselves. They may refuse to eat because of paranoid thoughts, or may exhibit bizarre eating habits. Daily functions such as bathing, showering, and dressing may be overwhelming tasks requiring assistance.

Reality should be presented when caring for the patient who is disoriented. The nurse can do this by pointing out what would be appropriate behavior, that is, "I'd like you to put your shoes on now." Recognizing the presence of hallucinations and delusions, but not reinforcing such behavior or thoughts is an appropriate response when interacting with patients. The nurse should observe for precipitating factors causing hallucinations and attempt to intervene before they occur. The delusional system should be ignored.

Safety measures may need to be incorporated to protect the patient who displays poor judgment, disorientation, destructive behavior, suicidal ideation, or agitation. Limit setting, acknowledging spatial territory (giving the patient "room to breathe") and providing protective safety measures are examples of such nursing interventions. The patient must be protected from himself because he may injure himself accidently, or may try to destroy himself or attack other patients as a result of auditory hallucinations or paranoid ideations.

Efforts should be made to plan activities to increase the patient's self-concept. Sincere compliments should be given as often as possible, focusing on positive aspects of the person's personality or capabilities. Encourage participation in activities.

The nurse must observe for extrapyramidal side-effects of psychotropic drugs and monitor the patient's willingness to take the drugs. Patients may refuse to take medication, pretend to take medication by palming it, or pretend to swallow the medication while retaining the pill in the mouth (only to get rid of it at the first possible moment).

The following are examples of nursing diagnoses and interventions for patients with schizophrenic disorders.

NURSING DIAGNOSES	NURSING INTERVENTIONS
Sensory perceptual alteration: Disoriented to place and person, disoriented in time	Call the patient by name. Present reality when talking to or working with the patient. Keep a calendar in clear view to orientate the patient daily. Provide a protective, safe environment.
Social isolation: Withdrawal	Assign one member of the health care team to establish a one-to-one relationship. Provide a structured list of activities such as time to awaken, shower, and eat. Spend a specific amount of time daily with the patient. Set limits regarding amount of time spent alone in room.
Alteration in thought process: Delusional	Present reality when talking to or working with the patient. Ignore the delusion but do not attempt to disprove it or argue with the patient. Set limits by instructing the patient not to discuss the delusion with others.

(continued)

NURSING DIAGNOSES	NURSING INTERVENTIONS
Alteration in thought process: Hallucinations	Decrease environmental stimuli such as loud music or television shows, extremely bright colors, or flashing lights. Present reality; for example, "The voices may be real to you but I don't hear anything." Attempt to identify precipitating factors by asking the patient what happened before the onset of the hallucination.
Ineffective individual coping: Regression	Assess the patient's present developmental level. State expected behavior to the patient. Set limits to discourage regressive behavior.
Dysrhythmia of sleep–rest activity: Agitation and unpredictable behavior	Recognize signs of increasing agitation. Decrease environmental stimuli that could be upsetting to the patient. Attempt to "talk down" the patient; give the patient an opportunity to verbalize his feelings. Administer p.r.n. medication to decrease agitation. Limit setting may be necessary to keep the patient within a confined area that is, seclusion or restraints.
Sensory perceptual alteration: Suspiciousness	Be sincere and honest when talking with the patient. Avoid making promises that cannot be fulfilled. Face the patient while talking. Avoid whispering or any other behavior that may cause the patient to feel that you are talking about him. Give detailed explanations of tests, procedures, and so forth to the patient. Allow the patient to help to prepare food or have food brought from home if he refuses to eat (because he thinks it is poisoned).

SUMMARY

Schizophrenic disorders are categorized into five clinical types according to the presence of psychotic behavior, including impaired communication, loss of contact with reality, and deterioration in function related to work, social relations, or self-care. The primary and secondary symptoms of psychosis developed by Bleuler also are used to describe these clinical types. The psychodynamics of schizophrenic disorders are considered a result of psychological, biologic, environmental, organic, or deficiency factors. The following clinical types of schizophrenic disorders were discussed: disorganized, catatonic, paranoid, residual, and undifferentiated. The three subclassifications of schizophrenic like disorders also were described. These are schizoaffective disorder, schizophreniform disorder, and brief reactive psychosis. The four treatment modalities for schizophrenia presented are psychotherapy, milieu therapy, chemotherapy, and somatic therapy. Nursing diagnoses and interventions were presented, focusing on abnormal behavior, impaired communication, and impaired thought processes.

LEARNING ACTIVITIES

I. Clinical activities
   A. Begin a relationship with a person experiencing schizophrenia.
   B. Identify any primary and secondary symptoms that the patient exhibits.
   C. Identify examples of symptoms included on the terminology sheet.
   D. List the therapies used and discuss the patient's responses.
   E. Identify any antipsychotic drugs prescribed. State the rationale for their use; observe for side-effects; evaluate effectiveness.
   F. Identify nursing interventions used in caring for the patient.

II. Schizophrenia: Situations for discussion
   A. JW, 58 years old, has been admitted to the psychiatric unit and diagnosed as schizophrenic, paranoid type. He blames his wife for his losing his job and states his employer "bugged" his telephone in the office. He confides in you that he "sees" Jesus frequently and that Jesus tells him everything is okay. JW keeps to himself and rarely shows any emotion.
      1. Name the defense mechanisms that JW is using.
      2. List the primary and secondary symptoms present.
      3. List the behaviors JW displays.
      4. State the appropriate nursing interventions in response to this behavior.
   B. MC has been admitted to the hospital with the diagnosis of schizophrenia, undifferentiated type. She is hostile, aggressive, and verbally abusive. She tells you she hears voices, acts inappropriately at times, and is regressive in her behavior. She tells you her "phillies have covered the thung."
      1. Why is the patient diagnosed as undifferentiated schizophrenia?
      2. List all symptoms, including primary and secondary symptoms.
      3. State the nursing problems presented by MC.
      4. List the appropriate nursing interventions.

III. Terminology related to psychosis

The following is a list of terminology related to psychosis not identified in the chapter on schizophrenic disorders.

Apathy: Devoid of feeling, emotion, interest or concern. A patient
may show a lack of interest when visited by relatives.

Automatic obedience: An impaired thought process in which one
does what one is told to do. The person responds to commands or
suggestions similar to a dog who has attended obedience school. He
does not appear to have a free will to act independently.

Blocking: Sudden loss of thought content due to an anxiety-
producing situation

Clang association: A speech pattern characterized by the use of a
series of sound-alike or rhyming words without regard to logic. May
be used to compensate for defects in memory or communication. The
sound of a word sets off a new train of thought.

Déjà vu (French for "already seen"): The sensation that a new situation has occurred previously

Depersonalization: Feelings of unreality or strangeness of self or the
environment, a sense of not being one's self

Dissociation: A coping mechanism used to protect oneself from
uncomfortable feelings by denying their existence

Echolalia: Repetition of another person's words or phrases (*e.g.,* a
parrot mimicking a person's spoken word). Echolalia is seen in catatonic schizophrenia.

Echopraxia: Repetition or imitation of another person's movements
(seen in catatonic schizophrenia).

Feelings of estrangement: The person feels detached or removed from
people, the environment, or concepts.

Flight of ideas: Ideas or thoughts occur quickly and are so fragmentary that no single thought can be expressed clearly (*e.g.,* "I like
money. Money is the root of all evil. Evil things have happened
lately.")

Folie à deux: Two closely related or associated persons, usually in the
same family, share psychopathologic conditions that are nearly
identical.

Ideas of reference: A person feels or believes that conversation and
gestures occurring around him have meaning intended especially for
him (*i.e.,* a patient observing nurses giving report at the change of
shift says, "They're plotting against me").

Neologisms: Coining or forming new words to express a complex idea

Word salad: Severe associative looseness characterized by meaningless and incoherent mixtures of words and phrases (*i.e.,* "Sky is a blue rainbow my father's barrel.")

IV. Independent activity

    A. Read "What to do when your patient lets slip his grip on reality" by Barbara Clark (Nurs 84: July, 1984).

    B. Review CEU test offering immediately following the article to test your knowledge base of delusions, hallucinations, and illusions.

SELF-TEST

1. The most common theory regarding the cause of schizophrenia is known as the _____ theory.

2. "I love him but can't stand him" is an example of _____.

3. "See that tree. I like coke. Up in the air" is an example of _____.

4. "The gown is nice. Gowns are expensive. Expenses should be lowered. Lower that flag." is an example of _____.

5. Stating that the flag reminds one of America is an example of _____.

6. Coining words that are not understood by others is referred to as _____.

7. A category of schizophrenia referring to "in partial remission" is known as _____.

8. Abnormal posturing and stupor or mutism are clinical symptoms of what type of schizophrenia?

9. The disorganized type of schizophrenia is said to be a result of _____.

10. A person who presents a variety of symptoms not consistent with any specific category of schizophrenia would most likely be classified as what type of schizophrenia?

11. State three examples of nursing interventions for hallucinations.

12. List three nursing interventions for agitated behavior.

13. State Bleuler's four As or primary symptoms.

14. State three nursing interventions for withdrawal.

15. State two nursing interventions for delusional behavior.

16. List three psychotropic drugs used to treat schizophrenia.

REFERENCES

A Psychiatric Glossary, 5th ed. Washington, DC, American Psychiatric Association, 1980

Alman D: Sergeant Caulder thought he was a POW . . . we played along. Nurs 79: Febr, 1979

Arnold H: A guide to one-to-one relationships. Am J Nurs: June, 1976

Banes J: An ex-patient's perspective of psychiatric treatment. J Psych Nurs: Mar, 1983

Dreyer S, Bailey D, Doucet W: Nursing approaches to psychotic behavior disorders. In: Guide to Management of Psychiatric Patients. St. Louis, CV Mosby, 1979

Freedman et al: Modern Synopsis of Comprehensive Textbook of Psychiatry, 3rd ed. Baltimore, Williams & Wilkins, 1981

Green H: I Never Promised You a Rose Garden. New York, Holt, Rinehart & Winston, 1964

Hallucinations (filmstrip). Trainex

Harris E: Antipsychotic medications: Psychotropic drug therapy. Am J Nurs: July, 1981

King L: Schizophrenia/chronic. In Case Studies of Nursing Intervention. New York, McGraw–Hill, 1974

Kolb L: Modern Clinical Psychiatry. Philadelphia, WB Saunders, 1977

Koontz E: Schizophrenia: Current diagnostic concepts and implications for nursing care. J Psych Nurs: Sept, 1982

Lancaster J: Adult Psychiatric Nursing. New York, Medical Examination Publishing, 1980

Lynne L: Lisa and the 2:00 miracle. Nurs 80: May, 1980

Mereness D, Taylor C: Essentials of Psychiatric Nursing. St. Louis, CV Mosby, 1982

Rowe CJ: An Outline of Psychiatry. Dubuque, William Brown, 1980

Rubin T: Jordi: Lisa and David. New York, Ballantine Books, 1962

Schizophrenia (pamphlet). New York, Roerig (division of Pfizer Pharmaceuticals), 1972

Schizophrenia: The Role of Allied Health Professionals (pamphlet). New York, Roerig (division of Pfizer Pharmaceuticals), 1972

Schizophrenia (filmstrip). Trainex

Schmidt CS: Withdrawal behavior of schizophrenics: Application of Roy's model. J Psych Nurs: Nov, 1981

Schultz J, Dark S: Manual of Psychiatric Nursing Care Plans. Boston, Little, Brown & Co, 1982

Schwartzman S: The hallucinating patient and nursing intervention. In Backer B, Dubbert P, Eisenman E (eds.): Psychiatric/Mental Health Nursing: Contemporary Readings. New York, D. Van Nostrand, 1978

Sechehaye M: Autobiography of a Schizophrenic Girl. New York, Grune & Stratton, 1951

Shirley R: I.C.U. psychosis: Helping your patient return to reality. Nurs 82: Jan, 1982

Sills G, Wise D: The withdrawn client (film). New York, American Journal of Nursing

Story B: The catatonic schizophrenic and relationship therapy. J Psych Nurs: Mar 1978

Walker JI: Everybody's Guide to Emotional Well-being. San Francisco, GP Putnam & Sons, 1982

Wilson H, Kneisl C: Psychiatric Nursing, 2nd ed. Menlo Park, Addison–Wesley, 1983

26

DYSFUNCTION DUE TO

ORGANIC MENTAL

DISORDERS

LEARNING OBJECTIVES

1. Define organic mental disorder.
2. Differentiate between acute and chronic organic brain syndrome (OBS).
3. State the clinical features of
   Delirium
   Dementia
   Alzheimer's disease
4. Explain the purpose of the JOMAC assessment tool.
5. State diagnostic tests used to identify the precipitating cause of an organic mental disorder.
6. Cite short- and long-term nursing goals for a person with an organic mental disorder.
7. List nursing interventions for the following nursing diagnoses of a person with dementia:
   Alteration of thought process related to disorientation of person, place, and time
   Self-care deficit owing to loss of independent functions of bathing and dressing
   Alteration in thought process due to memory loss for recent information
   Potential for injury because of sensorimotor deficits of impaired vision and unstable gait

THIS broad general classification is used to categorize disorders due to transient or permanent brain dysfunction caused by a disturbance of physiologic functioning of brain tissue. DSM-III divides this classification into organic mental disorders in which the etiology or pathophysiologic process is due to certain neurologic diseases or direct effects of various substances on the nervous system, and organic mental disorders in which the etiology or physiologic process is known.

Organic mental disorders may occur at any age from mechanical, thermal, or chemical damage to the brain, from aging, or from physical disorders. The onset may be sudden or may occur over a period of time; can be steadily or irregularly progressive; may be temporary due to metabolic disorders, substance intoxication, or systemic illnesses; or may be permanent due to pathological processes causing structural brain damage.

No single description can characterize organic mental disorders because a wide variety of different emotional, motivational, and behavioral abnormalities may be seen. Associated features include anxiety, depression, irritability, paranoid attitudes, illusions, delusions, obsessions, compulsions, phobias, impairment (of judgment, orientation, memory, affect or cognition), and behavioral acting out.

The term *organic brain syndrome* (OBS) is used to refer to a cluster of signs and symptoms without reference to cause, whereas *organic mental disorder* designates a particular organic brain syndrome in which the etiology is presumed or known.

ORGANIC BRAIN SYNDROME

OBS may be acute or chronic. Acute brain syndromes are temporary, usually develop suddenly, can occur at any age, affect both sexes, and are characterized by impaired affect, orientation, memory, intellectual functioning and judgment. Physical symptoms are related to specific causative factors because any organic system may be affected. Recovery generally occurs, unless there are physical complications that are nonresponsive to treatment. Chronic brain syndromes are permanent or nonreversible. The onset is generally slow and subtle or insidious owing to various factors such as Alzheimer's disease, Huntington's chorea, and arteriosclerosis. The age of onset ranges from 40 to 70 years or later. Physical symptoms are related to etiology. Speech impairment such as dysphasia or slurred speech may be present. Mental symptoms may include poor concentration, poor judgment, memory loss, and confusion. Emotional symptoms such as depression, anger, delusions, irritability, lability, flat affect, loss of spontaneity, or temper outbursts may be seen. Chronic brain syndromes may result in intellectual and physical deterioration that progress over a period of years, reduced life expectancy, or death.

Six categories of OBSs are included in the DSM-III:

1. Delirium or acute brain syndrome, which develops rapidly, and dementia or chronic brain syndrome, which occurs gradually. Global cognitive impairment occurs in both syndromes

2. Amnesic syndrome and organic hallucinosis, in which cognition is impaired in relatively selective areas (*i.e.,* alcohol amnesic disorder due to vitamin deficiency and prolonged, heavy use of alcohol; Korsakoff's disease due to thiamine deficiency)

3. Organic delusional syndrome and organic affective syndrome, which resemble schizophrenic and affective disorders

4. Organic personality syndrome, characterized by emotional liability and impairment in impulse control or social judgment

5. Intoxication and withdrawal from ingestion or reduction in use of a substance that does not meet the criteria for any of the first four syndromes

6. Atypical or mixed OBS, which is a residual category for syndromes not classifiable in the previous syndromes

Three of the more common syndromes will be discussed: delirium, dementia, and Alzheimer's disease, a form of dementia.

Delirium

This disorder is considered to be a clouding of one's consciousness, accompanied by disorientation, memory impairment, and a decreased ability to focus, shift, or sustain attention to environmental stimuli. Irrelevant environmental stimuli may easily distract a person with a diagnosis of delirium. The person may misinterpret the environment or exhibit perceptual disturbances such as illusions or hallucinations. A disordered stream of thought may occur, resulting in speech that is limited, sparse, pressured, incoherent, or unpredictable. Lucid periods are more common in the morning as the individual appears more attentive and coherent.

Insomnia or daytime drowsiness often occurs along with a disturbance of the sleep–wake cycle, resulting in a stupor, semicoma, hypersomnolence, vivid dreams, or nightmares.

Persons with delirium are often restless, hyperactive, sluggish, or stuporous. Such psychomotor activity can shift abruptly from one extreme to another. *Asterixis,* an abnormal movement in which the patient exhibits a peculiar flapping movement of hyperextended hands, is seen in various delirious states.

Clinical features of delirium generally develop over a short period of time, tend to fluctuate on a daily basis, and usually last about a week or less.

Causative factors include systemic infections, metabolic disorders, postoperative states, cardiovascular disorders, substance intoxication or withdrawal, hypertensive encephalopathy, convulsive disorders, head trauma, frontal lesions of the right parietal lobe, postoperative complications, or sleep deprivation.

Diagnosis of delirium is based on evidence of a specific organic factor identified by a history, physical examination, or laboratory tests. DSM-III diagnostic criteria also state

1. Clouding of consciousness

2. At least two of the following: a) perceptual disturbance; b) incoherent speech at times; c) disturbance of sleep–wake cycle with insomnia or daytime drowsiness, or d) increased or decreased psychomotor activity

3. Disorientation and memory impairment

4. Clinical features develop within hours or days and fluctuate over the course of a day

Dementia

Dementia is a form of global or diffuse brain dysfunction that is characterized by a gradual, progressive, chronic deterioration of intellectual function. Judgment, orientation, memory, affect, emotional stability, cognition, and attention are affected either by a pattern of simple, gradual deterioration or by rapid, complicated deterioration. Impaired judgment, or the inability to make reasonable decisions, is one of the earliest signs of dementia and may occur in business dealings or social functions (*e.g.,* the person engages in a reckless business venture or displays a disregard for conventional rules of social conduct).

Disorientation to person, place, and time is one of the most common signs of brain dysfunction. The more extensive the dysfunction, the more severe the disorientation. A minimally impaired person may misjudge the date by weeks or months. Moderate impairment generally involves confusion about geographic location such as city or state as well as time, whereas severe impairment is demonstrated by disorientation with respect to time, place, and person. Short-term memory, attention, and concentration deficits are observable in this disorder since the person loses his train of thought, forgets what was said just a few minutes earlier, and may be unable to repeat the information just communicated.

Other characteristics or associated features include confabulation, perseveration, concrete thinking, and emotional lability. Confabulation is the filling-in of memory gaps with false but sometimes plausible content to conceal the memory deficit. Perseveration is the inappropriate continuation or repetition of a behavior such as giving the same details over and over even when told one is doing so. Abstraction skills are impaired; therefore, the person tends to think in concrete terms. The tendency to manifest rapid, inappropriate, exaggerated mood swings often occurs, and marked anxiety or depression may be seen in mild cases.

Personality changes are often seen in persons with dementia. The normally active person may become withdrawn and apathetic when social involvement narrows.

Although dementia may occur at any age, generally it is seen in elderly persons. The major causes of dementia are as follows: 1) Alzheimer's disease, 2) space-occupying lesions, 3) myxedema or other chronic endocrine disorders, 4) pernicious anemia, 5) central nervous system (CNS) infection, 6) brain trauma, 7) toxic–metabolic disturbances, 8) vascular disease such as multi-infarct dementia, and 9) neurologic diseases such as Huntington's chorea, Parkinson's disease, or multiple sclerosis.

Diagnostic criteria of dementia include

1. Loss of intellectual abilities, resulting in interference of social or occupational functioning

2. Memory impairment

3. At least one of the following: a) impaired abstract thinking; b) impaired judgment; c) disturbed higher cortical function, such as aphasia (loss of language comprehension or production), apraxia (loss

of ability to perform skilled motor acts), agnosia (ability to recognize objects), constructional difficulty (inability to copy three-dimensional figures, assemble blocks, or arrange sticks), or d) personality change.

4. Unclouded state of consciousness

5. One of the following: specific organic factor related to the disturbance or, in the absence of evidence from the history, physical examination, or laboratory tests, an organic factor can be presumed

Alzheimer's Disease (Primary Degenerative Dementia)

The presenile brain disease termed Alzheimer's disease is considered to be the fourth or fifth most common cause of death in the United States. It is *not* a natural course of aging, hardening of the arteries, an aftermath of a stroke, brought on by alcoholism, trauma, or overmedication, a depressed state, communicable, or curable. It *is* considered to be a silent epidemic that begins with a slight and easily dismissed flattening of personality characterized by confusion, restlessness, speech disturbances, withdrawal, decreased interest in hobbies, inability to carry out purposeful movements, and possible hallucinations. The person is aware of the loss of mental abilities as they occur. Sudden personality changes, violent flashes of anger, episodes of wandering, symptoms of paranoia, a stooped gait, loss of involuntary functions, and seizures all may occur.

Death can result from neglect, malnutrition, dehydration, incorrect diagnosis, inappropriate treatment, or suicide.

TREATMENT AND NURSING INTERVENTIONS

Assessment of persons with organic mental disorders is important especially in the early diagnostic phase. The interview and the assessment of judgment, orientation, memory, affect, and cognition (JOMAC) are essential. Lancaster (1980) lists the following aspects that also should be considered during the assessment process:

1. Intellectual ability, past and present

2. Changes in personality (*i.e.,* depression, irritability, loss of interest, and decrease or loss of interest in personal appearance)

3. Past and present health status

4. Any evidence of confabulation, negativistic behavior, perseveration, feigning deafness, projection, or rationalization for lack of appropriate response

5. Ability to provide self-care

A variety of diagnostic tests are used to identify the precipitating cause of organic mental disorders. Following a complete history and physical examination, an electroencephalogram (EEG), brain scan, skull x-rays, blood chemistry tests, electrocardiogram (ECG), or arteriogram may be ordered.

Treatment of choice for OBS is the correction of the underlying medical or neurologic disorder. Small doses of psychotropic and nonpsychotropic drugs may be used but could precipitate or exacerbate symptoms; therefore, it is important to monitor the patient closely while administering medication.

Nursing interventions focus on identification and symptomatic management of the evident deterioration, as well as other factors noted during the assessment process. A calm, supportive approach is necessary when handling the patient's emotional responses or defenses against the acknowledgment of intellectual deficits. Smith (Lego, 1984) lists the following observable behavioral defenses frequently seen in persons with organic mental disorders:

1. Lability of affect or rapid fluctuations in emotional responses

2. Indifference or apathy

3. Lack of energy or anergia

4. Negativistic behavior

5. Impulsivity or assaultive behavior

6. Emotional incontinence or inability to control aggressive or sexual impulses

7. Depression

8. Refusal to communicate

Short-term nursing goals include maintaining the patient's contact with reality, preventing injury, promoting adequate nutritional and fluid intake, promoting adequate sleep and rest, encouraging expression of feelings, and stimulating the memory through various activities.

Long-term goals focus on promotion of optimal level of independence, decreasing socially inappropriate behavior, forming satisfactory social relationships within limitations, and assisting the patient to live in as nonrestrictive an environment as possible (Schultz, 1982). The environment should be simple and well-structured, providing the person with an opportunity to adapt to impairments by doing things in less complex ways than in the past. Meeting basic needs becomes more demanding as the physical deterioration occurs.

Remaining learning potential should be maximized while the person is made to feel comfortable both physically and emotionally. New material or devices to provide self-care should be introduced simply and gradually.

Delusional thought processes increase as the intellectual functioning deteriorates. Sudden deterioration may indicate a superimposed treatable disease.

Examples of common nursing diagnoses and nursing interventions for organic mental disorders are listed as follows:

NURSING DIAGNOSES	NURSING INTERVENTIONS
Alteration in thought process related to disorientation of person, place, and time	Assess level of disorientation. Use reality therapy: 1. Orient to person, place, and time by using clocks, calendars, or other visual aids. 2. Refer to date, time of day, and recent activities during interactions with the patient. 3. Address the person by name. 4. Correct errors in a matter-of-fact manner. Establish a set daily routine. Encourage the person to have familiar personal belongings or possessions in his room. Assign the same nursing personnel to care for the patient whenever possible.
Self-care deficit because of loss of independent functions of bathing and dressing	Encourage independent functions by giving verbal step-by-step instructions. Remain with the patient. Allow ample time to perform a given task to avoid frustration. Assist the patient if sensorimotor impairment prevents him from functioning without help.
Alteration in thought process because of memory loss for recent information	Provide the patient with clear, simple, step-by-step directions while performing ADL routines. Give verbal reminders if the patient refuses or forgets to perform a task. Use supportive statements if fabricated stories or untruths are given in defense of memory loss (*i.e.*, "It's hard to find your glasses when their location slips your mind.").
Potential for injury owing to sensorimotor deficits of impaired vision and unstable gait	Establish a safe environment by 1. Providing adequate lighting in the patient's room 2. Providing a night light 3. Placing the light switch close to the bed for easy accessibility 4. Assessing the patient's ability to ambulate independently, providing assistance as needed (*i.e.*, walker, cane, or assist with ambulation) 5. Providing adequate restraints such as a Posey or vest if patient is disoriented as well as physically unstable

SUMMARY

Organic mental disorders are due to certain neurologic diseases or direct effects of various substances on the nervous system. The term organic brain syndrome (OBS) is used to refer to a cluster of signs and symptoms in which the etiology or physiologic process is unknown. This chapter discusses the characteristics and essential features of organic mental disorders, focusing on the acute OBS of delirium and the chronic OBS of dementia. Presenting symptoms, causative factors, and the diagnostic criteria of each were described. Alzheimer's disease, or primary degenerative dementia, was explained. The importance of an interview, the use of JOMAC, a complete physical and history examination, and diagnostic tests as part of the assessment process were stressed. Short- and long-term nursing goals were cited. Examples of nursing diagnoses and nursing interventions were stated. They included alteration in thought process because of disorientation of person, place, and time; self-care deficit from loss of independent functions of bathing and dressing; alteration in thought process owing to memory loss for recent information; and potential for injury because of sensorimotor deficits of impaired vision and unstable gait.

LEARNING ACTIVITIES

I. Clinical activities
   A. Care for a patient with the diagnosis of an organic mental disorder.
   B. List the clinical features of symptoms evident during hospitalization.
   C. State the diganostic tests used to identify the cause of the disorder.
   D. Develop a nursing care plan for this assigned patient, focusing on sensorimotor deficits and behavioral symptoms.
II. Independent activities
   A. Research literature on the following chronic brain syndromes:
      1. Alzheimer's disease
      2. Huntington's chorea
   B. Compare the personality changes seen in these disorders.
   C. Discuss the impact of such syndromes on family members.
   D. Discuss the types of care available to persons with these chronic debilitating diseases.

SELF-TEST

Match the following:

1. OBS
2. Acute OBS
3. Chronic OBS
4. Primary degenerative dementia
5. Anergia
6. Emotional incontinence
7. Lability of affect

a. Inability to control aggressive or sexual impulses
b. Delirium
c. Alzheimer's disease
d. Cluster of signs and symptoms without reference to cause
e. Rapid fluctuations in emotional responses
f. Dementia
g. Lack of energy
h. Refusal to communicate

Define the following terminology (Nos. 8–11):

8. Aphasia

9. Apraxia

10. Agnosia

11. Constructional difficulty

12. List four causes of death for persons with organic mental disorders.

13. What are the diagnostic tests used to identify causative factors of organic mental disorders?

14. Name behavioral defenses frequently seen in persons with organic mental disorders.

15. State four short-term nursing goals for patients with dementia.

16. List nursing interventions for
Alteration in thought process related to disorientation
Self-care deficit from loss of independent functions of bathing and dressing
Alteration in thought process because of memory loss
Potential for injury from sensorimotor deficits of impaired vision and unstable gait

REFERENCES

Altrocchi J: Abnormal Behavior. New York, Harcourt Brace Jovanovich, 1980
Carpenito LJ: Nursing Diagnosis: Application to Clinical Practice. Philadelphia, JB Lippincott, 1983
Donlon T, Rockwell DA: Psychiatric Disorders: Diagnoses and Treatment. Bowie, Robert J. Brady, 1982

Haber J et al: Comprehensive Psychiatric Nursing, 2nd ed. New York, McGraw–Hill, 1982

Lancaster J: Adult Psychiatric Nursing. Garden City, NJ, Medical Examination Publishing, 1980

Lego S: The American Handbook of Psychiatric Nursing. Philadelphia, JB Lippincott, 1984

Murray R et al: The Nursing Process in Later Maturity. Englewood Cliffs, Prentice–Hall, 1980

Schultz JM, Dark SL: Manual of Psychiatric Nursing Care Plans. Boston, Little, Brown & Company, 1982

Stuart G, Sundeen S: Principles and Practice of Psychiatric Nursing. St. Louis, CV Mosby, 1983

Wilson H, Kneisl C: Psychiatric Nursing, 2nd ed. Menlo Park, Addison–Wesley, 1983

27

PSYCHOSOCIAL ASPECTS

OF AGING

WHAT DO YOU SEE?*

What do you see, nurses? What do you see?
Are you thinking, when you are looking at me?
A crabby old woman, not very wise,
Uncertain of habit, with faraway eyes,
Who dribbles her food, and makes no reply,
When you say in a loud voice, "I do wish you'd try."
Who seems not to notice, the things that you do.
And forever is losing, a stocking or shoe.
Who unresisting or not, lets you do as you will,
When bathing and feeding, the long day to fill.
Is that what you are thinking, is that what you see?
Then open your eyes, nurse,
YOU ARE NOT LOOKING AT ME.

I'll tell you who I am, as I sit here so still.
As I move at your bidding, as I eat at your will.
I'm a small child of ten, with a father and mother,
Brothers and sisters, who love one another.
A young girl of sixteen, with wings on her feet,
Dreaming that soon now a lover she'll meet.
A bride soon at twenty, my heart gives a leap,
Remembering the vows, that I promised to keep.
At twenty-five now, I have young of my own,
Who need me to build a secure happy home.
A woman of thirty, my young now grow fast.
Bound to each other, with ties that should last.

*Written by a 92-year-old woman. Found by niece in personal belongings after her death.

At forty my young sons now grow and will be gone,
But my man stays beside me to see I don't mourn.
At fifty, once more babies play round my knee,
Again we know children, my loved one and me.
Dark days are upon me, my husband is dead.
I look at the future I shudder with dread.
For my young are all busy, rearing young of their own.
And I think of the years, and the love that I've known.
I'm an old woman now, and nature is cruel.
It's her jest, to make old age look like a fool
The body it crumbles, grace and vigor depart.
There is now a stone, where I once had a heart.
But inside this old carcass, a young girl still dwells,
And now and again, my battered heart swells,
I remember the joy, I remember the pain,
And I'm loving and living life over again.
I think of the years, all too few—gone too fast,
And accept the stark fact, that nothing can last.
So open your eyes, nurses, open and see
Not a crabby old woman. Look closer—see ME.

Anonymous

... there are now five medical geropsychiatric programs in the United States; there are no geropsychiatric nursing programs. Psychiatric nursing in general has not accepted the challenge of care for the elderly, yet the need for geropsychiatric nursing becomes increasingly apparent as nurses grapple with the behavioral problems of their clients.

Burnside (1981, p. 59)

LEARNING OBJECTIVES

1. Describe the intrinsic and extrinsic factors that affect the aging process.
2. List Duvall's developmental tasks of the elderly.
3. Discuss factors influencing each of the identified developmental tasks.
4. Differentiate between ego transcendence and ego preoccupation.
5. State Kuhn's demands to improve the quality of life for aging persons.
6. Explain the causes of the following emotional reactions or behaviors seen in elderly patients:
   Anxiety
   Loneliness
   Guilt
   Depression
   Somatic complaints
   Dementia or cognitive dysfunction
7. Differentiate between geriatric and gerontologic nursing.
8. Plan nursing interventions for elderly persons who demonstrate needs for
   Psychological safety and security
   Loving and belongingness
   Self-esteem
   Self-actualization

WEBSTER defines elderly as a characteristic of later life; past middle age. Aging is an interaction of physical, mental, social, spiritual, and intellectual dimensions that begins at birth and ends with death (Wantz, 1981, p. 9). Age 65 is the chosen age to differentiate middle age from old age. Ages 65 to 74 are often referred to as early old age, whereas 75 and older is considered to be advanced old age.

THEORIES ABOUT AGING

Wantz (1981) describes the following aging theories: 1) cellular theory and 2) genetic theory. The cellular theory lists three possible causes of aging: an accumulation of insufficient proteins within the cells that causes cellular aging, an accumulation of defective cells with impaired cellular functions, and an accumulation of harmful wastes and by-products in the body that affect the cells (metabolic waste product theory). According to the genetic theory, longevity, or one's life span, is determined at conception because genetic factors may cause cellular irregularities and mutations to occur. These irregularities and mutations, as well as one's environment and any disease processes, can influence the aging process. Genetic factors are discussed in the next section.

Havinghurst (1968) discusses two theories of aging: 1) the activity theory and 2) the disengagement theory. The activity theory states that an older person experiences the same psychological and social needs as when he was younger. The disengagement theory states that an older person and society initiate a decrease in social interaction and activity. The older person accepts and may even desire this interrupted relationship to occur as he becomes increasingly self-centered.

Nurses caring for aging persons should be aware of these theories as they plan nursing interventions for patients.

FACTORS INFLUENCING THE AGING PROCESS

Factors thought to influence the aging process are referred to as intrinsic and extrinsic components of aging. Intrinsic factors are those biologic and physiologic components that influence one's aging process such as sex, race, intelligence, familial longevity patterns, and genetic diseases. According to statistics, women live longer than men by approximately 7 years. One only needs to attend a senior citizen retirement center, visit a nursing home, eat out in a restaurant, or attend a concert to notice the ratio of men to women in the age group of 65 and over. As one senior citizen stated, "Men have their choice of lovely female companions. We women have to stand in line to be noticed." Factors assumed to contribute to this longevity of women over men include endocrine metabolism during menopause that provides protection against circulatory or cardiovascular diseases, higher activity level, less stress from one's occupation, better weight control, and less use of tobacco. Wantz (1981) states that the movement for women's rights may close the life expectancy gap between men and women. Although the life expectancy for whites is approximately 5 years more than for all other races, the death rate for whites over age 75 is higher than all other races. Persons with a higher level of intelligence appear to live longer than persons with lower levels of intelligence. This fact may, in part, be due to the life-style selected by persons with higher intelligence quotients (IQs). Such persons may remain physically active by participating in events that promote physical, mental, and social well-being (Wantz, 1981, p. 9). Persons with type A personality seldom relax or enjoy themselves due to a drive-to-succeed quality. They are prime candidates for heart attacks. The type B personality is an easy-going type who takes life in stride. "Personality influences the adoption of abusive behaviors, such as overeating, tobacco dependence, and alcohol abuse" (Wantz, 1981, p. 10). These abuses definitely impair one's physical health and shorten a person's life span. Familial longevity patterns are indicators of a person's potential life span. A person who is from a family with a record of long-lived great-grandparents, grandparents, and parents probably will live longer than a 45-year-old man who has a family history of heart attacks by his father and grandfather at middle age. Genetic disease may cause a person to experience a short life span, for example, persons with Down's syndrome, cystic fibrosis, and Tay–Sach's disease. The mortality rate for Down's syndrome is high within the first few years. If the person survives to adulthood, he is prone to respiratory infections, pneumonia, and other lung disease. Life expectancy for cystic fibrosis has improved, and patients may live to reach adulthood, although death usually occurs during childhood because of respiratory complications. Children with Tay–Sachs disease generally die between ages 2 and 4. Although people have minimal if any control over these intrinsic factors influencing the aging process, a high quality of life possibly could promote one's sense of physical, mental, and social well-being.

Extrinsic components or factors of aging can be controlled to some degree by the person. Examples of these environmental factors include one's "employment and economic level, education, health practices, and related diseases, and societal attitude" (Wantz, 1981, p. 13). Income, economic level, and educational level definitely determine how one lives. For example, low socioeconomic level ghetto families may have difficulty eating well-balanced diets because of both financial problems and little education regarding nutritional needs. Health care may not be sought because of high medical–surgical costs, no insurance, or ignorance about contributing factors or symptoms of various diseases. Such people, who eat inadequate diets, have poor living conditions, ignore or minimize health problems, or experience financial stress are definitely at risk for a shortened life span. Substance abuse, lack of experience, and poor diets are seen in all age groups. These practices have a negative effect on health and have proven to contribute to earlier deaths. Societal attitudes affect persons psychologically and definitely have an impact on the aging process. "Older adults are expected to be unproductive, inflexible, senile, and asexual." (Wantz, 1981, p. 17). Most persons seek the approval of society and will behave the way they think society expects them to behave. Such thinking could lead to a life-style that is detrimental to one's health. "You're only as old as you feel" is an adage that an aging person should heed. Older adults should seek intellectual, emotional, and physical stimulation to maintain an optimal level of health and longevity.

DEVELOPMENTAL TASKS OF AGING

In addition to various factors that influence aging, consider how aging can affect one's psychosocial needs. Butler (1982) states that only 5% of older persons are institutionalized for health or emotional problems. The larger percentage of aging adults live in central parts of cities or in rural locations. Statistics in 1978 showed that Florida, California, and New York contained approximately 25% of the elderly population. These statistics may be relatively higher at this time.

Duvall (1977) lists the following developmental tasks of the elderly that influence one's emotional needs. They are summarized as follows.

ESTABLISHING SATISFACTORY LIVING ARRANGEMENTS. Many factors influence this developmental task. Is the person single, widowed, divorced, or married? Does the elderly person have an incapacitating illness or handicap? Does the person require assistance or supervision with the activities of daily living (ADL)? Are the grocery store, pharmacy, doctor's office, and church located close by or within walking distance? Is the person able to stay in his own home or does he need to be relocated? These are just a few questions that the family and the aging person consider when satisfactory living arrangements are made. Norling's article (1984) discusses the care of her 87-year-old mother-in-law and actions taken to ensure her satisfactory housing such as hiring a cleaning helper; using a service such as Meals on Wheels; scheduling a weekly visit by a nurse; and improvising with an amplifier on the telephone receiver. Loneliness, anxiety, or depression, as well as other emotional reactions, may occur if these needs are not met.

ADJUSTING TO RETIREMENT INCOME. Not all people are fortunate enough to have a savings account and receive social security, retirement benefits, or some other form of supplemental income. Retirement may be a planned time for relaxation and leisure activities or may pose a financial crisis. Adjusting one's standard of living to a reduced income can be quite stressful for the elderly when the cost of living continues to rise.

ESTABLISHING COMFORTABLE ROUTINES. Retirement, which provides a person with newfound leisure time, allows one to establish a comfortable routine such as going on a last-minute trip, participating in a weekly bowling league during the day, doing volunteer work, or developing new hobbies. Retirement may be stressful for the "workaholic," or type A personality, who needs to be busy all the time. "All my husband does is get in my way. He's always underfoot like a little puppy dog. I wish he was still working", "I thought we'd do things together such as golf, bowl, or play bridge. He's not interested in doing anything", and "I don't enjoy life any more. There's nothing to look forward to now that I am retired" are just a few comments by persons having difficulty adjusting routines during retirement. On the positive side, the following comment was made by a senior citizen thoroughly enjoying retirement: "I don't know how I managed to work before. I don't have enough time in the day to do everything." This

69-year-old person bowls in two leagues and golfs with his wife, does all the lawn care himself, and manages to travel several times a year.

MAINTAINING LOVE, SEX, AND MARITAL RELATIONSHIPS. "Most older people want— and are able to lead—an active, satisfying sex life . . . When problems occur they should not be viewed as inevitable, but rather as the result of the disease, disability, drug reactions, or emotional upset—and as requiring medical care" (National Institute on Aging, 1981). Walker states, "The notion that old age will be sexless has been proven false in study after study. Provided that they are healthy, elderly people are capable of an active sex life into their 80s and 90s. Sexual performance may be slowed somewhat with aging, but sexual pleasure and capacity remain intact" (1983, p. 171). Sexual problems can arise in later years from physiologic changes, fear of impotence, fear of a heart attack because of physical exertion, or boredom. Data published by the U.S. Department of Health, Education, and Welfare in 1979 stated that 77% of older men were married, whereas 52% of all older women were widowed. An older widowed man is able to maintain a marital relationship more readily than a woman due to the availability of women in his age group or younger. Older women are "frowned on" if they marry a man much younger.

KEEPING ACTIVE AND INVOLVED. Special characteristics of the elderly to keep active that demonstrate their ability to meet this developmental task have been identified by Butler (1982). These characteristics include the desire to leave a legacy, the desire to share knowledge and experience with younger generations, the ability to demonstrate an increased emotional investment in the environment, a sense of immediacy or "here and now" owing to the decreased number of years left, the ability to experience an entire life cycle, increased creativity and curiosity, and a satisfaction with life. Physical illness may prevent a person from being active and becoming involved with others. The theory of disengagement also refers to the aging person's lessened activity and interaction with society. Active senior citizens may participate in various volunteer employment programs such as Retired Senior Volunteer Program (RSVP), Service Core of Retired Executives (SCORE), Volunteers in Service to America (VISTA), Peace Corps, Foster Grandparents Programs, and Senior Opportunities and Service programs (SOS).

STAYING IN TOUCH WITH OTHER FAMILY MEMBERS. "I cry inside every day. Each time they come to visit me, I beseech them to take me home . . . All I want . . . is to hold my daughter's hand and be surrounded by those people and things I love" (Hahn, 1970). This statement was made by a 94-year-old woman placed in a nursing home by her family.

The following narrative appeared in a local newspaper along with the drawing of a forlorn-looking elderly woman sitting alone in her home:

"Next year.
  They said they'll
come down for Christmas
    next year.
  Excuses again.
    It's warm today.
  Too warm for Christmas anyway.
    I don't think I can wait
  another year."

Larry Moore (1983)

This scene depicts the loneliness experienced by many elderly people, especially at holidays, anniversary dates, and birthdays, because they do not have family or a substitute support system.

Loneliness can lead to depression and thoughts of suicide. The elderly are considered to account for approximately 25% of suicides reported yearly. Persons who meet the developmental tasks of maintaining love, sex, and marital relationships, as well as keeping active and involved probably would be able to cope with separation from family members more readily than those who choose to disengage themselves from society.

SUSTAINING AND MAINTAINING PHYSICAL AND MENTAL HEALTH. Walker (1983) states that 90% of those persons over age 65 exhibit no serious mental impairment. "Old folks are not children. Even though their reactions may appear similar, these are brought on by very different feelings. Their emotions are triggered not by the frustrations of growing up but by frustrations, fears, and anxieties of growing old" (Armour Pharmaceutical Company, 1971).

It is not easy to experience a slowing of one's mental and physical reactions and be unable to do anything about it; to look on as younger people perform one's job and assume one's role. Various emotional and behavioral reactions occur as one undergoes the physiologic changes of the aging process. These relations include anxiety, frustration, fear, depression, intolerance, stubbornness, loneliness, decreased independence, decreased productivity, low self-esteem, and numerous somatic complaints (also referred to as hypochondriasis). "Crankiness is not just a whim, but the expression of fear and uncertainty as the elderly person becomes less functional, more confined, and more dependent" (Armour Pharmaceuticals Co., 1971).

Imagine what your own emotional or behavioral reactions would be to the following physical impairments: loss of hearing or sight, inability to speak because of a stroke, inability to perform ADL because of a paralyzed left side or disorientation, and incontinency of stool or urine from loss of bladder and bowel control. "Loss is a predominant theme in characterizing the emotional experiences of older people" (Butler, 1982, p. 43). Johnson (1980) states that the aged person fears loss of control over daily routines, loss of identity, confinement (*e.g.,* placement in a nursing home or hospital), social isolation because of failing health, and death (20% to 25% of the elderly occupy nursing homes when they die).

FINDING MEANING IN LIFE. "Listen to the aged. They will teach you. They are a distinguished faculty who teach not from books but from long experience in living" (Burnside, 1975, p. 1800). The elderly reminisce frequently as they adapt to the aging process. They are eager to talk about "days gone by." Schrock (1980) refers to Roger C. Peck's concept of ego transcendence versus ego preoccupation in her discussion of the elderly person's outlook on life. *Ego transcendence* describes the aging person's positive approach to find meaning in life as he talks about past life experiences and realizes that he has the wisdom and knowledge to serve as a resource person. He is willing to share himself with others, remain active, and look to the future. The person exhibiting *ego preoccupation* resigns himself to the aging process, becomes inactive, feels he has no future, and waits to die. He does not feel his life has any significant meaning to himself or others.

Neugarten (Schrock, 1980) discussed five components of measuring the elderly's satisfaction with his life: 1) zest versus apathy, 2) resolution and fortitude versus passivity, 3) congruence between desired and achieved goals, 4) self-concept, and 5) mood tone. The following is a comparision of ego transcendence and ego preoccupation using Neugarten's five components of life satisfaction, which is a helpful tool to use in the nursing assessment of aging persons:

EGO TRANSCENDENCE	EGO PREOCCUPATION
Zest	*Apathetic*
Enthusiastic and personally involved in activities around him	Bored, lacks energy and interest in others and activities occurring around him
Resolution and fortitude	*Passivity*
Assumes an active responsibility for his life and actions. Maslow describes this self-actualized person as realistic; accepting of others; spontaneous in actions; displaying a need for privacy, autonomy, and independence; democratic; and humorous (Schrock, 1980).	Does not assume an active responsibility for his life and actions. Remains inactive and passive, allowing things to happen
Goal congruence (has achieved goals)	*Goal incongruence (has not achieved goals)*
Satisfied with the way goals have been met. Feels successful as a person	Regrets actions taken to achieve goals. Dissatisfied with the way life is treating him.

(continued)

EGO TRANSCENDENCE	EGO PREOCCUPATION
Positive self-concept	*Negative self-concept*
Likes his physical appearance and cares about how he presents himself to others. Feels competent. Is able to socialize with others without feeling like a "third party."	Does not place much emphasis or concern on physical appearance. Feels incompetent. Is unable to relate to others socially without feeling as if he is imposing
Positive mood tone	*Negative mood tone*
Has the ability to appreciate life, displays a sense of humor, is optimistic and happy	Is unable to appreciate life, displays a pessimistic attitude, may be irritable, bitter, or gloomy in emotional reactions

Kuhn (1982), founder and leader of the Gray Panthers, who seek to restore power to the elderly person, lists eight demands to improve quality of life for aging persons. These demands address some of the developmental tasks just described. Summarized, the demands state

1. The elderly should be permitted to be involved in society as older persons have continued potential and abilities.

2. Do away with poverty among the aged.

3. Social Security benefits should be more equitable for women. Women outlive men and generally have lower incomes.

4. The elderly should be permitted to work instead of forced into retirement or discriminated against because of their age. Continued employment provides relief to the social security system and reduces feelings of uselessness among the elderly.

5. Public transporation should be improved to meet the needs of aging persons who prefer to have others transport them or are physically unable to transport themselves.

6. A health system that promotes preventive medicine should be developed.

7. Safe, decent housing should be readily available for the elderly. "Unattractive housing, pollution, noise, and social tension too often characterize urban living" for the elderly in the inner city (Wantz, 1981, p. 77). Aging persons are prey for youth gangs or burglars and lock themselves in their apartments or homes when they should be taking advantage of their newfound leisure time. Social security checks may disappear from mailboxes in rural or urban areas because criminals familiarize themselves with the persons who receive social security benefits.

8. The aged should not be stereotyped by the news media, film industries, or commercial ads. (A positive approach to this demand occurred when Sea World in Florida used a 70-year-old, well-known actor, Eddie Albert, for promotional advertisement. Old and young alike

were able to identify with this active, physically and mentally well-adjusted senior citizen.)

EMOTIONAL REACTIONS OR BEHAVIORS

Walker (1982) adds a little humor in referring to the emotional problems of the older adult as "surviving being old." He cites the following stressful situations as percursors to emotional illness: retirement, loss of loved ones, slowing of responses, physical disability, and the inevitability of death. According to statistics stated by Walker, "Under the age of 15 there are 2.3 new cases of psychiatric disorders per 100,000 each year, while over 65 there are 236.1 cases per 100,000" (p. 155). These statistics are quite startling when one realizes that the elderly compose approximately 10% of the United States population of 230 million people.

Morgan (1973) lists three categories of older adults who have successfully adjusted to the aging process:

1. The mature older adult—This person is ego transcendent because he remains active and involved, accepts the aging process, adjusts well to various losses, faces life realistically, and is able to face death as the final stage of growth.

2. The armored older adult—This person protects himself or is armored with well-developed defenses such as denial and suppression, attempting to remain a middle-aged person although he is aging physically and chronologically.

3. The "rocking-chair" adult—This rather passive person leans on others and becomes more leisure oriented. He is able to "sit and rock without feeling guilty about it" (p. 168).

Emotional problems of the elderly have been classified from minor mental problems to the development of major psychotic disorders such as late-life schizophrenia. This chapter discusses the more common emotional reactions and behaviors of the elderly: anxiety, loneliness, guilt, depression, somatic complaints, paranoid reactions, and senility.

Anxiety

"Anxiety is common in old age and may be present intermittently or chronically" (Burnside, 1981, p. 62). Loss of mental acuity, admission to a nursing home, loss of a spouse, emergency surgery, confinement to bed because of a physical illness, and the diagnosis of a terminal illness are but a few causes of anxiety during old age. Aged persons may not be accustomed to expressing their feelings openly, for example: "I am angry with my son," "My husband upsets me when he criticizes me all the time," or "I don't want to move into a nursing home. I want to live with my daughter." Pent-up feelings, concerns or reactions to loss may manifest themselves as numerous physical or somatic complaints, insomnia, restlessness, fatigue, hostility, dependency, and isolation.

Loneliness

Loneliness is considered to be the "reactive response to separation from persons and things in which one has invested oneself and one's energy" (Burnside, 1981, p. 66). She lists five causes of loneliness in the elderly:

1. *Death of a spouse, relative, or friend.* A 93-year-old man was invited to ride in his hometown's centennial day celebration parade as the town's oldest citizen. His comment to the request was "All my friends have died. I have no one to visit with. It's lonely being the oldest person in town." This man felt there was no one left to care about him or his needs.

2. *Loss of a pet.* Some elderly persons relate to pets as though they were people, and the death of a long-time pet can be very traumatic. Occasionally one will read in the newspaper about an elderly person willing his estate to a pet rather than a family member or favorite charity. Lavish funeral arrangements have been held by persons wishing to communicate their feelings for their pets.

3. *The inability to communicate in the English language.* People feel isolated and lonely if they are in a foreign environment or are unable to understand what is being said. The influx of Cubans, Vietnamese, and other foreign persons is a contributing factor to this cause. Just recently, a student nurse cared for an elderly Spanish-speaking woman on a medical–surgical unit. The patient was admitted for possible surgical removal of her gallbladder. Nursing personnel were having difficulty communicating with her. Once an interpreter was located, the student nurse was able to converse with the patient. The woman told the interpretor she had just arrived in the United States to visit her son and daughter-in-law and that she was quite lonely because no one spoke her language.

4. *Pain.* People often complain of loneliness when pain occurs during the late evening or early morning hours because no one is around to provide comfort. Pain does not have to be a normal part of the aging process, although the elderly may feel that certain pains are "a part of growing old." For example, many elderly persons stoically endure pain because of rheumatism or arthritis, rather than take over-the-counter medication.

5. *Certain times of the day or night.* Changes in living habits due to institutionalization in a nursing home may cause loneliness since the elderly are no longer able to perform daily or nightly rituals. Daily

activities generally provide some stimulation for the elderly, whereas quiet evenings can seem quite long especially if no relatives or friends visit. The term "sundown syndrome" is used to describe behavioral changes that occur in the elderly at dusk. This is a pathologic symptom indicative of chronic cognitive dysfunction. Confusion, disorientation, agitation, and loneliness have all been described as symptoms present in one patient or another.

Guilt

As the elderly experience the "life-review process," reminiscing about the past, guilt feelings may emerge from past conflicts or regrets. For example, an elderly man revealed guilt feelings about not lending his son-in-law and daughter money several years ago when they were in a financial bind. At the time of the request, the man felt that the couple should be able to support themselves. "Young people don't appreciate things given to them on a silver platter. They need to work for what they get. Then they'll take care of it" were his words of advice at the time they asked for help. He went on to state that the had plenty of money now, but "money doesn't keep one company." Guilt feelings may also occur when one considers past grudges, actions taken against others, outliving others, or unemployment or retirement.

Depression

Depression can occur at any time during the life span but appears to increase in degree and frequency during old age. Although loss is the most common causative factor; unresolved grief, anger, loneliness, declining health, and guilt can result in feelings of mild to severe depression. Medications taken by the elderly also may precipitate or enhance a depressive reaction. As stated earlier, 25% of all suicides committed yearly are persons 65 years of age or over. Those at risk are white men over age 85, isolated elderly persons, older persons experiencing increased dependency and changes in body function, and those persons with the diagnosis of a terminal illness.

Somatic Complaints

Hypochrondriasis, or preoccupation with one's physical and emotional health resulting in bodily or somatic complaints, is common in the elderly patient. The aging person is rechanneling stress and anxiety into bodily concerns as he assumes the "sick" role described earlier in this text. Secondary gains of support, concern, and interest are conveyed to the patient reinforcing a sense of control (Stuart, 1983). All complaints should be assessed thoroughly and matter-of-factly, avoiding stereotyping the person as a "chronic complainer." Common somatic complaints include insomnia, anorexia, and pain.

Paranoid Reactions

Loss of sight or hearing, sensory deprivation, or physical impairments often contribute to suspiciousness in elderly persons. The aging person may feel others are talking about him or conspiring against him. Medication such as diazepam (Valium) or a strange environment also may contribute to confusion and suspicious behavior among the elderly.

Dementia (Senility) or Cognitive Dysfunction

Dementia is described as impaired memory from a physical cause. The person forgets recent events more readily than past events, as well as names, telephone numbers, and conversations. Attempts to compensate for memory loss include social withdrawal, keeping lists, and confabulation, or the fabrication of material to fill gaps in stories in response to questions about situations or events one is unable to recall. As mental deterioration or cognitive dysfunction occurs, personality changes are seen, including angry accusations, suspiciousness, vulgar language, poor personal hygiene, disregard for rules and regulations, and vague, incomprehensible speech.

The causative factor in 50% to 60% of all senile persons is an irreversible deterioration of the brain, termed Alzheimer's disease. Other factors include a series of ministrokes due to high blood pressure, chronic substance abuse, neurologic diseases, brain tumors, and metabolic diseases (Walker, 1983).

NURSING INTERVENTIONS

The American Nurses' Association Division on Gerontological Nursing Practice has published an informational and educational tool for the registered nurse entitled *The Registered Nurse Consultant to the Intermediate Care Facility* (1977). Two chapters of special interest to the student nurse are gerontologic nursing and the application of the nursing process. Geriatric nursing is defined as "meeting the needs for nursing that are created by disease and the medical treatment of disease in older people. It is often intuitive and custodial in nature . . ." (p. 41). Gerontologic nursing is described as "the assessment of health care needs of older people, planning and implementing health care to meet these needs, and evaluating the effectiveness of such care. Emphasis is placed on maximizing the older person's independence in the activities of everyday living; on preventing illness or disability; on promoting, maintaining, and restoring health; or on maintaining life in dignity and comfort until death ensues" (pp. 41–42). The booklet further states that an effort should be made to keep older people healthy, rather than just treating them as an illness occurs. This statement agrees with Kuhn's request to foster preventive medicine.

One approach to gerontologic nursing interventions focuses on Maslow's theory of motivation in which he identified five levels of basic human needs (Maslow, 1968). Beginning with the lower level or basic needs and progressing to the higher level needs they include: 1) physiologic needs of survival; 2) safety and security needs (physical and psychological); 3) love and belonging needs; 4) self-esteem needs; and 5) the need for self-actualization. Using Maslow's concept enables the care-giver to meet more than just survival needs, a condition that occurs too frequently in nursing care. The highest need of self-actualization refers to the mature person's need for self-development and self-fulfillment. The elderly should be encouraged to meet this need, not denied it.

The following are statements about the aging process that may be helpful as one plans nursing care to meet the psychological or emotional needs of elderly patients, whether they are seen as outpatients or inpatients:

1. People who suffer great difficulty in the process of aging have been somewhat emotionally frail all their lives. Such frailty may be due to unmet needs of psychological safety and security. Nursing care should be planned to meet these needs by

   Minimizing the amount of change to which the person is exposed

   Determining the person's previous life-style and encouraging the continuance of that life-style as much as possible

   Explaining new routines, medications, or treatments

   Introducing change gradually

   Including the person in decision making

   Encouraging relocated, hospitalized, or institutionalized patients or family members to bring familiar items from home

2. The older person has a need for love and belonging as well as a need to maintain his status in society. As he becomes older, it may be increasingly difficult for him to remain active or make contributions to society. If the person feels unwanted, he may resort to telling stories about earlier achievements. Nursing interventions to meet the need for love and belongingness include

   Encouraging expression of affection, touch, and human sexuality

   Permitting the person to select a roommate when appropriate

Providing opportunities to form new friendships and relationships with persons of varying ages

Permitting flexible visiting hours with family or friends

Providing privacy when desired

Encouraging expression of feelings such as loneliness and the need to be loved

3. Irritating behavior generally is related to the elderly person's frustration, fear, or awareness of limitations rather than a physiologic deficit or the actual issue at hand. "The older person needs a sense of self-worth, to take pride in his abilities and accomplishments, and to be respected by others" (American Nurses' Association, 1977, p. 162). Nursing interventions are planned to restore, preserve, and protect the elderly person's self-esteem by

Encouraging participation in decision making pertaining to ADL

Identifying strengths to promote self-confidence and independence

Encouraging the person to take pride in personal appearance

Communicating clearly with the elderly person at an adult level

Occasionally seeking the older person's advice

Listening thoughtfully as he reminisces about his life's experiences.

4. Self-actualization or self-fulfillment occurs only after the lower needs of survival, safety, and security, love and belonging, and a positive sense of self-esteem have been met.

Peck's concept of ego transcendence discussed earlier in this chapter describes the self-actualized person. Nursing interventions to promote self-fulfillment in the elderly include

Promoting decision making and independence. The elderly person is encouraged to take responsibility for actions.

Encouraging participation in activities or the development of hobbies to promote socialization, productivity, and creativity, as well as fostering a sense of accomplishment.

Encouraging the person to be a resource person as well as a teacher of skills or crafts to younger generations. Such activities serve a useful purpose and earn the elderly person recognition.

Working with the elderly person to meet the developmental task of dying (see Chap. 10). As he prepares to meet this task, the aging person experiences a life-review process in which he attempts to put his life in order. He reflects on what life means and on the finiteness of life. He may read philosophy, study religion, or discuss his accomplishments and failures. Discussing the person's accomplishments enhances his self-respect and prestige. Eliot (1984) states "hundreds of thousands of older Americans . . . could live full, productive lives, . . . could teach us and our children about the past and thus prepare us for the future, if we would just let them" (p. 150).

The following comments were made by student nurses who cared for residents of a nursing home during their geriatric nursing clinical rotation. They were asked to assess their assigned patients' needs as well as degree of independence. The comments address the needs just discussed:

The first day I walked into Mrs. K's room she was responsive to questions but volunteered no speech on her own. The second day I asked her if she remembered me and she stated "Yes, you are the one who made me laugh" . . . She responded to the radio and talked about different programs. I think she might have enjoyed my reading to her . . . She definitely wanted to maintain her independence.

My patients taught me to live today to the best of my ability; accept where I am in life; do the best I can at all times; and don't worry about tomorrow . . . I tried to give them a little extra attention and let them know they were special, worthwhile people.

Mrs. D. made a lot of progress while I cared for her. She attended activities, began talking more, enjoyed going outside, and would tell me her likes and dislikes. A person working with the elderly has to be a very patient and caring individual.

BC showed me a positive outlook on life. She appeared happy that she had fulfilled all her goals and was satisfied with the way the years have gone by. She said she had her memories and that's what she treasured most . . . Working with the elderly taught me something important . . . We must realize that every elderly person was once a young person who had ambitions, dreams, and goals . . . We need to take care of their emotional as well as physical needs.

The time to prepare people for the adjustment to growing older is during the middle years. Emphasis should be placed on the development of new interests, hobbies, and friendships that will assist them in filling extra hours available due to retirement, widowhood, or an illness. This primary prevention can be done by nurses assisting persons in the community, working with family members, or caring for patients in acute care settings.

The following examples of nursing diagnoses and nursing interventions pertain to the care of elderly patients with unmet psychosocial needs:

NURSING DIAGNOSES	**NURSING INTERVENTIONS**
Anxiety, mild because of retirement	Refer to Chapter 12 for suggested nursing interventions.
Diversional activity deficit because of postretirement inactivity	Assess causative factors (*i.e.,* social isolation, loneliness, boredom, or depression).

(continued)

NURSING DIAGNOSES	NURSING INTERVENTIONS
	With the patient's help, state ways to reduce or eliminate causative factors. If depressed, assess for suicidal ideation. (Refer to Chap. 24.)
	Identify factors that promote diversional activity (*i.e.,* socialization with peers, increased feelings of self-worth, or encouragement of the person to challenge himself with a new learning skill).
Impaired home management maintenance following hospitalization owing to insufficient finances	Assess knowledge of resources available for financial assistance or support and refer to social services whenever necessary.
	Assess type of housing, including appearance and presence of physical facilitites (*i.e.,* apartment vs single family house, sanitary vs unsanitary conditions, and adequate or inadequate lighting, heating, and ventilation).
	Assess the safety features of the patient's home environment (*i.e.,* Is there a telephone present? Is there a "grab" bar present in the bathroom?) Contact homemaker services and community nursing services whenever necessary.

SUMMARY

This chapter focused on the psychosocial aspects of aging by defining aging, briefly stating the cellular and genetic theories of aging, and listing intrinsic and extrinsic factors influencing the aging process. Duvall's eight developmental tasks of aging and the impact on one's emotional needs were discussed. They include establishing satisfactory living arrangements; adjusting to retirement income; establishing comfortable routines; maintaining love, sex, and marital relationships; keeping active and involved; staying in touch with other family members; sustaining and maintaining physical and mental health; and finding meaning in life. Common emotional reactions or behaviors, such as anxiety, loneliness, guilt, depression, somatic complaints, paranoid reactions, and senility were explained. Maslow's theory of motivation, identifying five levels of basic human needs was presented. Nursing interventions were discussed, focusing on the need for psychological safety and security, love and belonging, self-esteem, and self-actualization. Examples of nursing interventions also were given for anxiety, mild due to retirement; diversional activity deficit due to postretirement inactivity; and impaired home management maintenance following hospitalization owing to insufficient finances.

LEARNING ACTIVITIES

I. Clinical activities
    A. Care for an elderly patient.
        1. Identify any unmet developmental tasks as described by Duvall.
        2. State identified emotional needs of the patient.
        3. Plan nursing interventions for unmet needs and tasks.
    B. Assess the patient's satisfaction with his life. Does he appear to be ego transcendent or ego preoccupied? Why?
II. Independent activities
    A. Research the community to identify volunteer employment programs for the elderly.
    B. Contact a local senior citizen's club. What activities are available to members of the community? Are special discount rates for dining, attending movies, bowling, and other activities available to senior citizens?
    C. Read the following articles listed in the references to develop personal and professional insight regarding the aging process:
        1. Emma Elliot, "My Name is Mrs. Simon."
        2. Donna Norling, "Please Take Care of Mother."
        3. Mildred Hogstel, "While Growing Old: How Do the Elderly View Their World?"
        4. Irene Burnside, "Listen to the Aged."

SELF-TEST

1. Define the aging process.

2. List the intrinsic factors that influence aging.

3. Describe the extrinsic factors that influence aging.

4. Compare the cellular and genetic theories of aging.

5. Describe Duvall's eight developmental tasks of the elderly.

6. State the components of ego transcendence.

7. Describe Morgan's three categories of well-adjusted older adults.

8. List causative factors of the following emotional reactions or behaviors in the elderly person:
    Anxiety
    Loneliness
    Guilt
    Depression
    Somatic complaints
    Paranoid reactions
    Dementia or cognitive dysfunction

9. State the goals of gerontologic nursing.

10. List the five levels of basic human needs identified by Maslow.

11. List at least two nursing interventions for each of the needs listed in question No. 8 in relation to elderly persons.

REFERENCES

Altrocchi J: Abnormal Behavior. New York, Harcourt Brace Jovanovich, 1980

American Nurses' Association Division on Gerontological Nursing Practice: The Registered Nurse Consultant to the Intermediate Care Facility. Kansas City, American Nurses' Association, 1977

Armour Pharmaceutical Company: What Makes Old Folks Cranky and How to Cope With It (pamphlet). Scicom, 1971

Bowers J: Caring for the elderly. Nur 78: Jan, 1978

Burnside I: Listen to the aged. Am J Nurs: Nov, 1975

Burnside I: Nursing and the Aged, 2nd ed. New York, McGraw–Hill, 1981

Butler R, Lewis M: Aging and Mental Health: Positive Psychosocial and Biomedical Approaches, 3rd ed. St. Louis, CV Mosby, 1982

Duvall EM: Marriage and Family Development, 5th ed. Philadelphia, JB Lippincott, 1977

Elliott E: My name is Mrs. Simon. Ladies' Home Journal: Aug, 1984

Hahn A: It's tough to be old. Am J Nurs: Aug, 1970

Havinghurst RJ: Personality and patterns of aging. Gerontologist: Aug, 1968

Hogstel MO: While growing old: How do the elderly view their world? Am J Nurs: Aug, 1978

Johnson E, Williamson J: Growing Old: The Social Problems of Aging. New York, Holt, Rinehart, & Winston, 1980

Kozier B, Erb G: Fundamentals of Nursing: Concepts and Procedures, 2nd ed. Menlo Park, Addison–Wesley, 1983

Kuhn M: Powers to the elderly people. Family Week: Jan 3, 1982

Lore A: Supporting the hospitalized elderly person. Am J Nurs: Mar, 1979

Maslow AH: Toward a Psychology of Being. New York, D. Van Nostrand, 1968

Maslow AH: Motivation and Personality. New York, Harper & Row, 1970

Miles H, Hayes D: Widowhood. In Backer B, Dubbert P, Eisenman E (eds.): Psychiatric/Mental Health Health Nursing: Contemporary Readings. New York, D. Van Nostrand, 1978

Morgan A, Moreno J: The Practice of Mental Health Nursing: A Community Approach. Philadelphia, JB Lippincott Co., 1973

Murray R et al: The Nursing Process in Later Maturity. Englewood Cliffs, Prentice–Hall, 1979

National Institute of Aging: Age page: Sexuality in later life. Washington, DC, U.S. Department of Health and Human Services, October, 1981

Neugarten BL et al: The measurement of life satisfaction. J Gerontology, Vol 16: 1961

Norling D: Please take care of mother. The Lutheran Standard: May, 1984

Roberts S: Behavioral Concepts and Nursing Throughout the Life Span. Englewood Cliffs, Prentice–Hall, 1978

Schrock MM: Holistic Assessment of the Healthy Aged. New York, John Wiley & Sons, 1980

Sontag S: The double standard for aging. Focus: Aging. Guilford, Duskin Publishing Group, 1978

Stuart G, Sundeen S: Principles and Practice of Psychiatric Nursing. St. Louis, CV Mosby, 1983

Walker JI: Everybody's Guide to Emotional Well-Being. San Francisco, Harbor Publishing, 1982

Wantz M, Gay J: The Aging Process: A Health Perspective. Cambridge, Winthrop Publishers, 1981

28

CHILD ABUSE AND NEGLECT

PLEASE, MOM AND DAD

My hands are small—I don't mean to spill my milk.

My legs are short—Please slow down so I can
keep up with you.

Don't slap my hands when I touch something
bright and pretty—I don't understand.

Please look at me when I talk to you—it lets
me know you are really listening.

My feelings are tender—don't nag me all day—let
me make mistakes without feeling stupid.

Don't expect the bed I make or the picture I
draw to be perfect—just love me for trying.

Remember I am a child not a small adult—sometimes
I don't understand what you are saying.

I love you so much. Please love me just for being
me—not just for the things I can do.

By Richardson J, Richardson J.
(Funded by Health and Rehabilitative Services, State of Florida)

LEARNING OBJECTIVES

1. Discuss the elements that generally create an environment for abuse to occur.
2. Describe the characteristics of potentially abusive or neglectful parents.
3. Define the following:
   Child abuse
   Child neglect
   Discipline
4. List physical, behavioral, and environmental indicators of
   Physical abuse of a child
   Child neglect
   Emotional maltreatment of a child
   Sexual abuse of a child
5. Discuss the multidisciplinary treatment approach of child abuse.
6. List community support services available to help prevent the repetition of abuse.
7. State how the nurse may help prevent child abuse.
8. List the steps in reporting child abuse or neglect.
9. Develop a nursing care plan for a victim of child abuse.

HILD abuse has become increasingly frequent since the onset of the industrial revolution. Terms used to describe child abuse include "battered child syndrome" and "nonaccidental injury to children." Barker (1983) states that the cause of child abuse is complex and can occur at three levels: 1) in the home, where the abusers are parents or parent substitutes; 2) in the institutional setting, such as day-care centers, child-care agencies, schools, welfare departments, correctional settings, and residential centers; and 3) in society, which allows children to live in poverty or be denied the basic necessities of life. This chapter focuses on child abuse and neglect occurring within the home setting.

Statistics reveal that children who are abused physically are generally under 2 years of age, whereas victims of sexual abuse are usually 6 to 9 years old at the onset of abuse. Most reported cases of sexual abuse involve girls. Physical abuse may be carried out by a father or stepfather, mother, babysitter, or guardian. Sexual abuse generally occurs between a father and child (Stuart and Sundeen, 1983).

Numerous factors are involved in defining child abuse and neglect. They include cultural and ethnic backgrounds, attitudes concerning parenting, social factors, and environmental or circumstantial factors. Abuse is considered an act of commission in which intentional physical, mental, or emotional harm is inflicted on a child by a parent or other person. It may include repeated injuries or unexplained cuts, bruises, fractures, burns or scars; harsh punishment; or sexual abuse or exploitation. Abuse is not to be confused with discipline. Discipline is a purposeful action to restrain or correct a child's behavior. It is done in a reasonable manner to teach, not punish, and it is not designated solely to hurt the child or result in injury. Neglect is an act of omission and refers to a parent's or person's failure to meet a dependent's basic needs such as proper food, clothing, shelter, medical care, schooling, or attention; provide safe living conditions; provide physical or emotional care; or provide supervision, thus leaving him unattended or abandoning him.

CAUSES OF ABUSE AND NEGLECT

Anyone can neglect or abuse a child under certain circumstances such as stress due to illness, marital problems, financial difficulties, or during parent–child conflict. Parents or other persons may lose control of their feelings of anger or frustration and direct such feelings toward a child.

Three elements that generally create the environment for an incident of abuse to occur include the abuser, the abused, and a crisis. The abuser is generally a parent or caretaker who has certain characteristics and a behavior pattern not representative of good parenting. Many abusers have a history of having been brought up in very strict families and being abused themselves. Abusive parents generally are young; pick a mate who is indifferent, passive, or of little help to them; keep to themselves; and move from place to place. In general, they display a poor self-concept, immaturity, fear of authority, lack of skills to meet their own emotional needs, belief in harsh physical discipline, fear of spoiling a child, poor impulsive control, and unreasonable expectations for a child. The mate, who usually knows about the abuse, either ignores it or may even participate in it. The abused or child victim is usually under 6 years of age, more vulnerable to abuse than others, and may have a physical or mental handicap. Emotionally disturbed, temperamental, hyperactive, or adopted children also demonstrate a higher incidence of abuse. The child may irritate the parent to the point of loss of control or may provoke abuse while attempting to get attention. A crisis (*e.g.,* loss of a job, divorce, illness, or death in the family) is generally the precipitating factor that sets the abusive parent in motion. The parent overreacts because he is unable to cope with numerous or complex stressors, becomes frustrated and anxious, and suddenly loses control, abusing the child.

OTHER CHARACTERISTICS OF POTENTIALLY ABUSIVE OR NEGLECTFUL PARENTS

Characteristics of potentially abusive or neglectful parents are warning signals but do not mean that abuse or neglect will inevitably occur. They are often present in high-risk families and may be noticeable before the birth of a child. Such characteristics (described below) displayed for a short period of time may indicate the result of anxiety in a new mother or father; however, if they persist, the parent should seek help.

The profile of abusive or neglectful parents of a soon-to-be or newborn child include:

1. Denial of a pregnancy by a mother who has made no plans for the birth of the child and refuses to talk about the pregnancy

2. Depression during pregnancy

3. Fear of delivery

4. Lack of support from husband or family

5. Undue concern about the unborn child's sex and how well it will perform

6. Fear that the child will be one of too many children

7. Giving birth to an unwanted child

8. Resentment toward the child by a jealous parent

9. Indifference or a negative attitude toward the child by the parent after delivery

10. Inability to tolerate the child's crying, views it as being too demanding

There are no physical characteristics that automatically identify the potential child abuser; the person may be rich or poor, of any racial origin, and male or female.

AREAS OF CHILD ABUSE OR NEGLECT

Maltreatment of children generally falls into the following general areas: 1) physical abuse; 2) neglect; 3) emotional maltreatment; and 4) sexual abuse. Physical, behavioral, and environmental indicators often afford clues to a child's needs and treatment by parents. They will be discussed in reference to each of the four general areas of maltreatment.

Physical Abuse

The most common physical indicators seen in child abuse are bruises in which there is no breakage of the skin. They are generally seen on the posterior side of the body or on the face, in unusual patterns or clusters, and in various stages of healing, making it difficult to determine the exact age of a bruise. Burns also are frequently seen and generally are due to immersion in hot water, contact with cigarettes, tying with a rope, or the application of a hot iron. Areas of the body where burns are seen include the buttocks, palms of hands, soles of feet, wrists, ankles, or genitals. Lacerations, abrasions, welts, and scars may be noted on the lips, eyes, face, or external genitalia. Other physical indicators include missing or loosened teeth; skeletal injuries such as fractured bones, and epiphyseal separation or stiff, swollen, enlarged joints; head injuries; and internal injuries. Such physical injuries should be considered with respect to the child's medical history, developmental ability to injury himself, and behavioral indicators.

Behavioral indicators of physical abuse are dependent on the age at which the child is abused, as well as the frequency and the severity of abuse. The behavioral profile of a physically abused child includes

1. Fear of parents as well as fear of physical contact with an adult

2. Extremes in behavior such as passivity or aggressiveness, or crying very often or very little

3. Sudden onset of regressive behavior such as thumb sucking, enuresis, or encopresis

4. Learning problems that cannot be diagnosed

5. Truancy or tardiness in school

6. Fatigue causing the child to sleep in class

7. Inappropriate dress to hide burns, bruises, or other marks of abuse

8. Inappropriate dress, resulting in frostbite or illness due to exposure to inclement weather

9. Overly compliant to avoid confrontation

10. Sporadic temper tantrums

11. Hurting other children

12. Demanding behavior

If such behaviors are present in a child, he should be observed for physical injuries.

Environmental indicators that indicate the increase of the likelihood for physical abuse in children include severe parental problems such as drug addiction, alcoholism, and mental illness; family crisis; and geographic or social isolation of the family.

Child Abuse: Examples

Parents of an 8-month-old girl hired two babysitters ages 14 and 12 to watch their daughter while they celebrated their wedding anniversary. The young sitters physically abused the child by tossing her back and forth in a game of catch and suspended her from a ceiling light fixture, allowing her to fall on the floor. She sustained several internal injuries and was hospitalized in serious condition. The babysitters were charged with delinquency and the parents were found guilty of child abuse and neglect by placing her in the care of two minors.

In another case of child abuse, a man was accused of beating his girl-friend's 5-year-old girl severely enough to cause permanent brain damage. The child was beaten with a stick and forced to drink dishwashing liquid because she was "too sassy." After the beating, the child was kept on the floor of the apartment because she appeared to be unconscious at times. The mother force-fed her daughter oatmeal and bananas in an effort to revive her. Two days later the child was taken to the hospital and was found to have burn marks on her buttocks, a head injury, and bruises on her body. The mother was charged with child abuse, and the boyfriend was sentenced to 15 years in prison due to aggravated child abuse.

Neglect

As stated earlier, neglect is an act of omission and includes abandonment; lack of adequate supervision; and failure to meet the child's basic human needs of shelter, adequate nutrition, good hygiene, adequate clothing, and proper medical or dental care. Financial status, cultural values, and parental capacity should be considered before a parent or adult is accused of neglecting a child.

Behavioral indicators of neglect commonly seen include failure to thrive; learning difficulties due to poor attention span, inability to concentrate, or autistic behavior; use of drugs or alcohol; delinquency; and sexual misconduct.

Neglected children may live in an environment characterized by poverty, come from a large family with marital conflict, lack material resources, or experience indifferent parental attitudes.

Characteristics of neglectful parents include lack of understanding of the child's physical and emotional needs, lack of interest in the child's activities, poor parenting skills, and poor personal hygiene.

Child Neglect: Examples

A fundamentalist mother and father denied medical care to their infant son, resulting in the child's death due to suffocation from pneumonia. The parents, who were convicted of reckless homicide and child neglect, were sentenced to 5 years in prison.

A second case of child neglect occurred when a young divorced working mother entrusted the care of her 1- and 2-year-old children to her 8-year-old daughter while she worked as a waitress from approximately 7 PM to midnight. Before she left for work each evening she locked the younger children in their bedrooms and instructed the older daughter to stay indoors and "keep an eye on the children." One evening a fire began on the second floor of the apartment, killing the two younger children by smoke inhalation. The 8-year-old was able to escape the fire. The mother told the authorities she made minimum wages and was unable to afford to pay a babysitter, so that she worked at night while her older daughter was home.

Emotional Maltreatment (Abuse or Neglect)

Emotional maltreatment or psychological abuse may consist of verbal assaults or threats that provoke fear; poor communication that may send double messages; and blaming, confusing, or demeaning messages. Inappropriate discipline, immature parenting, continuous friction or conflict in the home, rejecting parents, discriminatory treatment of children in the family, and abuse of drugs or alcohol are examples of environmental indicators or pathologic, destructive parenting patterns. Such parents may tell the child that he is unwanted, unloved, or unworthy of care. He may become the scapegoat of the family; that is, accused of causing family problems. "If it weren't for your bad habits, Daddy wouldn't leave us!", "It's all your fault we don't have any money. You're sick all the time" and "The family got along fine until you started to act so selfish." The child often develops a low self-concept as he hears such negative comments and may exhibit behavioral indicators such as

1. Stuttering
2. Enuresis or encopresis
3. Delinquency, truancy, or other disciplinary problems
4. Hypochondriasis
5. Autism or failure to thrive
6. Overeating
7. Childhood depression
8. Suicide attempts

Emotional neglect occurs when parents or a responsible adult fail to provide an emotional climate that fosters feelings of love, belonging, recognition, and an enhanced self-esteem. Examples of emotional neglect include ignoring the child, providing minimal human contact, and failure to provide opportunities to foster growth and development.

Emotional Maltreatment and Sexual Abuse: Example

Two brothers, ages 5 and 7, were found on several occasions acting as if they were dogs. Their mother stated they would walk, eat, bark, and carry objects in their mouths. At times they would drop their heads in their cereal bowls or soup and lap their food like a dog. They had to be reminded continually that they were little boys. When questioned by the police, the young boys stated that their father hooked them to a chain and harness and told them to act like dogs. Their father and other men also performed sexual acts on the boys. The father was sentenced to 2 years imprisonment.

Sexual Abuse

Sexual abuse is not easy to identify because the physical signs of abuse generally are not seen outside a clinical or medical setting. The child victim is usually reluctant to share information about the abuse, which may include anything from fondling to forcible rape.

Incest, or sexual intercourse between family members who are so closely related as to be legally prohibited from marrying one another due to consanguinity, is generally a well-guarded secret. Approximately 100,000 cases of incest occur each year but fewer than 25% are reported, according to the American Psychological Association and the National Center on Child Abuse and Neglect.

Physical indicators of sexual abuse that may be present during an examination include:

1. Itching, pain, bruises, or bleeding in the external genitalia, vagina, or anal area
2. Edema of the cervix, vulva, or perineum
3. Torn, stained, or bloody undergarments
4. Stretched hymen at a very young age
5. Presence of semen or of a sexually transmitted disease
6. Pregnancy in an older child
7. Bladder infections

Behavioral indicators or characteristics exhibited by a sexually abused child are quite numerous. The more commonly seen behaviors include

1. Difficulty in walking or sitting
2. Reluctance to participate in recreational or physical activities
3. Poor peer relationships
4. Delinquency, truancy, acting out, or runaway behavior
5. Preoccupation with sexual organs of self or others (occurs with younger children)
6. Sexual promiscuity or prostitution in older children

7. Use of drugs and alcohol

8. Confiding in a friend, teacher, or to the authorities

Environmental indicators or elements common in cases of child sexual abuse are as follows:

1. Overcrowding in the home

2. Prolonged absence of a parent

3. Social and/or geographical isolation of a family

4. Intergenerational pattern of incest

5. Alcoholism

6. Extremely protective attitude toward the child by a jealous parent who refuses to allow the child to have any social contact, distrusts the child and accuses the child of sexual promiscuity

7. Marital difficulties

8. Personality disorders in the parents

Sexual Abuse: Examples

A 6-year-old girl, daughter of a well-liked and respected member of the community, was forced by her father to have oral sex with him when her mother was away at club meetings. The sexual encounters lasted only a few months but had a profound effect on the young girl, whose parents divorced when she was 14. She loved her father but also hated him and swore that she would never tell anyone about the incest. A few years after she married, her deteriorating sexual relationship with her husband prompted her to admit the incest and to seek therapy.

Another case of sexual abuse involved several children in an unlicensed babysitting service. The owner was arrested on charges of violating his probation from a previous child molestation conviction, filming infants and toddlers during incidents of child abuse, and having oral sex with some of the children under his care. One child was found to have gonorrhea of the throat.

TREATMENT

Treatment of victims of child abuse or neglect is considered to be a multidisciplinary process, frequently beginning with crisis intervention. Members of the treatment team may include doctors, nurses, psychologists, psychiatrists, social workers, teachers, and law enforcement officers. Once child abuse is established, the child welfare agency is responsible for the child's immediate welfare and decides whether to remove the child from his natural environment by placing him in a hospital or foster home.

A social worker from the child welfare agency usually investigates the family and recommends whether psychiatric treatment is needed for the child, family, or both. Barker (1983) recommends that a nonpunitive, empathetic approach be used when the parents or responsible adults are questioned about the child's abuse. The helping person or interviewer should not become overinvolved or display anger toward them because such approaches negate the development of a therapeutic relationship. He also recommends temporary or permanent removal of abused children from their natural environment, depending on the details of the abuse during psychiatric evaluation and treatment of the child. Child abuse may result in a serious injury, permanent brain or physical damage, growth failure, personality or behavioral problems, or intellectual retardation.

Support services available in the community to help prevent the repetition of abuse may include the following:

1. Visiting or public health nurses
2. Protective services
3. Emergency shelter for children
4. Day care centers or nurseries
5. Self-help groups
6. Telephone hot-lines
7. Home maker services
8. Financial assistance
9. Employment counseling
10. Parent education classes
11. Foster home care
12. Transportation services
13. Counseling
14. Assertiveness training

NURSING CARE OF ABUSED CHILDREN

Nursing personnel generally respond to child abuse with feelings of shock, anger, rage, or revulsion. People who have abused children anticipate such responses from helping persons and authority figures, thus resisting efforts to involve them in therapy. If the nurse displays negative responses such as frustration, hopelessness, sadness, or sympathy, she is unable to be objective and to plan competent nursing interventions. Nurses should realize that abusive parents as well as abused children have severe, unmet dependency needs, and accept abusive parents as worthwhile people.

Parents of physically abused children brought to emergency room settings generally give a predictable history, namely, falling out of bed, against a piece of furniture or household appliance, or down a flight of stairs. They are generally inconsistent in giving details that are nearly always incompatible with the child's injuries. The child may appear guarded or afraid of any physical contact with the examiner or parents while receiving treatment. Such victims of sexual abuse generally try to protect the offender and may act in a pseudoadult manner.

ASSESSMENT

The assessment process includes a thorough physical and x-ray examination, including inspection of the genitals and anus. Play therapy and art therapy also serve as assessment tools when child abuse is suspected. A mature, patient, empathetic approach should be used, while focusing on physical, behavioral, and environmental indicators of abuse as well as family dynamics. Evidence of malnutrition, dehydration, old fractures, bruises, internal injuries, or intracranial hemorrhage may be present. The child's behavioral characteristics may include withdrawal, low self-esteem, oppositional behavior, compulsive behavior, hypervigilance, or an increased awareness of the environment, and a fearful attitude toward the parents.

The results of the assessment process should be well documented, with particular emphasis on the child's physical status, emotional status, developmental level or stage, interpersonal skills, and behavioral response to the family.

NURSING DIAGNOSIS

Once the data are analyzed, nursing diagnoses are formulated. The following are examples of nursing diagnoses commonly seen in victims of child abuse or neglect:

1. Alterations in comfort: pain from physical abuse by parents
2. Impaired verbal communication owing to the psychological barrier of fear
3. Ineffective individual coping because of developmental delays
4. Ineffective family coping because of parental child abuse
5. Fear due to history of child abuse
6. Potential for less than adequate nutritional requirements due to parental neglect
7. Disturbance in self-concept due to a sense of inferiority

INTERVENTION

Nursing intervention may occur in a variety of settings such as in the school, by the school nurse; the home, by the public health nurse; the hospital, by the emergency room or staff nurse; or the doctor's office, by the office nurse.

The hardest task for the nurse is to develop a trusting relationship with the abused child and family. Immediate care should focus on meeting physical and emotional needs to promote homeostasis and comfort, and to reduce fear. Once these needs are met, problems such as impaired verbal communication, ineffective individual coping, ineffective family coping, and disturbance in self-concept can be addressed. Ideally, during this time, intervention also may focus on treating the family as a unit to facilitate a healthy, safe environment for the child later.

PREVENTION OF CHILD ABUSE AND NEGLECT

The nurse may help prevent child abuse by recognizing early signs of abuse, supporting and working for legislation to interrupt the child abuse syndrome, promoting educational courses on family interpersonal relationships and child raising practices, promoting community awareness programs, participating in continuing educational courses, and participating in nursing research of child abuse and effective treatment measures.

In most states, certain professional people are required by law to report suspected child abuse, neglect, or sexual abuse. Even if the law does not require a nurse to report such a case, she has an ethical obligation to protect a child from harm. It is not the intent of the law to remove a child from his home unless he is in danger. Parents are not punished unless undue harm has occurred. In most situations, the family is helped so that the parents and child can stay together. Directions on how to report child abuse follow. Such a report may be made by telephone, in person, or in writing to a local welfare department children's services board or the local police department. The nurse should state the following information:

1. Name and address of the suspected victim
2. Child's age
3. Name and address of the child's parent or caretaker
4. Name of the person suspected of abusing or neglecting the child
5. Why abuse or neglect is suspected
6. Any other helpful information
7. Her name, if she wishes

The case will be investigated whether the reporter remains anonymous or gives a name.

SUMMARY

Child abuse can occur at three levels: in the home, in institutional set-tings, and in society. Physical abuse generally occurs in children under 2 years of age, whereas sexual abuse usually begins between the ages of 6 and 9 years. This chapter discussed the factors contributing to child abuse and neglect; defined abuse, discipline, and neglect; and listed the three elements necessary for abuse to occur. Characteristics of potentially abu-sive or neglectful parents were stated. The four areas of child abuse or neglect were described and examples of each were given. They include physical abuse, neglect, emotional maltreatment, and sexual abuse. Phys-ical, behavioral, and environmental indicators of child abuse were explored. The multidisciplinary treatment approach was explained, and support services available to abusive families were listed. Nursing care of abused children focused on the nurse's reponse to an abused child, the assessment process, and prevention of abuse. Information on how to report child abuse was detailed.

LEARNING ACTIVITIES

   I. Clinical activities
      A. Care for a victim of physical abuse, neglect, emotional maltreat-ment, or sexual abuse if possible.
      B. Assess the victim's physical, behavioral, and environmental stressors.
      C. Develop a nursing care plan, stating appropriate diagnoses and interventions.
  II. Independent activities
      A. Obtain data from the local child welfare agency regarding its role and function in child abuse.
      B. Investigate the law on reporting child abuse in the state in which you reside.

SELF-TEST

Answer the following questions with a statement to support your choice of true or false:

1. Child abuse and neglect occur rarely.
2. Many neglected or abused children become neglectful or abusive parents themselves.
3. Abuse may be directed toward only one child in a family.

4. Most abusive and neglectful parents suffer from severe mental illness.

5. You must have concrete evidence of abuse or neglect before you report it.

6. An anonymous report of abuse and neglect will not be investigated.

Complete the following statements:

7. Reasons why parents do not take care of their children (neglect them), include _____.

8. Children are physically abused because _____.

9. The most common physical indicators seen in child abuse are _____.

10. Behavioral symptoms of child abuse include _____.

11. Examples of child neglect include _____.

12. Examples of emotional maltreatment include _____.

13. Physical indicators of sexual abuse include _____.

14. Characteristics of potentially abusive or neglectful parents include _____.

15. The multidisciplinary team approach for child abuse includes _____.

16. Support services available in the community to prevent the repetition of abuse include _____.

17. The attitude of a nurse dealing with child abuse victims should be one of _____.

18. Examples of nursing diagnoses commonly seen in victims of child abuse or neglect include _____.

19. Settings in which nursing interventions for child abuse may occur include _____.

20. Examples of prevention of child abuse include _____.

REFERENCES

Barker P: Basic Child Psychiatry, 4th ed. Baltimore, University Park Press, 1983

Burgess AW: Psychiatric Nursing in the Hospital and the Community, 3rd ed. Englewood Cliffs, Prentice–Hall, 1981

Burgess AW et al: Sexual Abuse of Children and Adolescent. Lexington, Mass.: D.C. Heath and Co, 1977

Carpenito LJ: Nursing Diagnosis: Application to Clinical Practice. Philadelphia, JB Lippincott, 1983

Chase N: A Child Is Being Beaten. New York, Holt, Rinehart & Winston, 1975

Child abuse rate called 'epidemic'. New York Times: Nov 30, 1975

Gagnon J: Female child victims of sexual offenses. J Sociological Problems: 1978

Haber J et al: Comprehensive Psychiatric Nursing, 2nd ed. New York, McGraw–Hill, 1982

Jacoby S: Nothing really happened. McCall's: Nov, 1981

Justice B, Justice R: The Abusing Family. New York, Human Services Press, 1976

Keanon K: The sexually abused child. Nurs 77: May, 1977

Kempe CH et al: The Battered Child Syndrome. JAMA: July, 1962

Kempe R, Kempe C: Child Abuse. Boston, Harvard University Press, 1978

Leaman K: The sexually abused child. Nurs 77: May, 1977

Lego S: The American Handbook of Psychiatric Nursing. Philadelphia, JB Lippincott, 1984

Maurer A: 1001 Alternatives to Corporal Punishment, Vol 1. Berkeley, CA, Generations Books, 1984

McNeese MC, Hebeler JR: The abused child. Clin Symp: Sept, 1977

Murray R, Heulskoetter M: Psychiatric Mental Health Nursing: Giving Emotional Care. Englewood Cliffs, Prentice–Hall, 1983

Stuart G, Sundeen S: Principles and Practice of Psychiatric Nursing, 2nd ed. St. Louis, CV Mosby, 1983

Wathey R, Densengerber J: Incest: An analysis of the victim and the aggressor. New York, Odyssey Institute, 1976

29

THE ABUSED PERSON

WITHIN THE FAMILY UNIT

LEARNING OBJECTIVES

1. Discuss how a person can be abused physically, psychologically, economically, socially, or sexually.

2. Describe the dynamics of spouse abuse.

3. Explain how elderly persons are abused.

4. Discuss the assessment process of a physically abused person.

5. Cite nursing interventions for the following diagnoses of a physically abused person:

Disturbance in self-concept

Anxiety due to a physical assault

Ineffective family coping because of abusive behavior by a spouse

BUSIVE or battering behavior is one of the most underreported crimes because of fear, embarrassment, and humiliation by the victim, who may be abused physically, psychologically, economically, socially, or sexually. Studies by Strauss in 1975 reveal that 16% of middle-aged couples had abused each other physically. Benedek reports spouse abuse in one out of every two couples (Friedman, 1981). The term *spouse* refers to a partner in a marriage or a partner in a heterosexual common-law marriage, in which both partners share the same household. Lau and Cosberg report that approximately 1 out of 10 persons aged 60 or older are abused or neglected (Wilson and Kneisl, 1983). This chapter centers on abuse of adults within the family unit: spouses and elderly parents.

THEORIES REGARDING ABUSIVE BEHAVIOR

Various theories describe the causative factors for abusive behavior toward spouses and elderly parents. These theories are classified as 1) psychodynamic, 2) social learning, 3) psychosocial, 4) enviornmental, 5) family structure, and 6) family systems theories. The following is a summary of such causative factors:

1. The abuser is deprived of nurturing and mothering as a child; therefore, he is unable to do so as an adult. Such a person may be a victim of physical or sexual abuse and unable to trust others.

2. The abuser may have a history of antisocial behavior, including drug and alcohol abuse, and is unable to control impulsive behavior owing to frustration or anxiety. Persons often act more violently when they are under the influence of alcohol or drugs.

3. Specific behaviors learned during various developmental stages become part of a person's interactions with spouse and family. For example, a child who lives in an environment in which spouse or parental abuse occurs probably will believe that abuse is normal unless intervention occurs to prohibit such behavior.

4. Poor socioeconomic conditions resulting in increased stress, anxiety, or frustration may precipitate abusive behavior within the family unit.

5. Poor communication skills may result in the use of verbal or physical abuse.

6. Abusive behavior may increase after the death of a significant family member, the loss of a job, a geographic move, the onset of physical or mental illness, a developmental change, or family change such as pregnancy or the birth of a child.

TYPES OF ABUSE

Physical abuse involves a willful, nonaccidental attempt to injure a person by way of a direct, overtly aggressive attack. Morton (Lego, 1984) cites various levels of battering behavior by physically abusive persons. The least injurious level is referred to as mild physical abuse (*e.g.,* throwing objects at a family member); the most serious type, lethal abuse, includes threatening, torturing, or strangling one's spouse or parent.* Men generally push, shove, grab, slap, hit repeatedly, torture, or threaten with a lethal object during physical abuse. Women hit with or throw objects, use fists, kick, bite, or scratch. An estimated 2 million women are battered yearly. No statistics are yet available on the number of men who are victims of battery.

Physical battering may be accomplished by psychological abuse as a spouse or elderly parent is verbally degraded and threatened with hostile or vicious language. The abused person may feel rejected, embarrassed, stupid, or unloved when self-worth is threatened. Abusers may prohibit victims from socializing with others, force victims to engage in unwanted sexual activity, use the act of sex as a form of punishment or reward, or control the abused person's source of income.

Psychological, Social, and Sexual Abuse: Clinical Example

SJ, a 27-year-old mother of two children, confided in the nurse that her husband constantly "put her down" in the presence of family and friends by calling her stupid, ignorant, and lazy. Although they were financially stable, he refused to give her a weekly allowance for groceries or miscellaneous expenses. He also refused to let her use the family car to visit friends or relatives. When she asked for money to replace a bicycle tire, she was told there was no money for such an unnecessary request. SJ also related that her husband decided when and where they would engage in sexual activity. She stated her husband withheld marital sex as a form of

*Although men are victims of abuse, most commonly victims are women. In this chapter the portrayed victims are female.

punishment whenever he felt she was not "performing her duties as a model wife and mother." She denied any physical abuse, although she commented that at times her husband appeared to be on the verge of hitting her as he verbally abused her.

Abuse as experienced by SJ: 1) may occur in any socioeconomic, religious, or racial group; 2) occurs within various cultures; 3) increases during pregnancy; 4) generally occurs between the hours of 8 PM to 11:30 PM; and 5) occurs most frequently on weekends. The most common setting for physical abuse is the kitchen. The batterer, or abuser, frequently appears to be possessive, suspicious, jealous, dependent, and believes in the traditional male-dominant role. He usually blames others for his actions when he appears depressed, anxious, contrite, remorseful, or guilty. His low self-esteem may result in the use of alcohol, drugs, or violence to cope with increased stress, and he may use sex to establish dominance in interpersonal relationships. The battered partner is viewed as a submissive, passive, dependent person with low self-esteem, who is guilt-ridden and accepts the responsibility for another's actions. Feelings of anxiety, depression, or helplessness may result in the use of alcohol or drugs, the expression of somatic complaints, or suicidal behavior. The battered person also believes in the traditional male and female roles and uses sex to establish an intimate relationship.

Dynamic of Physical Spouse Abuse

Spouse abuse generally occurs as a tension-releasing mechanism precipitated by the inability to cope with an increase of daily stressors. Disagreements may occur between a couple as the battered person is unable to assert herself and withdraws in an attempt to display any anger verbally or nonverbally. The spouse becomes possessive, jealous, and fearful as he senses the partner's anger, causing emotional distancing to occur. Such nonassertiveness on the part of the battered person is rationalized by the spouse as acceptance and permission to vent tensions. Minor physical abusive incidents may cause the battered person to cope with abuse by somatizing while the spouse attempts to reduce tension by taking drugs or drinking alcohol, which further decreases inhibitions and precipitates abusive episodes.

During an acute battering incident, the spouse loses control of behavior because of blind rage. The battered person also loses control and is unable to stop the physical abusiveness experienced. Both persons are in a state of shock immediately after the incident. The spouse is unable to recall his behavior; the battered person depersonalizes during the abusive incident and is able to recall in detail what occurred. As both calm down, the spouse may exhibit feelings of remorse, beg forgiveness, promise not to control in the future, and state that he cannot live without the battered partner. The abused person believes her spouse's promises and forgives him because she then feels less helpless. Such behavior on her part is interpreted by the spouse as an act of love and acceptance. She generally does not take assertive action to stop the abuse because she believes her husband will change; is afraid of more violence; lacks self-confidence; feels trapped; feels guilty, ashamed, embarrassed, helpless, or powerless; is dependent emotionally and financially on her spouse; feels that her child or children need their father; or rationalizes that life is "not so bad." (Lego, 1984 and Altrocchi, 1980).

Family Violence Due to Spouse Abuse: Clinical Example

JW, a 43-year-old housewife, was beaten, bruised, and afraid. She stood in her bedroom pointing a pistol at her angry, abusive husband. Both her eyes were swollen, choke marks were on her neck, and bruises were evident on several areas of her body. She killed her husband with the pistol. When questioned by police, she stated that he was totally out of control after drinking beer. His blood alcohol level was 0.236. (A person is considered legally intoxicated if the level is above 0.10!) JW described her husband as a hard worker and good father who was a loving person when he was sober but a totally different person when he was intoxicated. He had beaten her on several occasions in the past 6 months but never to the point of choking and punching her. In the past, JW's husband would wake up in the morning after physically abusing her and ask "Did I do that?" He would promise such behavior "wouldn't happen again" and she would believe him.

ABUSE OF THE ELDERLY

According to some estimates, approximately 1 in 10 elderly individuals (*i.e.,* 60 years of age or older) living with their families are subject to some type of abuse or neglect and the incidence is increasing. Causative factors eliciting abusive behavior include severe physical or mental disabilities, financial dependency, personality conflicts, societal attitudes toward aging (*e.g.,* considering the elderly person to be a burden), and frustration while caring for an impaired elderly person. Many times elderly persons are expected to meet the needs of their grown children. These family members may become abusive if the elderly parent is unable to communicate clearly with them or meet their emotional needs.

The abuse of elderly persons can occur in a variety of settings, such as nursing homes, general hospitals, retirement centers, in their homes, or in the homes of adults who care for them. Many states are presently advocating the adoption of laws similar to child abuse laws to prevent the abuse of the elderly.

Types and examples of abuse of the elderly are given below:

TYPES	EXAMPLES
Physical	Direct beatings Lack of or withholding food or medical care Lack of supervision Overmedication Withholding life-sustaining medication
Psychological	Verbal assault or threats Intentional isolation of the elderly by refusing to transport the person who is unable to leave home unattended
Violation of rights	Placing the elderly person in a nursing home against his wishes when he is not dangerous to himself or others
Material abuse	Misuse of money or property by children or legal guardians Stealing of social security checks Robbery

Elderly persons may not report abusive behavior because of fear of retaliation by the abuser, fear of rejection, a low self-esteem (whereby they feel they deserve such treatment), loyalty to caretakers, or lack of contact with helping persons.

ASSESSMENT OF ABUSED OR ASSAULTED PERSONS

Clinical assessment by the nurse and attending physician is done to determine if the abused or assaulted victim is in any physical or life-threatening danger due to injuries requiring emergency medical care. The battered person may present with multiple bruises or injuries, somatic complaints or symptoms associated with trauma that may not be observable, or characteristic behavioral reactions such as acute anxiety reaction, depression, suicidal ideation, or crisis. Determining the emotional status of the victim is imperative. Obtaining a medical history is also important to obtain additional clues to battering and to make a tentative medical, psychological, and nursing diagnosis. The person may describe a history of multiple injuries, psychiatric problems, medical problems, or self-abusive behavior (*e.g.,* substance abuse, drug abuse, or suicidal gestures).

Interview questions directed at possible battered persons should be carried out in a supportive and sensitive manner. Inquiries focus on any suspicious-looking injuries; how the injuries occurred; whether the battered person is living with the abuser; the victim's emotional response to the abuser; a safe place for the victim and any children to go such as a shelter; and whether the victim wants to press charges.

NURSING INTERVENTIONS

The physician's primary concerns center on immediate care of physical injuries, prevention or alleviation of psychological damage, and proper medical examination.

The nurse's role is to give emergency medical care and to plan appropriate intervention as an acute anxiety reaction may occur after abuse. Crisis intervention skills are used to reduce anxiety and provide supportive care. (See Chaps. 6 and 12). It is important that arrangements are made for someone to stay with the battered or abused person. If an in-depth formal interview is necessary, the assault victim is informed of her rights and arrangements are made for the story to be told in detail only once so that the victim does not have to relive the incident psychologically by unnecessary repetition.

Other initial nursing interventions after abuse include: providing privacy and respecting the rights to confidentiality, displaying a nonjudgmental attitude, encouraging verbalization of feelings and thoughts about the assault, explaining the examination process, and assisting with an examination.

After the person has been examined and crisis intervention has been employed, the abused person may benefit from one or more of the following therapeutic interventions: 1) individual psychotherapy; 2) family or couple therapy; 3) group psychotherapy; 4) temporary emergency housing, such as a shelter for battered persons, hospitalization, boarding house, or community church facility; 5) emergency financial assistance for food, shelter, or clothing; 6) vocational counseling; 7) legal counseling; and 8) referral to a crisis hot-line, self-help group, or social worker.

Older adults may benefit from additional services such as alternative housing, nursing care by the visiting nurse or public health nurse, food from Meals on Wheels, assistance from a visiting home-maker program, visits by persons involved in a foster grandparent program, and transportation for the elderly provided by community organizations.

Following are examples of nursing diagnoses and nursing interventions for persons who have been abused. Emphasis is placed on meeting the psychological needs of the people.

NURSING DIAGNOSES	NURSING INTERVENTIONS
Disturbance in self-concept because of severe trauma of physical abuse	Establish trust and rapport by encouraging expression of feelings, avoiding negative criticism or judgmental comments, providing a safe, protective environment. Display acceptance. Assess the person's physical and psychological needs. Provide emergency medical care as needed.

NURSING DIAGNOSES	NURSING INTERVENTIONS
	Employ crisis intervention if necessary (see Chap. 6).
	Assess the need for emergency housing following medical care and financial assistance.
Anxiety because of actual threat to biologic integrity (physical assault)	Assess level of anxiety (see Chap. 12).
	Provide reassurance and comfort.
	Decrease environmental stimulation.
	Support present coping mechanisms.
	Explore alternative coping mechanisms such as relaxation techniques.
Ineffective family coping because of abusive behavior by a spouse	Provide an opportunity for expression of feelings in a safe environment.
	Encourage a realistic perception of the situation.
	Assess support systems.
	Provide a list of community agencies to obtain emergency and long-term support (*c.g.*, individual, group, or family therapy; legal counseling; crisis hot-line or support groups).

SUMMARY

Abusive or battering behavior can result in feelings of fear, embarrassment, and humiliation, thus making it one of the most underreported crimes. This chapter discussed physical, psychological, economical, social, and sexual abuse. Theories regarding abusive behavior were summarized. Examples of battering behavior were cited, and a clinical example of psychological, social, and sexual abuse was given. The dynamics of physical spouse abuse were explained, followed by an example of family violence from spouse abuse. Abuse of the elderly person was discussed, including types of abuse and examples of each. Assessment of abused or assaulted persons was described, and examples of nursing diagnoses and nursing interventions were given, focusing on disturbance in self-concept because of severe trauma of physical abuse; anxiety due to actual threat to biologic integrity; and ineffective family coping because of abusive behavior by a spouse.

LEARNING ACTIVITIES

I. Clinical activities
   A. If possible, spend a day of observation in a shelter for abused persons or in an emergency room of a large metropolitan hospital.

    B. Discuss the support systems made available to abused persons at this shelter or in the emergency room.

II. Independent activities

    A. Obtain a list of community agencies available to abused persons.

    B. Discuss the services provided by each agency.

    C. Contact the National Clearinghouse on Domestic Violence, P.O. Box 2309, Rockville, Maryland 20852, for additional information on family violence.

    D. Review the daily newspaper for a week and collect data on the types of domestic or family violence reported. Discuss the reported intervention for each case of abuse. Was it appropriate?

SELF-TEST

1. Describe abusive or battering behavior.

2. Give examples of
   Psychological abuse
   Social abuse
   Sexual abuse

3. Describe the personality of an abusive person.

4. State the dynamics of spouse abuse.

5. State why an abused spouse may not take assertive action to stop abuse.

6. State why elderly persons may be abused.

7. Cite examples of abuse of elderly persons.

8. State the rationale for clinical assessment of abused or assaulted victims.

9. List nursing interventions for a victim of spouse abuse who has experienced physical trauma.

10. List nursing interventions for an elderly parent whose daughter has withheld food, medication, and medical care.

REFERENCES

Altrocchi J: Abnormal Behavior. New York, Harcourt, Brace, Jovanovich, 1980

Backer BA et al: Psychiatric/Mental Health Nursing: Contemporary Readings. New York, D. Van Nostrand, 1978

Burgess AW: Psychiatric Nursing in the Hospital and the Community, 3rd ed. Englewood Cliffs, Prentice–Hall, 1981

Donlon PT, Rockwell DA: Psychiatric Disorders: Diagnoses and Treatment. Bowie, Robert J. Brady, 1982

Drake VK: Battered women: A health care problem in disguise. Image: June, 1982

Friedman MM: Family Nursing: Theory and Assessment. Norwalk, Appleton–Century–Crofts, 1981

Haber J et al: Comprehensive Psychiatric Nursing, 2nd ed. New York, McGraw–Hill, 1982

Lancaster J: Adult Psychiatric Nursing. Garden City, NJ: Medical Examination Publishing, 1980

Lego S: The American Handbook of Psychiatric Nursing. Philadephia, JB Lippincott, 1984

Mitchell JT, Resnik HLP: Emergency Response to Crisis, Bowie, Robert J. Brady, 1981

Murray RB, Huelskoetter MM: Psychiatric/Mental Health Nursing: Giving Emotional Care. Englewood Cliffs, Prentice–Hall, 1983

Stuart GW, Sundeen SJ: Principles and Practice of Psychiatric Nursing, 2nd ed. St. Louis, CV Mosby, 1983

Urdang L (ed): Mosby's Medical Nursing Dictionary. St. Louis, CV Mosby, 1983

Wilson HS, Kneisl CR: Psychiatric Nursing, 2nd ed. Menlo Park, Addison–Wesley, 1983

30

SEXUAL ABUSE: RAPE

LEARNING OBJECTIVES

1. Define rape.
2. State various motives for rape.
3. Differentiate between *blitz rape* and *confidence rape*.
4. Describe the following emotional reactions to rape:
   Rape trauma syndrome
   Maladaptive stress reaction
5. State the assessment process of a sexually abused person.
6. List nursing interventions for an acute stress reaction to rape.

RAPE is considered to be a universal crime against women: a violent sexual act committed against a woman's will involving the threat or use of force.

According to FBI statistics, in 1981, approximately 220,000 rapes occurred in 1 year, although only about 40% actually were reported. Sexual assault is considered a major unforgettable crisis and the most seriously underreported crime, in which the victim experiences an overwhelming, frightening experience of powerlessness and hopelessness (Mitchell and Resnik, 1981).

Three essential elements are necessary to define rape legally: 1) the use of force, threat, intimidation or duress; 2) vaginal, oral, or anal penetration; and 3) nonconsent by the victim. Rape statutes vary from state to state, and in some states a wife may charge her husband with rape. Attempted rape is defined as an assault on a woman in which oral, vaginal, or anal penetration is intended but does not occur. Statutory rape is the act of sexual intercourse with a girl under the age of consent (usually 16) *with* her consent. This chapter focuses on the rape of the adult female.

MOTIVES FOR RAPE

There is no typical rape victim profile. Every woman is a potential victim regardless of age, race, or socioeconomic status. Men who commit rape are from all walks of life and ethnic backgrounds; often victims of broken homes; young, usually under age 25, and often married, leading normal sex lives. Persons at high risk as rape victims include single females between the ages 11 and 25 who are black and come from a low socioeconomic background. Although most victims are women, men also have experienced sexual assaults.

Several motives for rape or sexual assault have been described by theorists: 1) anger rape, 2) power rape, 3) sadistic rape, and 4) impulsive or opportunistic rape. In the first pattern, anger rape, sex is used as a means of expressing rage, hatred, and contempt toward the victim. The rapist exhibits physical brutality by beating, kicking, or choking while he views the victim as a symbol of those women who wronged him at some point in life. Power rape is generally committed by persons with low self-esteem and a history of poor relationships with women, and is done in an attempt to prove manhood, competency, and strength. The offender forces the victim to become weak, helpless, and submissive, the exact qualities he despises in himself. Sadistic rape occurs because the person feels a need to inflict pain and torment on his victim to achieve sexual satisfaction. He misinterprets the victim's emotional anguish as sexual excitation rather than a refusal of his advances. Bizarre ritualistic behavior may occur during a sadistic rape. Impulsive, opportunistic rape may occur in conjunction with another antisocial act, such as a robbery. A person who is so antisocial takes what he wants whenever he desires it; rape therefore becomes a form of stealing.

Sexual attacks are considered to be one of the following: 1) blitz rape, in which an unexpected surprise attack occurs in the absence of prior interaction with the victim; 2) confidence rape, in which the offender and victim have had a prior interaction; 3) marked victim rape, in which the offender assaults a women he has been acquainted with in some way; 4) accessory-to-sex rape, which refers to a vulnerable victim's inability to give consent (as in the case of a mentally retarded person); and 5) "date-rape" after consent initially was given to participate in sexual relations but one partner exploits the other's initial friendliness or behavior.

EMOTIONAL REACTIONS TO RAPE

Rape trauma syndrome is a diagnosis used to describe the result of one's being raped, including an acute phase of disorganization and a longer phase of reorganization in a victim's life. The DSM-III recognizes rape as a post-traumatic stress disorder (see Chap. 12). The acute phase of rape trauma occurs when the victim is disrupted by the crisis and displays emotional reactions of anger, guilt, embarrassment, humiliation, denial, shock, disbelief, or fear of death; multiple physical or somatic complaints; or a wish for revenge. After a period of several weeks, the acute phase reactions give way to deeper, more long-term feelings of reorganization that cause the victim to change daily life patterns, experience recurring dreams and nightmares, seek support from friends and family, feel the need to talk about the sexual assault or refuse counseling, or develop irrational fears (phobias). One or more of six major phobic reactions may occur: 1) fear of being indoors if the rape occurred in the bedroom; 2) fear of the outdoors if the victim was sexually assaulted outside the home; 3) fear of crowds; 4) fear of being alone; 5) fear of people around the victim while the person engages in daily activities; and 6) fear of sexual activity if the person had no prior sexual experience. Long-term reactions to rape generally take a year or so to resolve, especially if the person goes through legal court action. During this time the victim may move into a new residence, change the telephone number, change jobs, or move to a new state. If the victim is married, severe marital conflict may occur.

A maladaptive stress reaction referred to as "silent rape syndrome" may occur. The victim fails to disclose information about the rape to anyone, is unable to resolve feelings about the sexual assault, experiences increased anxiety, and may develop a sudden phobic reaction. Behavioral changes may include depression, suicidal behavior, somatization, and acting out (*e.g.,* alcohol or drug abuse or sexual promiscuity).

ASSESSMENT OF SEXUALLY ABUSED PERSONS

Assessment by the nurse, attending physician, or other health care professional is done to determine if any physical or life-threatening danger exists. Emergency medical care may be given while the assessment process occurs if multiple bruises or injuries are present. The abused person may have somatic complaints or symptoms associated with trauma that are not readily observable.

Characteristic behavioral reactions that may be identified during a psychological assessment include an acute anxiety reaction, depression, suicidal ideation, or crisis. Other assessment data that should be collected if the patient can be questioned is a history of the rape, or attempted rape; legal information, including the names of persons who have been notified, such as the police; what evidence has been preserved; and support persons or systems available to the abused person.

If the victim gives consent and is able to tolerate the procedure, generally a gynecologic examination, pregnancy test if indicated, and laboratory tests are performed following a rape situation. The date of the victim's last menstrual period should be obtained.

Evidence the nurse should be aware of includes the presence of semen, stains, fiber, or hair on clothing or the body; fingernail scrapings; and pieces of torn clothing. If the victim has any of these in her possession or on her body, the evidence or specimens must be saved to be analyzed and documented, according to hospital protocol.

Foley (Lego, 1984) states that "competent and sensitive assessment of rape victims requires knowledge of rape myths and facts, an understanding of victims at risk as well as rape offender characteristics, and an awareness of both the victim's and nurse's personal responses to rape" (p. 477). The more common myths and facts about rape are presented herein:

RAPE MYTHS	RAPE FACTS
Attractive women provoke men into raping them.	Over 70% to 80% of all rapes are violent, planned aggressive acts not based on physical attractiveness or age. Statistics show rape victims range in age from approximately 3 months to over 90 years.
If a woman struggles, rape can be avoided; no woman can be raped against her will.	Rapists frequently overpower smaller and physically weaker women and carry weapons to harm, mutilate, or kill their victims. Counterattack by the victim may cause more injury to occur.
Only women with bad reputations or who are friendly to strangers outside their homes are raped.	All women are potential sexual assault victims. The rapist's desire is control, not sex. Approximately one third to one half of all rapes occur in a victim's home. Rapists include husbands, ex-husbands, neighbors, lovers, and boyfriends.
Women "cry rape" to get revenge.	Rape is an underreported crime owing to feelings of guilt. Approximately 2% of all reported rape cases are false (Lego, 1984, p. 478).
Most sexual assaults involve black men raping white women.	The rapist and victim tend to be of the same race (intraracial) in most cases of sexual assault.

Emotional responses by the victim to abuse or sexual assault vary according to the person's developmental level; therefore, the nurse needs to be familiar with developmental stages of the life cycle. Foley (Lego, 1984) gives excellent examples of reactions to rape according to developmental levels from infancy to older adulthood. Reactions cited include trust in adults shaken during infancy (0–3 yrs); preoccupation with wrong or bad acts during childhood (4–7 yrs); misperception of rape as a sexual act during latency (7 yrs to puberty); confusion over normal sexual behavior and concern about pregnancy or venereal disease as an adolescent (puberty to 18 yrs); concern over credibility, life-style, morality, and character as a young adult (18–24 years); concern over how rape will affect family and life-style during adulthood (25–45 yrs); and concern over physical safety, fear of death, reputation, and respectability as an older adult (45 years and older).

During the initial assessment process, the nurse may experience strong reactions to the sexual assault including conflict over who is to blame; anxiety about the possibility of becoming a sexual assault victim herself; anger and hostility toward the victim, the rapist, and society for allowing such an act to occur; or a desire to learn more about rape to resolve personal feelings.

Identification of the victim's response to the assault as acute stress reaction, maladaptive stress reaction, or reorganization stress reaction is important because not all rapes are reported immediately after the assault occurs.

NURSING INTERVENTION

The physician's primary concerns center on immediate care of physical injuries, prevention or alleviation of psychological trauma, and referral for gynecological, medical, or psychological follow-up. Documentation of the patient's physical and emotional status, and any evidence, including stained clothing, fingernail scrapings, and mouth or anal smears containing semen, are important. Prevention of venereal disease and pregnancy also are concerns of the attending physician. The victim has the right to request medical treatment only and to refuse examination for the collection of legal evidence, so that a consent for examination and treatment is necessary *before* the examination.

The nurse's role is to plan appropriate interventions to help the victim recover from the physical, emotional, social, or sexual disruption that she is experiencing. During the acute stress reaction phase of rape, the nurse employs crisis intervention skills to reduce anxiety and to provide supportive care. (See Chaps. 6 and 12). It is imperative that arrangements be made for a nurse to stay with the victim. She should be calm and supportive, listen carefully to what the victim has to say, encourage the victim to speak distinctly and clearly when describing the rape incident, and reassure her that the information given will be confidential and handled discreetly. The victim should be treated with respect and dignity while receiving care.

Other interventions after abuse or during the acute stress reaction include providing privacy; displaying a nonjudgmental attitude; explaining the examination process; and if rape occurred, assisting with a rape examination according to hospital protocol. When preparing the victim for a physical and gynecologic examination, the nurse should find out if the patient has ever been examined. She should arrange for physical comfort such as drinks of water to relieve thirst and a place to wash after the initial examination has been completed. It is not unusual for the victim to feel "dirty" or "contaminated."

Treatment of maladaptive stress reactions following rape should include a psychiatric referral once the rape has been discovered to help with the victim's unresolved feelings and reactions resulting in increased psychological distress.

During the reorganization phase of the rape syndrome, nursing interventions vary according to individual needs of the victim, generally focusing on 1) providing a community resource list for medical and legal assistance; 2) providing written information about examinations, test results, or medications for the person to refer to once the state of anxiety decreases following delayed treatment; 3) documenting conversations and observations for possible legal action; and 4) arranging for follow-up medical care and counseling until the patient has recovered.

Patient education includes stating the rationale for medication (*e.g.,* penicillin as a prophylaxis for infection or venereal disease, and the "morning-after pill" to prevent pregnancy). Tranquilizers or antianxiety agents may be prescribed. Emphasis should be placed on follow-up appointments to repeat serology, cultures, pregnancy tests, and to provide counseling services as necessary. Concerns immediately after treatment include safety, transportation home, and attendance or absence from work or school.

Emergency room personnel should ask the victim for permission to provide a crisis center with her telephone number, with the understanding that a follow-up person will take the initiative in contacting the victim. The establishment of ongoing support systems is important if the person is to resolve an abuse or rape experience. Such support groups include crisis hot-lines, self-help groups, counseling, or shelters if the person requests a protective environment.

Examples of nursing diagnoses and nursing interventions for rape victims are discussed here, with emphasis on the psychological or emotional needs of the patient. Short-term goals focus on decreasing symptoms, describing treatment procedures, and identifying and using support systems. Returning to a precrisis level of functioning, with optimal psychosocial adjustment, is a long-term goal.

NURSING DIAGNOSES	NURSING INTERVENTIONS
Rape trauma syndrome: Acute phase resulting in emotional trauma	Assess the patient's psychological responses. Establish a trusting relationship by staying with the patient or arranging for other support. Encourage verbalization of feelings. Maintain a nonjudgmental attitude. Provide crisis intervention as soon as possible. Explain all procedures during the examination. Provide follow-up care to help the patient or victim control reactions and feelings (*i.e.,* telephone number of local crisis counseling center, legal counseling, referral to mental health clinic).
Ineffective individual coping: Depression due to rape	Assess level of depression. Assess for suicidal ideation (see Chaps. 23 and 24). Identify present coping mechanisms or skills. Discuss alternative coping mechanisms. Identify support systems.

NURSING DIAGNOSES	NURSING INTERVENTIONS
Disturbance in self-concept because of rape	Establish a trusting relationship. Encourage verbalization of feelings about self. Avoid negative criticism. Offer praise whenever possible (*e.g.,* for courage). Encourage participation in activities to increase self-worth.

SUMMARY

This chapter focuses on the definition of rape, motives for rape, and classification of sexual attacks. Emotional reactions to rape were described, with emphasis on the rape trauma syndrome. "Silent rape syndrome" was defined. The assessment process was explained, including physical, psychological, and behavioral assessment. Rape myths and facts were stated. Medical and nursing interventions were listed for both phases of the rape trauma syndrome and maladaptive stress reactions following rape. Examples of nursing diagnoses and nursing interventions given include rape trauma syndrome: acute phase resulting in emotional trauma; ineffective individual coping: depression due to rape; and disturbance in self-concept because of rape.

LEARNING ACTIVITIES

I. Clinical activities
   A. Spend a day in the emergency room of your clinical facility if possible, and obtain information regarding their rape treatment protocol. Share this information in postclinical conference.
   B. Identify support systems made available to rape victims *while* they are receiving treatment in the facility.
II. Independent activities
   A. List measures suggested for preventing rape relevant to
      1. Environmental protection
      2. Physical protection
      3. Self-protection as an attack occurs
   B. Read one or more of the following articles or books for professional growth:
      1. "Assessing Trauma in the Rape Victim" by Lynda Holmstrom.
      2. "The Rape Victim" by D. Sredl.
      3. *Rape: Crisis and Recovery* by Ann Burgess.

SELF-TEST

1. List the three essential elements necessary to legally define rape.
2. State the motives for rape or sexual assault.
3. Differentiate between blitz and confidence rape.
4. Explain the phases of rape trauma syndrome.
5. Describe maladaptive stress reaction to rape.
6. Discuss the following myths about rape.
   Attractive women provoke men into raping them.
   Women cry rape to get revenge.
   Women avoid rape by struggling with the rapist.

REFERENCES

Backer B et al: Psychiatric/Mental Health Nursing: Contemporary Readings. New York, D. Van Nostrand, 1978

Burgess AW: Psychiatric Nursing in the Hospital and the Community, 3rd ed. Englewood Cliffs, Prentice–Hall, 1981

Burgess AW, Holmstrom LL: Rape: Crisis and Recovery. Bowie, Robert J. Brady, 1979

Burgess AW, Laszlo AT: Courtroom use of hospital records in sexual assault cases. Am J Nurs: 1977

Donlon PT, Rockwell DA: Psychiatric Disorders: Diagnoses and Treatment. Bowie, Robert J. Brady, 1982

Gagnon JH: Human Sexualities. Glenview, Scott, Foresman & Co, 1977

Haber J et al: Comprehensive Psychiatric Nursing, 2nd ed. New York, McGraw–Hill, 1982

Holmstrom LL, Burgess AW: Assessing trauma in the rape victim. Am J Nurs: Aug, 1975

Jacoby S: Nothing really happened. McCalls: Nov, 1981

Lancaster J: Adult Psychiatric Nursing. Garden City, NJ Medical Examination Publishing, 1980

Lego S: The American Handbook of Psychiatric Nursing. Philadelphia, JB Lippincott, 1984

Mitchell JT, Resnik HLP: Emergency Response to Crisis. Bowie, Robert J. Brady, 1981

Murray RB, Huelskoetter MM: Psychiatric/Mental Health Nursing: Giving Emotional Care. Englewood Cliffs, Prentice–Hall, 1983

Sredl D, Klenke C: The rape victim. Nurs 79: July, 1979

Stuart GW, Sundeen SJ: Principles and Practice of Psychiatric Nursing, 2nd ed. St. Louis, CV Mosby, 1983

Urdang L (ed): Mosby's Medical Nursing Dictionary. St. Louis, CV Mosby, 1983

Warner C: Conflict Intervention in Social/Domestic Violence. Bowie, Robert J. Brady, 1981

Wilson HS, Kneisl CR: Psychiatric Nursing, 2nd ed. Menlo Park, Addison–Wesley, 1983

APPENDIX

DSM-III CLASSIFICATION—
AXES I AND II CATEGORIES AND CODES*

All official DSM-III codes and terms are included in ICD-9-CM. To differentiate those DSM-III categories that use the same ICD-9-CM codes, unofficial non–ICD-9-CM codes are provided in parentheses for use when greater specificity is necessary.

The long dashes indicate the need for a fifth-digit subtype or other qualifying term.

Disorders Usually First Evident in Infancy, Childhood, or Adolescence

MENTAL RETARDATION

(Code in fifth digit: 1 = with other behavioral symptoms [requiring attention or treatment and that are not part of another disorder], 0 = without other behavioral symptoms.)

317.0(x)	Mild mental retardation	_____
318.0(x)	Moderate mental retardation	_____
318.1(x)	Severe mental retardation	_____
318.2(x)	Profound mental retardation	_____
319.0(x)	Unspecified mental retardation	_____

*From American Psychiatric Association: Diagnostic and Statistical Manual of Mental Disorders, 3rd ed. Washington, DC, American Psychiatric Association, 1980
Axes I and II are used to constitute an official diagnostic assessment in the evaluation of persons with mental disorders. Axis I is used to classify clinical syndromes and conditions not attributable to a mental disorder that are a focus of attention or treatment. Axis II is used to classify personality disorders and specific developmental disorders.

ATTENTION DEFICIT DISORDER

314.01   With hyperactivity
314.00   Without hyperactivity
314.80   Residual type

CONDUCT DISORDER

312.00   Undersocialized, aggressive
312.10   Undersocialized, nonaggressive
312.23   Socialized, aggressive
312.21   Socialized, nonaggressive
312.90   Atypical

ANXIETY DISORDERS OF CHILDHOOD OR ADOLESCENCE

309.21   Separation anxiety disorder
313.21   Avoidant disorder of childhood or adolescence
313.00   Overanxious disorder

OTHER DISORDERS OF INFANCY, CHILDHOOD, OR ADOLESCENCE

313.89   Reactive attachment disorder of infancy
313.22   Schizoid disorder of childhood or adolescence
313.23   Elective mutism
313.81   Oppositional disorder
313.82   Identity disorder

EATING DISORDERS

307.10   Anorexia nervosa
307.51   Bulimia
307.52   Pica
307.53   Rumination disorder of infancy
307.50   Atypical eating disorder

STEREOTYPED MOVEMENT DISORDERS

307.21   Transient tic disorder
307.22   Chronic motor tic disorder

307.23   Tourette's disorder
307.20   Atypical tic disorder
307.30   Atypical stereotyped movement disorder

OTHER DISORDERS WITH PHYSICAL MANIFESTATIONS

307.00   Stuttering
307.60   Functional enuresis
307.70   Functional encopresis
307.46   Sleepwalking disorder
307.46   Sleep terror disorder (307.49)

PERVASIVE DEVELOPMENTAL DISORDERS

Code in fifth digit: 0 = full syndrome present, 1 = residual state.
299.0x   Infantile autism _____
299.9x   Childhood onset pervasive developmental disorder _____
299.8x   Atypical _____

SPECIFIC DEVELOPMENTAL DISORDERS

Note: These are coded on Axis II.
315.00   Developmental reading disorder
315.10   Developmental arithmetic disorder
315.31   Developmental language disorder
315.39   Developmental articulation disorder
315.50   Mixed specific developmental disorder
315.90   Atypical specific developmental disorder

Organic Mental Disorders

SECTION 1

Organic mental disorders whose etiology or pathophysiological process is listed below (taken from the mental disorders section of ICD-9-CM).

DEMENTIAS ARISING IN THE SENIUM AND PRESENIUM

Primary Degenerative Dementia, Senile Onset
290.30   With delirium

290.20   With delusions

290.21   With depression

290.00   Uncomplicated

Code in fifth digit: 1 = with delirium, 2 = with delusions, 3 = with depression, 0 = uncomplicated.

290.1x   Primary degenerative dementia, presenile onset _____

290.4x   Multi-infarct dementia _____

SUBSTANCE-INDUCED

Alcohol

303.00   Intoxication

291.40   Idiosyncratic intoxication

291.80   Withdrawal

291.00   Withdrawal delirium

291.30   Hallucinosis

291.10   Amnestic disorder

Code severity of dementia in fifth digit: 1 = mild, 2 = moderate, 3 = severe, 0 = unspecified.

291.2x   Dementia associated with alcoholism _____

Barbiturate or Similarly Acting Sedative or Hypnotic

305.40   Intoxication (327.00)

292.00   Withdrawal (327.01)

292.00   Withdrawal delirium (327.02)

292.83   Amnestic disorder (327.04)

Opioid

305.50   Intoxication (327.10)

292.00   Withdrawal (327.11)

Cocaine

305.60   Intoxication (327.20)

Amphetamine or Similarly Acting Sympathomimetic

305.70   Intoxication (327.30)

292.81   Delirium (327.32)
292.11   Delusional disorder (327.35)
292.00   Withdrawal (327.31)

Phencyclidine (PCP) or Similarly Acting Arylcyclohexylamine

305.90   Intoxication (327.40)
292.81   Delirium (327.42)
292.90   Mixed organic mental disorder (327.49)

Hallucinogen

305.30   Hallucinosis (327.56)
292.11   Delusional disorder (327.55)
292.84   Affective disorder (327.57)

Cannabis

305.20   Intoxication (327.60)
292.11   Delusional disorder (327.65)

Tobacco

292.00   Withdrawal (327.71)

Caffeine

305.90   Intoxication (327.80)

Other or Unspecified Substance

305.90   Intoxication (327.90)
292.00   Withdrawal (327.91)
292.81   Delirium (327.92)
292.82   Dementia (327.93)
292.83   Amnestic disorder (327.94)
292.11   Delusional disorder (327.95)
292.12   Hallucinosis (327.96)
292.84   Affective disorder (327.97)
292.89   Personality disorder (327.98)
292.90   Atypical or mixed organic mental disorder (327.99)

SECTION 2

Organic brain syndromes the etiology or pathophysiologic process of which is either noted as an additional diagnosis from outside the mental disorders section of ICD-9-CM or is unknown.

  293.00   Delirium
  294.10   Dementia
  294.00   Amnestic syndrome
  293.81   Organic delusional syndrome
  293.82   Organic hallucinosis
  293.83   Organic affective syndrome
  310.10   Organic personality syndrome
  294.80   Atypical or mixed organic brain syndrome

Substance Use Disorders

Code in fifth digit: 1 = continuous, 2 = episodic, 3 = in remission, 0 = unspecified.

  305.0x   Alcohol abuse _____
  303.9x   Alcohol dependence (alcoholism) _____
  305.4x   Barbiturate or similarly acting sedative or hypnotic abuse _____
  304.1x   Barbiturate or similarly acting sedative or hypnotic dependence _____
  305.5x   Opioid abuse _____
  304.0x   Opioid dependence _____
  305.6x   Cocaine abuse _____
  305.7x   Amphetamine or similarly acting sympathomimetic abuse _____
  304.4x   Amphetamine or similarly acting sympathomimetic dependence _____
  305.9x   Phencyclidine (PCP) or similarly acting arylcyclohexylamine abuse _____(328.4x)
  305.3x   Hallucinogen abuse _____
  305.2x   Cannabis abuse _____
  304.3x   Cannabis dependence _____
  305.1x   Tobacco dependence _____
  305.9x   Other, mixed or unspecified substance abuse _____
  304.6x   Other specified substance dependence _____
  304.9x   Unspecified substance dependence _____

304.7x   Dependence on combination of opioid and other nonalcoholic substance _____

304.8x   Dependence on combination of substances, excluding opioids and alcohol _____

Schizophrenic Disorders

Code in fifth digit: 1 = subchronic, 2 = chronic, 3 = subchronic with acute exacerbation, 4 = chronic with acute exacerbation, 5 = in remission, 0 = unspecified.

SCHIZOPHRENIA

295.1x   Disorganized _____
295.2x   Catatonic _____
295.3x   Paranoid _____
295.9x   Undifferentiated _____
295.6x   Residual _____

Paranoid Disorders

297.10   Paranoia
297.30   Shared paranoid disorder
298.30   Acute paranoid disorder
297.90   Atypical paranoid disorder

Psychotic Disorders Not Elsewhere Classified

295.40   Schizophreniform disorder
298.80   Brief reactive psychosis
295.70   Schizoaffective disorder
298.90   Atypical psychosis

Neurotic Disorders

These are included in affective, anxiety, somatoform, dissociative, and psychosexual disorders. To facilitate the identification of the categories that in DSM-II were grouped together in the class of neuroses, the DSM-II terms are included separately in parentheses after the corresponding categories. These DSM-II terms are included in ICD-9-CM and are therefore acceptable as alternatives to the recommended DSM-III terms that precede them.

Affective Disorders

MAJOR AFFECTIVE DISORDERS

Code major depressive episode in fifth digit: 6 = in remission, 4 = with psychotic features (the unofficial non–ICD-9-CM fifth digit 7 may be used instead to indicate that the psychotic features are mood incongruent), 3 = with melancholia, 2 = without melancholia, 0 = unspecified.

Code manic episode in fifth digit: 6 = in remission, 4 = with psychotic features (the unofficial non-ICD-9-CM fifth digit 7 may be used instead to indicate that the psychotic features are mood incongruent), 2 = without psychotic features, 0 = unspecified.

Bipolar Disorder

    296.6x Mixed _____
    296.4x Manic _____
    296.5x Depressed _____

Major Depression

    296.2x Single episode _____
    296.3x Recurrent _____

OTHER SPECIFIC AFFECTIVE DISORDERS

    301.13 Cyclothymic disorder
    300.40 Dysthymic disorder (or depressive neurosis)

ATYPICAL AFFECTIVE DISORDERS

    296.70 Atypical bipolar disorder
    296.82 Atypical depression

Anxiety Disorders

PHOBIC DISORDERS (OR PHOBIC NEUROSES)

300.21   Agoraphobia with panic attacks
300.22   Agoraphobia without panic attacks
300.23   Social phobia
300.29   Simple phobia

ANXIETY STATES (OR ANXIETY NEUROSES)

300.01   Panic disorder
300.02   Generalized anxiety disorder
300.30   Obsessive compulsive disorder (or obsessive compulsive neurosis)

POST-TRAUMATIC STRESS DISORDER

308.30   Acute
309.81   Chronic or delayed
300.00   Atypical anxiety disorder

Somatoform Disorders

300.81   Somatization disorder
300.11   Conversion disorder (or hysterical neurosis conversion type)
307.80   Psychogenic pain disorder
300.70   Hypochondriasis (or hypochondriacal neurosis)
300.70   Atypical somatoform disorder (300.71)

Dissociative Disorders (or Hysterical Neuroses, Dissociative Type)

300.12   Psychogenic amnesia
300.13   Psychogenic fugue
300.14   Multiple personality
300.60   Depersonalization disorder (or depersonalization neurosis)
300.15   Atypical dissociative disorder

Psychosexual Disorders

GENDER IDENTITY DISORDERS

Indicate sexual history in the fifth digit of transsexualism code: 1 = asexual, 2 = homosexual, 3 = homosexual, 0 = unspecified.

302.5x   Transsexualism _____
302.60   Gender identity disorder of childhood _____
302.85   Atypical gender identity disorder _____

PARAPHILIAS

302.81   Fetishism
302.30   Transvestism
302.10   Zoophilia
302.20   Pedophilia
302.40   Exhibitionism
302.82   Voyeurism
302.83   Sexual masochism
302.84   Sexual sadism
302.90   Atypical paraphilia

PSYCHOSEXUAL DYSFUNCTIONS

302.71   Inhibited sexual desire
302.72   Inhibited sexual excitement
302.73   Inhibited female orgasm
302.74   Inhibited male orgasm
302.75   Premature ejaculation
302.76   Functional dyspareunia
306.51   Functional vaginismus
302.70   Atypical psychosexual dysfunction

OTHER PSYCHOSEXUAL DISORDERS

302.00   Ego-dystonic homosexuality
302.89   Psychosexual disorder not elsewhere classified

Factitious Disorders

300.16 Factitious disorder with psychological symptoms
301.51 Chronic factitious disorder with physical symptoms
300.19 Atypical factitious disorder with physical symptoms

Disorders of Impulse Control Not Elsewhere Classified

312.31 Pathological gambling
312.32 Kleptomania
312.33 Pyromania
312.34 Intermittent explosive disorder
312.35 Isolated explosive disorder
312.39 Atypical impulse control disorder

Adjustment Disorder

309.00 With depressed mood
309.24 With anxious mood
309.28 With mixed emotional features
309.30 With disturbance of conduct
309.40 With mixed disturbance of emotions and conduct
309.23 With work (or academic) inhibition
309.83 With withdrawal
309.90 With atypical features

Psychological Factors Affecting Physical Condition

Specify physical condition on Axis III.
316.00 Psychological factors affecting physical condition

PERSONALITY DISORDERS

Note: These are coded on Axis II.
301.00 Paranoid
301.20 Schizoid
301.22 Schizotypal
301.50 Histrionic
301.81 Narcissistic

301.70 Antisocial
301.83 Borderline
301.82 Avoidant
301.60 Dependent
301.40 Compulsive
301.84 Passive–aggressive
301.89 Atypical, mixed or other personality disorder

V Codes for Conditions Not Attributable to a Mental Disorder That Are a Focus of Attention or Treatment

V65.20 Malingering
V62.89 Borderline intellectual functioning (V62.88)
V71.01 Adult antisocial behavior
V71.02 Childhood or adolescent antisocial behavior
V62.30 Academic problem
V62.20 Occupational problem
V62.82 Uncomplicated bereavement
V15.81 Noncompliance with medical treatment
V62.89 Phase of life problem or other life circumstance problem
V61.10 Marital problem
V61.20 Parent–child problem
V61.80 Other specified family circumstances
V62.81 Other interpersonal problem

Additional Codes

300.90 Unspecified mental disorder (nonpsychotic)
V71.09 No diagnosis or condition on Axis I
799.90 Diagnosis or condition deferred on Axis I
V71.09 No diagnosis on Axis II
799.90 Diagnosis deferred on Axis II

GLOSSARY

Acute dystonic reaction: Irregular, involuntary spastic muscle movements; wryneck; facial grimacing; abnormal eye movements or backward rolling of eyes in the sockets. May occur anytime after the first dose of an antipsychotic drug.

Addiction: A state of chronic or recurrent intoxication characterized by psychologic dependence, tolerance, and physical dependence. The person is emotionally dependent on a drug, is able to obtain a desired effect from a specific dosage, and experiences withdrawal symptoms after he stops taking the drug.

Adjustment disorder: A maladaptive reaction in response to an identifiable event or situation that is stress producing and not the result or part of a mental disorder. The reaction generally occurs within 3 months of the onset of the stressor, manifests itself as impaired social or occupational functioning, and is exaggerated beyond the normal reaction to an identified stressor. Remission of the reaction generally occurs when the stressor diminishes or disappears.

Affect: A person's mood, feelings, or tone observable as an outward manifestation. Often referred to as *emotion*. Affect may be referred to as inappropriate, flat or blunt.

Affective disorder: A mental disorder exhibiting prominent and persistent mood changes of elation or depression accompanied by symptoms such as fatigue and insomnia. An abnormality of affect, activity, or thought process is noted. The mood changes appear to be disproportionate to any cause.

Affective disturbance: Inappropriate mood. The person lacks the ability to show appropriate emotional response.

Akathisia: Motor restlessness. The person experiences a constant state of movement, characterized by restlessness, difficulty sitting still, or a strong urge to move about.

Akinesia: Motor retardation or reduced voluntary motor movement

Alcoholism: The inability to stop drinking that seriously alters a normal living pattern. Cessation of drinking or a reduction in intake results in withdrawal symptoms.

Alzheimer's disease: A presenile brain disease that begins with a slight and easily dismissed flattening of personality characterized by confusion, inability to carry out purposeful movements, and possible hallucinations. Sudden personality changes, violent flashes of anger, episodes of wandering, symptoms of paranoia, a stooped gait, loss of involuntary functions, and seizures may occur.

Ambivalence: Contradictory or opposing emotions, attitudes, ideas, or desires for the same person, thing, or situation

Amnesia: Loss of memory that may be organic or emotional in origin

Anhedonia: The inability to experience pleasure while engaged in activities that normally produce pleasurable feelings.

Antidepressant: Drug used to treat depressive disorders caused by emotional or environmental stressors, frustrations, or losses

Antiparkinsonism drugs: Drugs used to treat extrapyramidal effects of antipsychotic drugs. Anticholinergic agents are the drugs of choice.

Anxiety: A term used to describe feelings of uncertainty, uneasiness, apprehension, or tension that a person experiences in response to an unknown object or situation

Associative disturbance or looseness: An inability to think logically. Ideas expressed have little connection, if any, and shift from one subject to another.

Autism: A thought process defined as a retreat from reality. The person may feel unrelated to others or to the environment and appears to be emotionally detached from others.

Barbiturates: Drugs used for sedative effects by depressing the central nervous system

Behavior therapy: Treatment that focuses on modifying observable, quantifiable behavior by manipulation of the environment and behavior

Bestiality: Sexual contact with animals to produce sexual excitement

Bipolar disorder: A major affective disorder characterized by episodes of mania and depression

Blocking: A sudden stoppage in the spontaneous flow or stream of thinking or speaking for no apparent external or environmental reason. May be due to preoccupation, delusional thoughts, or hallucinations

Bulimia: An eating disorder characterized by episodic eating binges or the excessive intake of food or fluids beyond voluntary control

Catatonia: Muscular rigidity or inflexibility, resulting in immobility. Such a person may respond to stimuli and suddenly become extremely agitated.

Child abuse: An act of commission in which intentional physical, mental, or emotional harm is inflicted on a child by a parent or other person

Child neglect: An act of omission in which a parent or person fails to meet a dependent's basic needs, or to provide safe living conditions, physical or emotional care, or supervision, thus leaving the child unattended or abandoned

Circumstantiality: A pattern of speech in which the person gives much unnecessary detail that delays meeting a goal or point

Compensation: The act of making up for a real or imagined inability or deficiency with a specific behavior to maintain self-respect or self-esteem

Compulsion: An unwanted, insistent, repetitive urge to perform or engage in an activity contrary to one's wishes or standards

Conversion: Transferring a mental conflict into a physical symptom to release tension or anxiety

Coping mechanisms: Conscious and unconscious methods of adjusting to environmental stress without changing or altering one's goals

Crisis intervention: An attempt to resolve an immediate crisis when a person's life goals are obstructed and usual problem-solving methods fail. The four steps in the process of crisis intervention include assessment, planning therapeutic intervention, implementing techniques of intervention, and resolution of the crisis, including anticipatory planning.

Cyclothymic disorder: A disorder characterized by periods of depression and hypomania, (a mood somewhere between euphoria and excessive elation). Symptoms include rapid or accelerated speech, increased activity, and a decreased need for sleep.

Defense mechanism: An intrapsychic reaction to protect oneself from stressful situations, resolve a mental conflict, reduce anxiety or fear, or protect one's self-esteem or sense of security. Common defense mechanisms include compensation, conversion, denial, displacement, rationalization, repression, and suppression. Defense mechanisms are considered unconscious, with the exception of suppression, and are often referred to as *coping mechanisms.*

Déjà vu: The sensation of seeing what one has seen in the past

Delirium: An acute brain syndrome that develops rapidly, characterized by cognitive impairment. Symptoms include clouding of the consciousness, disorientation, memory impairment, and a decreased ability to focus, shift, or sustain attention to environmental stimuli.

Delusion: False belief not true to fact and not ordinarily accepted by other members of the person's culture

Dementia: Diffuse brain dysfunction characterized by a gradual, progressive, and chronic deterioration of intellectual function. Judgment, orientation, memory, affect or emotional stability, cognition, and attention all are affected.

Denial: Unconscious refusal to face thoughts, feelings, wishes, needs, or reality factors that are intolerable

Depression: A mood state characterized by a feeling of sadness, dejection, despair, discouragement, or hopelessness

Disorientation: A level of consciousness in which a person is unaware of the position of self in relation to time, surroundings, or other persons

Displacement: The transference of feelings such as frustration, hostility, or anxiety, from one idea, person, or object to another

Dissociation: The act of separating and detaching a strong emotionally charged conflict from one's consciousness

Echolalia: Pathologic, parrotlike repetition of phrases or words of another person

Echopraxia: Pathologic repetition or imitation of observed movements

ECT: Electroconvulsive therapy. Convulsive seizures induced by the passage of electrical current through electrodes applied to both temporal areas of the head. Used in the treatment of severe depression

Ego: The part of the personality that meets and interacts with the outside world as an integrator or mediator and is the executive function of the personality that functions at all three levels of consciousness

Encopresis: Fecal incontinence

Enuresis: Urinary incontinence

Euphoria: An exaggerated sense of physical and emotional well-being inconsistent with reality

Exhibitionism: Obtaining sexual gratification by repeatedly exposing the genitals to unsuspecting strangers such as women and children who are involuntary observers. The male has a strong need to demonstrate masculinity and potency.

Extrapyramidal side-effects: Adverse neurologic effects that may occur during the early phase of drug therapy. These effects are classified as parkinsonism, akathisia, and acute dystonic reactions.

Family therapy: Treating family members in a modified group therapy is referred to as *family* or *systems* therapy. Such therapy attempts to establish open communication and healthy interactions within the family.

Fantasy: Imagined events or fabricated series of mental pictures such as daydreaming to express unconscious conflicts, gratify unconscious wishes, or prepare for anticipated future events

Fear: The body's physiologic and emotional response to a known or recognized danger

Fetishism: Sexual contact with an inanimate article (fetish), resulting in sexual gratification (*e.g.,* a piece of clothing). Its occurrence is almost exclusive with men who fear rejection by members of the opposite sex.

Flight of ideas: Overproductivity of talk characterized by verbal skipping of one idea to another. The ideas are fragmentary and connections between parts of speech often are determined by chance associations.

Folie à deux: Sharing of the same delusion or false belief by two closely related persons

Free-floating anxiety: Anxiety that is always present and accompanied by a feeling of dread. The person may exhibit ritualistic avoidance or phobic behavior.

Fugue: A rare occurrence in which a person suddenly and unexpectedly leaves home or work and is unable to recall the past or his identity. Assumption of a new identity usually occurs after relocation to another geographic area.

Gender identity disorder: The feeling of discomfort about one's own sexuality while one is experiencing conflict between anatomic sex and gender identity. The person has difficulty achieving normal heterosexual relations.

Geriatric nursing: Meeting the needs, created by disease, of older people. Such care is often intuitive and custodial in nature.

Gerontologic nursing: The assessment of health care needs of older people, including planning and implementing health care, and evaluating the effectiveness of such care. An effort is made to promote independence, prevent illness, promote health, and maintain life with dignity and comfort.

Grandiose: An exaggerated belief in one's importance or identity

Group psychotherapy: Application of psychotherapeutic techniques in a group setting of approximately six to ten persons. Group therapy provides the opportunity for each member to examine interactions, learn and practice successful interpersonal communication skills, and explore emotional conflicts.

Hallucinations: Sensory perceptions that occur in the absence of an actual external stimulus. They may be auditory, visual, olfactory, gustatory, or tactile.

Holistic health care: Treating the patient's physical, psychological, and spiritual needs. The person receiving holistic health care attempts to identify any stressor(s) related to the present physical condition, discusses ways to modify or eliminate any stressors, and states specific changes that can be made.

Homosexual: Sexual preference by which a person prefers to have sexual relations with members of the same sex.

Homosexual panic: An acute reaction that occurs when a person with dormant or latent homosexual tendencies is exposed to members of the same sex in settings such as a military barracks or penal institution. The person experiences severe anxiety, then panics, becomes confused, and may hallucinate.

Hyperkinetic: An attention deficit disorder characterized by restlessness, short attention span, distractibility, overactivity, difficulty in learning, and difficulty with perceptual motor function

Hypnotic: Any drug or agent that induces sleep

Hypochondriasis: A diagnosis used to describe persons who present unrealistic or exaggerated physical complaints. Minor symptoms are of great concern to the person and often result in impairment of social or occupational functioning.

Id: That part of the personality that is an unconscious reservoir of primitive drives and instincts dominated by thinking and the pleasure principle

Ideas of reference: A thought process by which a person believes he is the object of environmental attention

Identification: A defense mechanism by which a person attempts to be like someone or to resemble the personality and traits of another to preserve one's ego

Illusion: A false interpretation or perception of a real environmental stimulus that may involve any of the senses

Intellectualization: A defense mechanism by which a person transfers emotional concerns into the sphere of the intellect. Reasoning is used as a means of avoiding confrontation with unconscious conflicts and their stressful emotions.

Introjection: A defense mechanism by which a person attributes the good qualities of others to self; symbolically taking on the character traits of another person by "ingesting" the person's philosophy, ideas, and so forth

Isolation: A defense mechanism by which a person separates an unacceptable feeling, idea, or impulse from his thoughts

La belle indifference: An inappropriate lack of concern; indifference

Labile: Unstable, rapidly shifting emotions; moody

Libido: Emotional energy; psychic drive (often referred to as psychosexual energy)

Lithium: A salt that is considered the treatment of choice for the manic phase of a bipolar disorder; also used as maintenance medication to treat recurrent affective episodes

Major tranquilizer: Antipsychotic drug or neuroleptic agent used in the treatment of disorders such as schizophrenia, mania, paranoid disorders, and acute brain syndrome

Mania: A mood disorder characterized by psychomotor overactivity or excitement, insomnia without fatigue, euphoria or a state of elation, distractibility, and pressured speech

Masochism: Experiencing pleasure or sexual arousal as a result of emotional or physical pain inflicted by oneself or by others

Mental health: A state of being in which a person is simultaneously successful at working, loving, and resolving conflicts by coping and adjusting to the recurrent stresses of everyday living

Mental illness: A state of being characterized by a disturbance of emotional equilibrium, manifested in maladaptive behavior or impaired functioning due to a biologic, genetic, social, psychological, physical, or chemical disturbance

Mental retardation: A disorder characterized by the onset of subaverage intellectual functioning associated with or resulting in impairments in adaptive behavior before age 18. Such a person is unable to think abstractly, adapt to new situations, learn new information, solve problems, or profit from experience.

Methadone: A synthetic narcotic used as a substitute for heroin during detoxification or the withdrawal from heroin

Milieu therapy: A therapeutic or structured environment that encourages persons to function within the range of social norms through modification of the person's life circumstances and immediate environment

Multiple personality: A disorder in which a person is dominated by at least one of two or more definitive personalities at one time. Emergence of various personalities occurs suddenly and often is associated with psychosocial stress and conflict.

Mutism: Refusal to speak even though the person may give indications of being aware of the environment

Neologism: A new word or combination of several words coined or self-invented by a individual and not readily understood by others

Neuroleptic: Major tranquilizer or antipsychotic drug

Neurosis: A descriptive term used to differentiate nonpsychotic clinical symptoms (No longer used as a separate DSM-III classification)

Nihilism: A veiwpoint that existence is senseless and useless

Obsession: An insistent, painful, intrusive thought, emotion, or urge that arises from within oneself, is considered absurd and meaningless, and cannot be suppressed or ignored

Occupational therapy: The use of creative techniques and purposeful activities, as well as a therapeutic relationship, to alter the course of an illness. Focuses on vocational skills and activities of daily living to raise self-esteem and promote independence

Organic mental disorder: A disorder of transient or permanent brain dysfunction caused by a disturbance of physiologic functioning of brain tissue. Causes include mechanical, thermal, or chemical damage to the brain, in addition to aging or physical illness.

Paranoia: A rare condition characterized by a delusional system that develops gradually, becomes fixed, and is based on the misinterpretation of an actual event. The thought process appears clear and orderly, reality testing is intact, affect remains appropriate, sociability is maintained, and delusions are persecutory or grandiose in content.

Paranoid disorder: A psychotic state characterized by moderately impaired reality testing, affect, and sociability. Delusions may be persecutory, grandiose, erotic, or jealous in thought content.

Paraphilia: A disorder in which unusual or bizarre sexual acts or imagery arc enacted to achieve sexual excitement

Parkinsonism: An extrapyramidal side-effect characterized by motor retardation or akinesia, a masklike face, rigidity, tremors, "pill rolling," and salivation. Can occur after the first week of psychotropic drug therapy

Pedophilia: The use of prepubertal children to achieve sexual gratification

Personality disorder: A nonpsychotic illness characterized by maladaptive behavior that the person uses to fulfill his or her needs and bring satisfaction to self. As a result of the inability to relate to the environment, the person acts out conflicts socially.

Phobia: An irrational fear of an object, activity, or situation that is out of proportion to the stimulus and results in avoidance of the identified object, activity, or situation. Clinical categories of phobia include agoraphobia with or without panic attacks, social phobia, and simple phobia.

Play therapy: Used with children between ages 3 and 12. Various toys, puppets, or other materials are used to encourage a child to act out feelings such as anger, hostility, frustration, and fear.

Post-traumatic stress disorder: A category reserved for persons who experience a psychologically traumatic event that is considered to be outside the realm of usual human experience. Examples include rape or assault, military combat, and natural disasters.

Primary gain: Obtaining relief from anxiety by using a defense mechanism to keep an internal need or conflict out of awareness

Projection: A defense mechanism in which a person rejects unwanted characteristics of self and assigns them to others

Psychalgia: Psychogenic pain disorder in which severe, prolonged pain is due to psychological factors

Psychiatric nursing: A specialized area of nursing that focuses on the prevention and cure of mental disorders by employing theories of human behavior and the purposeful use of self

Psychoanalysis: A lengthy method of psychotherapy in which the patient talks in an uncontrolled, spontaneous manner termed *free association*. Exploration of repressed anxieties, fears, and childhood images occurs by the interpretation of dreams, emotions, and behaviors.

Psychodrama: A form of group therapy by which persons use dramatization to express their own or assigned emotional problems

Psychosis: A mental disorder in which a person experiences an impairment of the ability to remember, think, communicate, respond emotionally, interpret reality, and behave appropriately. Examples include schizophrenia, bipolar depression, and paranoia.

Psychotropic drugs: Chemicals that alter feelings, emotions, and consciousness in various ways and are used therapeutically in the practice of psychiatry to treat a broad range of mental and emotional illnesses

Rape: A violent sexual act committed against a woman's will, involving the threat or use of force

Rape trauma syndrome: An acute phase of disorganization followed by a longer phase of reorganization experienced by a rape victim. The acute phase is exhibited by emotional reactions of anger, guilt, embarrassment, and humiliation, multiple physical or somatic complaints, or a wish for revenge. During the phase of reorganization the victim may change daily life patterns, experience recurring dreams and nightmares, seek support from friends and family, feel the need to discuss the sexual assault, or develop irrational fears or phobias.

Rationalization: The act of justifying ideas, actions, or feelings with acceptable reasons or explanations

Reaction–formation: The act of displaying the exact opposite behavior, attitude, or feeling of that which one would normally show in a given situation

Regression: Retreating to past levels of behavior to reduce anxiety and allow one to become dependent on others

Repression: The inability to recall painful or unpleasant thoughts or feelings since they are automatically and involuntarily pushed into one's unconsciousness

Restitution or undoing: The negation of a previous consciously intolerable action or experience to reduce or alleviate feelings of guilt

Sadism: The act of experiencing sexual gratification while inflicting physical or emotional pain on others

Scapegoating: Term used to describe the role of a person within a family who is the recipient of angry, hostile, frustrated, or ambivalent emotions experienced by various family members

Schizophrenia: A serious psychiatric disorder characterized by impaired communication with loss of contact with reality and deterioration from a previous level of functioning in work, social relations, or self-care. Clinical types include disorganized, catatonic, paranoid, residual, and undifferentiated schizophrenia.

Secondary gain: Any benefit or support that a person obtains as a result of being sick, other than relief from anxiety

Sedative–hypnotic: An agent used to induce a state of natural sleep, reduce periods of involuntary awakenings during the night, and increase total sleep time

"Silent rape" syndrome: A maladaptive reaction to rape, in which the victim fails to disclose information about the rape, is unable to resolve feelings about the sexual assault, experiences increased anxiety, and may develop a sudden phobic reaction

Somatoform disorder: A disorder characterized by physiologic complaints or symptoms that are not under voluntary control and do not demonstrate organic findings. Five categories include somatization disorder or Briquet's syndrome, coversion disorder, psychogenic pain disorder, hypochondriasis, and atypical somatoform disorder.

Stimulant: An agent that directly stimulates the central nervous system and creates a feeling of alertness and self-confidence in the user

Sublimation: The rechanneling of consciously intolerable or socially unacceptable impulses or behaviors into activities that are personally or socially acceptable

Substitution: The act of finding another goal when one is blocked

Superego: The censoring force or conscience of the personality composed of morals, mores, values, and ethics largely derived from one's own parents

Suppression: Willfully or consciously putting a thought or feeling out of one's mind, with the ability to recall the thought or feeling at will

Symbolization: An object, idea, or act represents another through some common aspect and carries the emotional feeling that is associated with the other

Tardive dyskinesia: Most frequent serious side-effect occurring during abrupt termination of an antipsychotic drug, reduction in dosage, or after long-term, high-dose therapy, characterized by involuntary rhythmic, stereotyped movements, protrusion of the tongue, puffing of the cheeks, and chewing movements

Therapeutic community: A specific type of milieu therapy using social and interpersonal interactions in the hospital as therapeutic tools to bring about change in the patient by encouraging active participation in treatment. It is democratic, rehabilitative, permissive, and communal in function.

Therapeutic window: The serum plasma level of a drug at which optimal therapeutic response occurs (*i.e.,* tricyclic antidepressants)

Transsexual: A type of gender identity disorder in which the person desires to live, dress, and act as a member of the opposite sex because of discomfort with his own anatomic sex

Transvestism: A type of paraphilia in which a heterosexual male achieves sexual gratification by wearing the clothing of a woman (cross-dressing)

Undoing: See *restitution*

Verbigeration: A severe form of perseveration in which a person repeats the same verbal or motor response to verbal stimuli despite efforts to produce another response

Voyeurism: The achievement of sexual pleasure by looking at unsuspecting persons who are naked, undressing, or engaged in sexual activity

Waxy flexibility: The catatonic person maintains the position in which he has been placed.

INDEX